5/1/15

To Glenn,

Congratulations on becoming a super judge!

Michael Miller MD

D1565066

HEAL YOUR HEART

THE POSITIVE EMOTIONS PRESCRIPTION TO PREVENT AND REVERSE HEART DISEASE

HEAL YOUR HEART

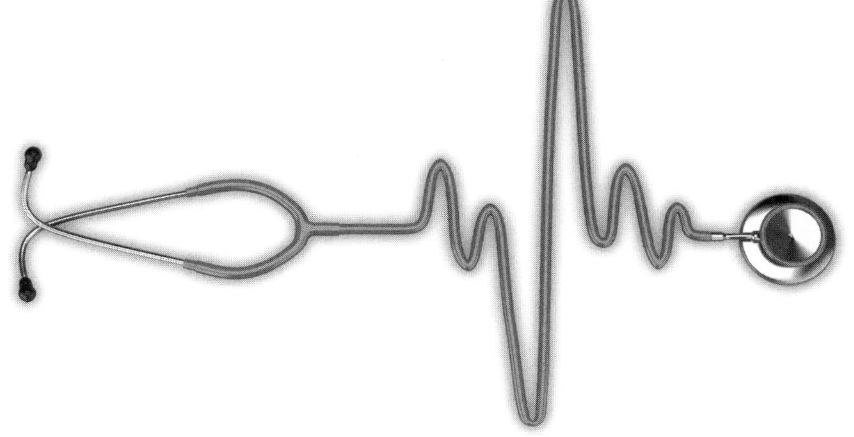

MICHAEL MILLER, MD

with CATHERINE KNEPPER

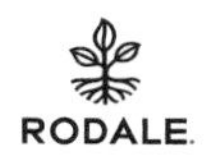

RODALE

This book is intended as a reference volume only, not as a medical manual. The information given here is designed to help you make informed decisions about your health. It is not intended as a substitute for any treatment that may have been prescribed by your doctor. If you suspect that you have a medical problem, we urge you to seek competent medical help.

Mention of specific companies, organizations, or authorities in this book does not imply endorsement by the author or publisher, nor does mention of specific companies, organizations, or authorities imply that they endorse this book, its author, or the publisher.

Internet addresses and telephone numbers given in this book were accurate at the time it went to press.

Printed in the United States of America

Rodale Inc. makes every effort to use acid-free ♾, recycled paper ♲.

Illustrations by Karen Kuchar

Book design by Elizabeth Neal

Library of Congress Cataloging-in-Publication Data is on file with the publisher.

ISBN 978-1-62336-362-8

2 4 6 8 10 9 7 5 3 1 hardcover

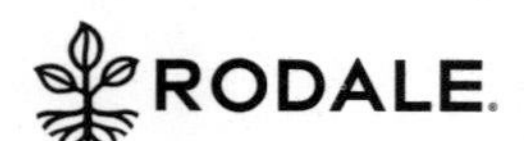

We inspire and enable people to improve their lives and the world around them.
For more of our products, visit **rodalestore.com** or call 800-848-4735.

To Lisa, "my teal-eyed girl," with gratitude and love

CONTENTS

Preface ix

Acknowledgments xi

Introduction xiii

CHAPTER 1—HEARTS AND MINDS
Comprehensive Medicine for Comprehensive Health 1

CHAPTER 2—EVERYBODY'S GOT A HUNGRY HEART
The Mood, Food, and Heart Health Connection 15

CHAPTER 3—LAUGHING MATTERS
The Best Medicine You'll Ever Take 65

CHAPTER 4—WITH A SONG IN YOUR HEART
The Healing Power of Music 85

CHAPTER 5—LIGHTHEARTED AND LIGHT ON YOUR FEET
Your Emotional Health and Physical Activity 95

CHAPTER 6—HAVING A HEART-TO-HEART
Positive Emotions and Your Personal Life 113

CHAPTER 7—MY JOB IS KILLING ME
Positive Emotions and Your Professional Life 127

CHAPTER 8—RECOVERING FROM A BROKEN HEART
Regaining Positive Emotions after a Life-Altering Event 141

CHAPTER 9—WHAT'S ON YOUR MIND IS ON YOUR HEART
A Survey of Integrative Therapies 151

CHAPTER 10—THE POSITIVE EMOTIONS PRESCRIPTION
Your Comprehensive 4-Week Plan for Whole-Body Wellness 165

CHAPTER 11—RECIPES FOR YOUR MIND AND YOUR HEART 213

Endnotes 289

Index 321

PREFACE

NEARLY 10 YEARS AGO, I was contacted by literary agent Jill Marsal to discuss the possibility of writing a book related to the effects of positive emotions on the heart. My colleagues and I had just completed a research project demonstrating that laughter dilates blood vessels, which was in direct contrast to the blood vessel constriction we observed after our volunteers watched the harrowing opening segment of the movie *Saving Private Ryan*. Although these research results were promising, and although the effect of stress on the heart had been known for quite some time, research was still lacking with regard to how positive emotions benefit the heart. As a physician/scientist and researcher, I decided to hold off on writing such a book until more studies became available.

That time has now arrived. As research in our new subspecialty, behavioral cardiology, has blossomed, we have begun to uncover new ways to improve and maximize mind-heart connections. Think of it as your positive emotions prescription to good health. That is what this book is all about—learning to heal your heart by actively engaging in positive emotions each and every day. And while good nutrition and physical activity are necessary components to good health, they are unlikely to be sufficient if the soul of your body's engine is ailing.

As a practicing physician with more than 25 years of experience, I have treated countless patients who time and again have beaten the odds by following a simple formula that combines good nutrition practices, daily activity, and perhaps most importantly, learning to foster positive emotions. You'll get to read about some of them in this book, and I'll guide you in how to use the same Positive Emotions Prescription they follow. This successful, proven plan, which combines the very best of traditional medicine with holistic practices that strengthen the mind-heart connection, has transformed my stressed-out patients at high risk for a heart attack and stroke into healthier women and men who have a more optimistic outlook and who have achieved sustained weight loss, lower blood pressure, and reduced cholesterol. Whether your heart is currently in need of healing, if you are at risk of heart disease, or if you simply want to keep your heart healthy, this book will show you how to get on—and stay on—the road to excellent heart health.

ACKNOWLEDGMENTS

I AM INDEBTED TO the thousands of patients whom I've had the privilege of taking care of at the University of Maryland Medical Center and the Baltimore Veterans Affairs Medical Center. Along the way, I've been extremely fortunate to have had the opportunity to conduct medical research with giants in the field. They include Drs. Peter L. Carlton, Robert Deutsch, and Arthur Kling at Rutgers Medical School, with whom I learned a great deal about the amygdala and its role in processing emotions. At Johns Hopkins, my mentor, Dr. Pete Kwiterovich, taught me everything I know about cholesterol; Dr. Tom Pearson generously provided his large database so that we could study the importance of HDL and triglycerides in patients with heart disease; and Dr. Myron (Mike) Weisfeldt encouraged my research efforts in heart disease prevention during cardiology training. At the University of Maryland School of Medicine, Dr. Bob Vogel provided invaluable expertise in our positive emotion and nutrition-based research studies. Dr. Steve Havas was a great partner in the development of a novel nutrition-based education program for our medical students.

In writing this book, I owe a great deal of gratitude to the talented Catherine Knepper, who brought each chapter to life. I'd like to gratefully acknowledge the assistance of Hannah S. Magram in drafting and editing the proposal to the publisher for the publication of this book. At Rodale, Lora Sickora has been an amazing editor who was encouraging from the outset and did a masterful job navigating the manuscript in a remarkably seamless manner. Finally, I have been very lucky to have Jill Marsal as my agent, as she has guided me through this process with unwavering support, a great deal of assistance, and extreme patience.

I am especially grateful to my children, Avery, Ilana, and Max, who provided much-needed positive emotions throughout this period. Finally, this book could not have been written without my wife's love and support, not to mention her delicious, mood-uplifting meals, recipes for many of which are included in this book. As I temporarily moved my office to the kitchen, no one was happier to have this project completed so that she could have her kitchen (and peace of mind) back!

INTRODUCTION

ONE BEAUTIFUL SUMMER EVENING in July 1963, my 31-year-old father met up with his friends for a game of baseball after work. Dad was a textile designer and a decorated veteran; tall and handsome and athletic, he was a man in the prime of his life. He loved those weekly baseball games, and he was a good player with a nice, compact swing. Back at our Brooklyn apartment, my mother had her hands full getting two rambunctious young boys bathed and ready for bed. (I had just turned 6, and my brother was 4½.) On baseball nights, Mom set aside a plate of dinner for Dad, which she'd warm and serve when he returned.

The phone rang and Mom left to get it, telling my brother and me to behave. She was back almost immediately, her face pale and afraid. "Hurry and get dressed, boys," she said. "Your father's sick." That's all she would say, but I knew it was serious. Later I would learn that my dad had collapsed on the baseball field and two of his teammates had rushed him to Coney Island Hospital.

By the time we arrived at the ER waiting room, most of the baseball team and some of my father's family were already there. My unease grew. Finally someone called us back to see him.

My father was alone in the hallway, lying on a gurney pushed up next to the wall. He didn't complain, but his deep blue eyes winced from pain, and when I held his hand it was ice cold. He gave my brother and me a weak smile and told us to be good boys.

Back in the waiting room just moments later, a doctor spoke to my mother and she began to cry. My 31-year-old father had died of a massive heart attack.

Today, my dad would have survived. He would've been taken to the catheterization lab to open up his blocked blood vessels, or he would've been given clot-busting medication. He would've been warned about the dangers of cigarette smoking long before heart disease had him in its lethal grip. But in 1963, scientists were in the early stages of testing clot-busting therapies, doctors had not yet learned coronary angioplasty (a procedure that widens an obstructed coronary artery), and defibrillators to resuscitate patients (by restoring normal heart rhythm via an electrical shock) were not yet commonly used. It was also a year before the US Surgeon General released the first statement alerting the public to the serious health risks of cigarette smoking. And my father, like so many in the armed services and 40 to 50 percent of the general adult population at that time, was a smoker.

Other, subtler medical knowledge that still lay years in the future would have made a lifesaving difference as well. A week before his heart attack, my father had doubled over in pain at work. His doctor treated him for an ulcer, never suspecting that such a young, physically fit man could be at risk for heart disease. Then, a couple of weeks after his death, coworkers told my mother that my father had been under enormous job-related stress. This was a surprise to her. Like many of his generation, he bottled up his negative emotions. Unaddressed and unexpressed, these negative emotions ate away at him, stimulating his heart into overdrive and triggering the steady release of toxic stress chemicals that took a toll on his cardiovascular system.

Fifty years after my father's tragically premature death, we enjoy incredible advances in interventional cardiology treatment therapies. Interventional cardiology, which treats heart disease that has *already* developed, has saved millions of lives. But despite these technological and medical advances, premature death from heart disease continues to strike down millions each year. Today, more than 15 million Americans will see heart disease when they look in the mirror,[1] and more than 2,150 will die of heart disease—that's one cardiac death every 40 seconds.[2] And over the course of their lifetimes, one of every two Americans will suffer a cardiovascular event that will end in heart attack, stroke, or death. In other words, at some point, *half* of us will experience a life-threatening cardiovascular event. As if these alarming statistics aren't enough, a stunning 120 million Americans already have risk factors for developing heart disease, and many of them don't even know it.

The Emotion Factor

Why, when we have so much accumulated knowledge and access to so many sophisticated medical interventions, does heart disease stubbornly remain the number one cause of death in the United States? And when I was a young cardiologist, why was I still seeing 40-year-olds who'd suffered heart attacks? Or nonsmokers with cholesterol levels well within the American Heart Association's guidelines who nonetheless showed clear signs of coronary artery disease?

There had to be something—and something critical—missing from the picture.

Thus, early in my career, I began to shift my focus from the cardiology training that included cardiac catheterization to detect artery blockages to *preventive* cardiology, which considers what we can do to prevent heart disease before it ever develops.

I've now devoted my entire academic career to this single question: How can we *prevent* heart disease? In cardiac research involving more than 10,000 patients, my colleagues and I performed 25 years of clinical trials and ongoing medical care to discover how we can best protect healthy hearts and prevent the onset of disease, rather than continuing with interventional cardiology's focus on treating hearts that are already unhealthy. What I discovered through my own research and through examining the research of other preventive cardiologists surprised a lot of people, including myself.

According to recent research, just nine factors account for more than 90 percent of heart attacks.[3] The first eight are well-known risk factors such as high blood pressure, high cholesterol, cigarette smoking, and obesity. But even though the medical community and the general public are well aware of these "egregious eight," half of all Americans can still expect to experience a cardiac event. Sure, plenty of people engage in risky behaviors like smoking and being sedentary despite knowing the negative repercussions for their health. But a disproportionate number of folks, despite having healthy BMIs (body mass indexes) and healthy habits, still have

Nine Factors That Explain More Than 90 Percent of Heart Attacks Worldwide

1. High cholesterol
2. Cigarette smoking
3. High blood pressure
4. Diabetes
5. Sedentary lifestyle
6. Abdominal obesity
7. Lack of vegetable and fruit intake
8. Total abstention from alcohol
9. STRESS

unhealthy hearts. It turns out that the ninth risk factor, a risk factor that runs rampant throughout our culture, sheds light on the mystery. And it's the very reason I'm writing this book.

The latest research indicates that an *inability to deal effectively with stress* is a direct contributor to heart disease. A recent review of all the medical and psychological literature on stress and coronary heart disease (CHD) published between 1995 and 2012 states unequivocally that "psychological factors, including depression, anxiety, and stress" constitute their own, "independent risk factors for CHD."[4] In other words, those negative psychological factors are equally as harmful as physical risk factors such as diabetes, or behavioral risk factors such as cigarette smoking. In my own lab, we've demonstrated that even short exposure to stressful situations—such as seeing a violent movie or listening to music that you find irritating—constricts and stiffens the blood vessels, which impedes blood flow and raises blood pressure, leaving you more vulnerable to stroke and heart attack. If isolated experiences of stress can have this kind of immediate negative impact, imagine the cardiovascular havoc that *chronic* exposure to stress can wreak!

The Power of Positive Emotions

Now, if all of this news is giving you heart palpitations, take a deep breath and relax: As harmful as the effects of negative emotions are on our cardiovascular health, they don't hold a candle to the power of positive emotions. We *can* learn simple ways to deal with the daily stresses of life in a healthy way. We *can* harness the power of positive experiences and emotions—things like optimism, confidence, joy, life satisfaction, a sense of purpose, laughter, social connections, and relaxation—to help our hearts get healthy and stay healthy. What's on your mind really does affect your heart.

Now, before I get into some of the specifics of what you can expect from *Heal Your Heart*, let me be clear on what this book is *not*. This is not a manual on how to be happy. It's not a diet book. It's not a manifesto on the power of positive thinking. And it's not going to suggest that positive emotions *alone* are enough to prevent or recover from heart disease. (In other words, you can't sit on your duff eating sugary foods all day and expect to reverse heart disease by "going to your happy place.")

What you *will* find within these pages is research-substantiated explanations of the direct and immediate impact of negative emotions on your cardiovascular health. You'll learn what happens on a cardiovascular level when you become hostile or lose your temper, when you experience stress in the workplace or in your relationships, and as a result of chronic, unresolved stress.

But of course, that's just one side of the story. I'll take you past the description of the problem and show you how to solve it. Remember: There's no damage caused by negative emotions that positive emotions can't heal.

To show you how to find and create the kind of positive emotions your heart requires, I'll offer you a new and proven guide for emotional and cardiovascular wellness called the Positive Emotions Prescription. Based on thousands of hours of clinical research, it's the same plan that I prescribe to all of my patients, and I'll give you step-by-step guidance in implementing this simple yet powerful prescription for health. You'll read stories of patients who've suffered a life-threatening cardiac event and who've used the Positive Emotions Prescription to get back on the road to overall health and wellness and remain there for years. If they can do this, you can do this!

The Positive Emotions Prescription works because it synergizes the latest clinical research in preventive and behavioral cardiology, the role of emotional well-being, and the proven connection between body and mind. You'll be surprised by many of the latest findings. I'll explain why you may be at risk for a heart attack—even if your cholesterol and blood pressure levels are perfectly normal. I'll debunk the myth that blood vessels naturally stiffen and narrow as a consequence of aging—and then show you how you can reduce the aging of your vessels with simple, fast-acting techniques that are actually fun. I'll show you why laughter is as effective at lowering blood pressure as a daily blood pressure medication, and I'll guide you in how to maximize positive, heart-healthy emotions in your life without ingesting vitamins or supplements that have not been proven to prevent a heart attack. I'll show you how to slow down and give yourself a daily dose of heart-healthy relaxation—even if you're an avowed type A personality. And I'll give you recipes for delicious, heart-healthy meals that are designed to boost your emotional well-being on a chemical level.

Heal Your Heart offers you all the newest breakthroughs about the critical role our emotions play in heart health so you can begin—right now—to protect yourself from heart disease. It doesn't matter if your heart is perfectly healthy, or if you're at risk for heart disease, or even if you're already suffering from heart disease: Learning to enhance positive emotions via the easily accessible avenues of lifestyle, diet, and stress-relieving practices is your gateway to optimal cardiac health and overall wellness.

And it just may bring you a little more happiness and peace of mind, too.

CHAPTER 1

Hearts and Minds

COMPREHENSIVE MEDICINE FOR COMPREHENSIVE HEALTH

BETWEEN MY TIME AS a medical student, intern, and resident in the late 1970s and early '80s and my cardiology training at the Johns Hopkins Hospital, which concluded in the early '90s, I received a world-class education in medicine and, specifically, in my specialty, cardiology. My colleagues and I were well schooled in what's known as the oculostenotic reflex. The standard procedure of the time, it meant that when a cardiologist saw (oculo, from the Greek *oculus,* meaning "eye") a blockage (stenosis) in a blood vessel, his or her immediate impulse (reflex) was to open it up with angioplasty or stenting.[1] Angioplasty, as you may know, is the technique of widening a narrowed or blocked vessel by inserting a balloon that is inflated and then removed. A stent, or mesh tube, is then inserted into the blood vessel to keep the vessel open. With the blockage "compressed," blood is once again able to flow freely, relieving the patient of pain and further damage to the heart muscle, which can be fatal. This procedure not only relieves symptoms of angina but also saves lives when performed immediately or soon after a heart attack.

Yet, believe it or not, it turns out that not all blockages benefit from stenting. The common presumption is that an 80 percent blockage means that you'd better open up that vessel ASAP or the person will drop dead from a heart attack. In fact, *up to 20 percent* of such blockages have no physiological relevance, meaning they will not benefit from intervention.[2] And whenever an angioplasty is performed or a stent is inserted, the inner lining of the blood vessels—an incredibly important organ known as the endothelium—inevitably receives some injury. This results in local inflammation and an increased clotting tendency, meaning an intervention may actually cause more harm than good.

Now, clearly the benefit of a stent exceeds the risk when a patient is in the throes of a heart attack, or if the patient experiences repeated symptoms of chest discomfort during physical activity. Also, in some cases, frequent episodes of shortness of breath or fatigue predominate, symptoms we refer to as an "anginal equivalent." If further testing reveals a physiological blockage of a coronary artery, a stent is then placed to relieve the symptoms.

But stenting is not without possible complications, the most feared of which is in-stent thrombosis. This potentially life-threatening condition occurs when a blood clot forms on the surface of the stent, and it is especially likely to occur if the prescribed antiplatelet medicines aren't taken every day. Restenosis—the reblockage of an opened vessel—is less common in the modern stent era, but it continues to be known as the Achilles' heel of angioplasty and stenting.

What if there were simpler, less invasive, and more effective solutions? My research team at the University of Maryland School of Medicine was part of two landmark studies that looked at whether medication may be just as effective as angioplasty and/or stenting. In the first study, patients who had at least a 50 percent coronary blockage were randomly assigned a statin—a drug used to lower cholesterol levels—versus the traditional interventional treatment of angioplasty.[3] In the second study, patients with an abnormal stress test and at least a 70 percent or greater blockage in one or more major coronary arteries were assigned to either a combination of stent placement and optimal medical therapy or optimal medical therapy alone.[4] Keep in mind that in both studies, the patients' medical conditions were fairly stable despite having significant blockages in their coronary arteries. When the results were analyzed, the group treated with medication only did just as well if not better than the angioplasty/stent group.

How could that be? In other words, why would medicines, most notably statins, work so well in these patients? The answer is quite instructive.

Stress and Inflammation

When our bodies make cholesterol, there are many steps involved. But well before cholesterol is churned out, inflammatory-like proteins are produced. What most people don't know is that statins work at the top of this chain reaction, so they not only block cholesterol from being made but also knock out "instigators of inflammation."[5] That is why statins can reduce the risk of a heart attack in someone who has a normal cholesterol level but also has high levels of inflammation or C-reactive protein (CRP).

Now when you normally think of inflammation, you probably picture a red, swollen wound or a sore muscle that you might treat with rest, your favorite homeopathic remedy, or an anti-inflammatory medicine like aspirin or ibuprofen. I want you now to think of a statin working in a similar manner, but instead of reducing inflammation in muscles, it reduces inflammation in blood vessels. The big difference is that inflammation of our muscles is usually very apparent early on, as we feel sore and achy, whereas inflammation of our blood vessels is silent until the later stages, when we have symptoms of heart disease.

What causes inflammation of our blood vessels? In addition to our stenting scenario and the usual cast of villains (cigarette smoking, high blood pressure, high cholesterol, and diabetes), you may be surprised to learn that stress plays a critically important role in causing our blood vessels to become inflamed. Research teams discovered this years ago when volunteers were asked to subtract 7 from 100, first slowly and then more rapidly.

Okay, close your eyes now and try it. Start with 100 and subtract 7, and then subtract 7 from that number, and on and on until you get to 2.

If you tried the exercise, I think you'll agree that unless you're a math whiz, it's not exactly easy. Now imagine that someone is holding a timer while you're saying "100, 93, 85—I mean 86," and so on. It can be quite a nerve-racking experience! In fact, scientists found that this stressful exercise caused the blood vessels to clamp down or constrict, a normal physiological response that allows us to respond in emergencies. You know this as the fight-or-flight response, where your heart races, your blood vessels constrict, your blood pressure goes up, and blood flow is diverted to your brain so that you can be alert, focus, and think and act quickly. The blood vessel constriction occurs because the inner lining of our blood vessels, the endothelium, releases toxic chemicals in response to stress. (The endothelium also releases good chemicals, which we will discuss in Chapter 4.) If we're stressed-out only occasionally, our bodies are well equipped to deal with these situations. That's because specialized white blood cells known as macrophages—literally, "big eaters"—seek out and engulf toxins and pathogens. Problem solved.

However, if we are exposed to stress over and over and over again, our bodies simply cannot keep up. Our once friendly macrophages now become "angry" because they are constantly scavenging toxins that continue to build up unabated. The blood vessel literally becomes hot because of the ongoing inflammation.

But there's more! As the blood vessels continue to release toxic chemicals in response to stress, which recruits more macrophages to the area, low-density lipoprotein (LDL) particles become oxidized as they react to free radicals released by the toxic stress chemicals. Now we're in real trouble, because oxidized LDL is even more dangerous than normal LDL. This is due to the macrophages' insatiable appetite for these toxins, which then attract even *more* macrophages to the surrounding area.

Now you have a group of angry and overfed macrophages that don't get around so well. They need more space, so they group together, invade the blood vessel lining, and voilà, you have "foam cells," the precursor of cholesterol plaque. If we do not effectively manage our stress or do not keep risk factors for heart disease at bay, this process gains momentum. So don't let their slouching around deceive you, because these angry macrophages will release inflammatory proteins that start to nibble away at the barrier separating plaque on the vessel wall from the bloodstream. The "hotter" the plaque, the more likely it is to rupture. And when a large plaque ruptures and an ensuing large blood clot forms to obstruct the artery, the result is—you guessed it—a heart attack.

Why LDL Is Very Toxic to Certain People but Not to Others

To prevent a heart attack, we really need to learn how to better manage stress for two critically important reasons. The first is that stress compounds the effect of other cardiovascular risk factors. We've already seen how stress can convert harmless LDL into a more harmful, toxic form. Well, it turns out that high triglyceride levels, diabetes, and cigarette smoking do the same thing! As I'll discuss in Chapter 2, one reason a high triglyceride level raises the risk of heart disease is its association with small LDL particles that are susceptible to oxidation. The elevated blood glucose levels in people with diabetes, as well as sugars contained in tobacco smoke, also convert LDL to a toxic form. And that's why LDL is especially toxic to smokers, diabetics, those with high triglycerides, and those suffering from chronic stress—even when LDL levels appear to be normal. Now throw in high blood pressure, too, because hypertension causes blood vessel stiffness, premature aging of the vessels, and excess wear and tear on the endothelium. Stress plus any of the traditional cardiovascular risk factors makes for a lethal double whammy.[6]

But even more sobering is the second reason we need to learn to better manage stress: You don't need *any* of these above-mentioned risk factors to have a heart attack. *All you need is stress.* This is so important that I'm going to repeat it in another way: *Stress alone* can cause an internal chain reaction that leads to a heart attack. You probably know or have read about someone who was the picture of perfect health, only to drop dead from a sudden heart attack. The scientific community recently lost a brilliant scientist, Bill Stanley, PhD, chair of cardiovascular physiology at the University of Sydney in Australia, who at the age of 56 died suddenly from a heart attack. Bill never smoked, nor did he have high blood pressure, high cholesterol, or diabetes. In fact, he was an avid cyclist who even biked to work when he was with us in Baltimore. But then he moved to Australia to take on additional responsibilities on top of an already overloaded plate. Some of my colleagues and I believe that the most plausible explanation for Bill's terribly unfortunate and premature death was overwork and the resulting internal stress that led to his heart attack.[7]

Although plaque rupture can occur without warning, in many cases an emotional trigger sets it off. We know this from the sudden surge in heart attacks and cardiac deaths that occurs in the aftermath of natural disasters such as earthquakes. Other emotional triggers include the death of a spouse or loved one; we'll cover this topic in greater detail in Chapter 8. Clearly, stress is an important trigger that can set off a heart attack, but the Positive Emotions Prescription will give you strategies that you can use to prevent an emotional trigger from causing damage to your heart.

The New Field of Behavioral Cardiology

Behavioral cardiology, a specialized branch of *preventive* cardiology that aims to prevent heart disease before it develops, marries the very best of traditional cardiology with groundbreaking research in how our *behaviors* and our *emotions* affect our heart health. Studies in behavioral cardiology have demonstrated conclusively that negative emotions such as chronic stress, anger, hostility, and cynicism have a deleterious effect on the heart and vasculature, both immediately and in the long term. (And that's true even if you're in excellent physical health.) We now know that there's far more to reversing heart disease and maintaining heart health than diet, exercise, and cholesterol levels. Without looking at a patient's psychosocial history, which would help physicians understand a patient's sources of stress and how well he or she is dealing with that stress, we're missing half the story.

Your heart isn't a stand-alone organ, after all. It's part of a vast, highly complex, and interconnected system. What you put into the system in the form of food, drink, and substances affects your heart; the positive and negative thoughts and emotions in your mind affect your heart; and other choices you make (level of activity, tobacco use, and so on) affect your heart.

As a result of the new knowledge we've gained from behavioral cardiology, a growing number of scientists and medical professionals—myself included—are recognizing that stress and other negative emotions play a crucial role in the onset of heart disease, as well as its progression, and thus deem stress as serious a risk factor as traditional risk factors such as high blood pressure, obesity, or high cholesterol. Thus, in addition to all of the regular physical examinations and lab work, behavioral cardiologists look at how a patient's emotional health is affecting his or her heart health, and we recommend behavioral changes that can reverse heart disease and prevent further injury to the heart. If a heart-healthy lifestyle that includes the support of emotional health were widely practiced, millions upon millions could be spared the misery of heart disease.

Let's take a look at some of the recent data from behavioral cardiology research. A study on anxiety and coronary heart disease (CHD) combined research data from 20 separate studies on nearly 250,000 subjects. The results? Anxiety was associated with a 26 percent increase in coronary heart disease and a 48 percent increased risk of cardiac-related death over an 11-year follow-up period. These results are independent of other variables such as biological risk factors (high blood pressure, obesity, etc.) and health behaviors (smoking, lack of exercise, etc.). In other words, anxiety is an independent risk factor for CHD and for death attributed to cardiac events.[8] People suffering from significant anxiety are far more susceptible to CHD and cardiac-related death.

Depression is as insidious as anxiety. In a study from the late 2000s, moderate to severe depression was found to *quadruple* the death rate in heart failure patients, and these patients were twice as likely to require emergency room visits or hospitalization compared to individuals who were not depressed. Even those who reported only mild depression experienced a nearly 60 percent increased risk of death![9] Additionally, a recent study out of Australia found that depressed middle-aged women are nearly twice as likely to have a stroke as their nondepressed counterparts.[10] Depression, like anxiety, is an independent risk factor for heart disease and has been shown to exert such a powerful role in cardiovascular disease that the American Heart Association now recommends that all cardiac patients be screened for it.

Then there's anger. People often wonder if some negative emotions are worse for their heart health than others. The answer is yes. Anger and hostility rank at the top of the list of heart-harmful emotions. Most of us have heard about the correlation between outbursts of anger and an increase in cardiovascular events—most notably, acute myocardial infarction (AMI), or heart attack. In one recent study, Harvard Medical School researchers asked nearly 4,000 patients who'd suffered AMI about their level of anger in the year prior to their heart attack, as well as any angry outburst that had occurred within 2 hours of the onset of symptoms. Nearly 40 percent reported significant anger within the previous year, and roughly 8 percent of that group reported experiencing rage within 2 hours of heart attack symptoms. What's more, as anger levels rose—when people were so angry that they were throwing things or screaming at others—so did the risk of cardiac events. This was true for both men and women. Researchers also asked subjects about the causes of their anger. The most common responses were family situations, work, and commuting.[11] In other words, these are normal, everyday life situations—things that most of us encounter on a daily basis. And a new study has shown that people who lose their tempers have a fivefold increased risk of a heart attack and threefold increased risk of a stroke within 2 hours of an angry outburst.[12]

Granted, not everyone responds to stressful situations with rage, and the more placid among us have much to teach us about heart health. While studies in behavioral cardiology reveal a great deal about the harm that negative emotions deliver to the heart, they also clearly demonstrate the amazing healing power of positive emotions. Want even better news? The effect of positive emotions is available to everyone, right now—even to the most cynical and anger-prone of us, and even to those whose hearts are already unhealthy—and that healing effect outlasts the harmful effect of negative emotions.

In my own lab, we demonstrated that the stress engendered from watching a violent movie immediately triggered a narrowing of the blood vessels, which raises blood pressure and increases the risk of vessel blockage. But the effect of watching a comical movie that inspired belly laughter immediately *dilated* blood vessels. A follow-up study conducted in Texas reproduced our results and found that this heart-healthy result of laughter lasted nearly 24 hours! In Chapter 3 we'll take an extended look at this study and how laughter can quite literally heal your heart.

Bottom line? The lifesaving knowledge you need today is that *our hearts require emotional health in order to maintain cardiovascular health.* When we learn to tap into positive emotional experiences, we can significantly reduce the risk of a host of illnesses commonly brought on or exacerbated by stress and other negative emotions—including heart attack, heart failure, arteriosclerosis, and stroke, which together afflict more than 25 million Americans a year. The simple yet profound assumption of behavioral cardiology is that the best possible outcomes for cardiac health are achieved when treatment encompasses physical, emotional, and behavioral wellness. Along with heart-healthy behavioral choices like exercise, not smoking, and maintaining a healthy weight, if we learn to seek out and cultivate positive emotions, millions could avoid the suffering and debilitating effects of heart disease. Millions of deaths could be prevented, and millions more could enjoy better quality of life for the longer term.

Before we move on to examine the effects of stress and how our current medical model deals with patient stress, I'd like to make it clear that behavioral cardiologists, myself included, are not against interventional therapies when they're deemed necessary. In addition, I recommend statins to my patients who are at highest risk of a heart attack. They include patients who have already had a heart attack or stroke or who have peripheral artery disease. They also include diabetic patients, those with a super-high LDL level (higher than 190 milligrams per deciliter or mg/dL), and those who have more than a 7.5 percent chance of having a heart attack over the next 10 years based on age, race, and risk factors for heart disease (like cigarette smoking and hypertension). Other patients may also benefit from statins, like those with a strong family history of heart disease, such as a nonsmoking parent who had a heart attack before the age of 60, patients who are known to have high levels of CRP (above 2 milligrams per liter), and those with evidence of calcium in their coronary vessels.

I agree with my good friend, Neil Stone, MD, professor of medicine, division of cardiology, Northwestern University Feinberg School of Medicine, who chaired the committee that wrote the recent ACC/AHA Cholesterol Guidelines.[13] He and his distinguished team recommended that statins be reserved for those who are most likely to benefit. But statins should not be given to those least likely to benefit, and I certainly do not recommend statins for every Tom, Dick, and Henrietta who walks into my office, even if he or she has mild or moderate increases in LDL (130 to 160 mg/dL). While statins are good drugs, they are not without side effects, and in my practice about one out of every five patients who takes them experiences some degree of muscle achiness. One of the best-kept secrets about statins is that some—atorvastatin (Lipitor) and rosuvastatin (Crestor)—can sometimes be taken only two or three times a week for nearly the same cholesterol-lowering effect.[14]

If behavioral cardiologists have a bias, it's to try and gain as many health benefits as possible through lifestyle changes *before* we turn to medications and surgery. A tremendous amount can be gained through exercise, healthy eating, and stress reduction. In subsequent chapters, we'll look at different ways we can make behavioral changes that boost our emotions and promote cardiovascular health. Behavioral cardiology aims for that win-win scenario of least invasive and most effective therapies—and for the goal of preventing heart disease before it ever develops.

Welcome to Your Local Behavioral Cardiology Clinic—Or Not

This all sounds great, right? And it just makes intuitive sense, doesn't it? Stressed-out individuals are less healthy and less happy. They're more vulnerable to illness and they recover more slowly. Reduce your stress and you reduce your risk not only of heart disease, but also of a host of other conditions caused or exacerbated by chronic stress: increased susceptibility to infection, headaches, backaches, gastrointestinal issues, muscle pain, even hair loss. In addition, some types of cancer and premature aging have been associated with high levels of stress.

If we all know that stress is damaging to our mental and physical well-being, why then are so many physicians ignoring stress, especially when the research overwhelmingly demonstrates that stress and other negative emotions affect physical health? Answering that question would take a book in itself. But here are a few brief responses.

First, remember that the majority of today's medical model is built to treat disease that's already present. The objective of interventional therapies is to treat and cure illness that's already developed and to alleviate symptoms. This is the basic model of treatment in the United States, and we've excelled at delivering interventional therapies.

Second, stress is difficult to quantify. People experience stress in very different ways; what may be a minor irritation to one person can be a major obstacle to another. What's more, the interventional model tends to separate mind and body. Physicians typically stick to the physical only, and they don't even ask about a patient's emotional well-being. When I ask my patients if their primary care physician has spent more than a few minutes talking with them about their stress or emotional state, the answer is almost invariably no. So not only have physicians not received training in how to quantify stress, many are not even aware that they should ask about it.

Third, physicians are crunched for time. On a typical day, the average primary care physician can see 30 or more patients. And specialists can see even more. With that kind of schedule, you're lucky if you can get 10 minutes of face time with your doctor.

Fourth, there's a general lack of training in terms of practicing truly comprehensive health care, or care that includes attention to psychosocial and emotional factors. This is true for nearly every branch of medicine. Just in my own field, training in the "strictly physical" tenets of interventional cardiology continues to be the goal for many cardiologists being trained today. Part of the reason I'm writing this book is to increase awareness—in the medical community and among the general public—of the profound impact our emotional health has on our physical health. Physicians from every discipline need training in the importance of psychosocial factors and how to incorporate them into routine evaluations. And on the other side of the stethoscope, informed and educated patients can take the initiative to express their concerns about stress to their doctors.

There really is a better way. In my office, we take a tailored approach to caring for patients' cardiovascular health. Patients meet with me and then, depending upon the initial assessment, may be referred to a dietitian, a smoking cessation clinic, an endocrinologist, a cardiac rehabilitation center, or a study coordinator if there is interest in participating in one of our clinical trials. Initial visits are scheduled for an hour, follow-up visits are generally half an hour, and staff members periodically check in with patients via phone and e-mail. All of my patients also receive a customized letter reviewing their visit and detailing recommendations to follow prior to their next visit.

During their office visits, patients receive not only a thorough physical exam, but a psychosocial and behavioral inventory, as well. The one we've developed for use in my clinic is called the Positive Emotions Prescription Inventory (PEPI). We use it to gather information about a patient's life situation, current sources of stress, the ways he or she deals with stress, the support network in place, and general lifestyle habits. Fully informed, we're able to give patients full access to the best possible care from everything medicine has to offer. Yes, we do want to know if a patient is smoking and how much, and if a patient is exercising and how much, but we also want to know when the last time was that Richard got out to do some sailboat racing. Is James still bird hunting? Is Cliff still enjoying his "mindless" car shows? Is Lee Ann still hitting the soccer field? These are all real activities from real patients of the University of Maryland's Center for Preventive Cardiology. These educated patients regularly practice enjoyable activities that engender relaxation and cultivate heart-protecting positive emotions tailored to their lifestyles.

Behavioral cardiology's approach can take more time at the *outset*, but there's so much more to health than what can be discovered during a boilerplate physical exam and the standard lifestyle inventory. Not asking patients about the stresses that are affecting their lives and their health is the same as neglecting to ask a patient if she smokes or failing to run a full cholesterol panel. Without taking a psychosocial history, doctors are missing one of the key components in keeping hearts—and every part of the body, for that matter—healthy.

And guess where healthy patients are? They're out enjoying life. They're not in the ER, not in the clinic, not in the hospital. Ultimately, that's the goal of behavioral and preventive cardiologists—to put ourselves out of business. Of course, I say this with tongue at least half in cheek because I've been in this business too long and know all too well that recent advances toward better heart health have been counterbalanced by the rise in diabetes and obesity, coupled with a 24/7 culture of stress. No doubt this is guaranteed to make many of our scavenger cells quite angry for years to come unless we make the same behavioral changes that many of my patients have already made, changes that enabled them to manage stress effectively and that have improved their overall outlook.

Good Stress, Bad Stress

Stress is an inevitable part of life. From sources of chronic, ongoing stress—such as divorce, illness, financial troubles, or a demanding job—to sudden, acute stress—such as the death of a loved one, an accident, a frightening diagnosis, or the loss of a job—to ordinary irritations like long lines or traffic, stress is a part of daily life. And one could make the case that Americans are especially vulnerable to stress. In the United States, productivity is highly valued, and going the extra mile—which often includes inherently stressful practices such as skimping on sleep, getting by on caffeine and maybe a microwaved meal, and spending long hours seated at a desk—is part of the lifestyle norm. Neither does our lifestyle encourage the healthy release of stress. There are exceptions, of course, but generally speaking our culture values those who can soldier on in the midst of life's difficulties, and it implicitly condones many unhealthy forms of stress release, such as drinking too much or overeating. In embracing the prevailing American lifestyle norm, we're really setting our hearts *and* minds up for trouble.

Now, what if you're thinking, *Hey, I like my type A personality—it fuels my ambition and competitive drive and it's helped me get ahead in life!* Or maybe you value the stress that comes from a short-term jolt of adrenaline—it's what helps you meet a tight deadline, push on for that last half mile, get in that last rep, or get the kids to school on time. Are you still at risk for negative effects on your cardiovascular system?

The answer is yes.

Here's the thing: Our bodies don't know the difference between the stress that's helping you cram for an exam by keeping you revved up and alert and the stress that comes from getting a flat tire on the freeway. The physiological and emotional effects are the same—and the negative effects are exponentially compounded as stress grinds on and becomes chronic.

But here's the good news. It's how we *deal* with stress that's the deal breaker—or not. Some people are naturally resilient and can bounce back from stressful events that would leave others shaken for days. It's this latter group that's more at risk for cardiovascular illness and more at risk for illness in general. But again, there's very good news: It doesn't matter how resilient or not you are right now. You *can* learn to deal with stress in healthy ways, and this book will show you how. Many of my recommendations may surprise and—I hope—delight you.

Revisiting the Fight-or-Flight Response

Let's take a look at what happens in our bodies when sudden stress occurs. This is the classic fight-or-flight response you may have heard about.

When we perceive a threat, the brain triggers an absolutely remarkable series of events. For our ancestors, the threat that cued a system-wide red alert could've been a tiger crouching in the grassy savanna, ready to pounce. For us, it could be anything from our car careening out of control on an icy road to being asked to give a toast at the company's holiday party. Whatever the threat, when the amygdala (a small, almond-shaped set of neurons that plays a key role in the processing of emotions) senses danger, it immediately sends a distress signal to the hypothalamus.

Now, think of the hypothalamus as the command center for the body. The hypothalamus communicates with the rest of the body through what's known as the autonomic nervous system. As its name implies, the autonomic nervous system controls the involuntary functions of the body such as breathing, heartbeat, and blood pressure. When the hypothalamus receives the SOS signal from the amygdala, it signals the adrenal glands to leap into action. The adrenal glands pump the hormone adrenaline (epinephrine) into the bloodstream, and it's the adrenaline coursing through our systems that sparks the very familiar physiological responses that allow us to sprint away from the crouching tiger (or the boss asking us to deliver a toast) or to perform headline-garnering superhuman feats such as lifting a car off a person who is trapped underneath.

Whatever the threat, our bodies are now in a state of high arousal, and lots of things happen all at once. The heart rate speeds up so oxygen-rich blood can be supplied to the muscles and other vital organs. Blood pressure rises. The breathing rate increases, and the small airways in the lungs dilate to allow maximum oxygen to the muscles and to the brain, which is now more alert than ever. Senses become sharper, and people in a state of high arousal will often report a sense of "time slowing down." The evolutionary advantage here is that the person under threat now enjoys a *Matrix*-like ability to perceive a high-stress, high-stakes situation in slow motion, allowing *what feels like* ample time for decision making and action. Adrenaline also triggers the release of glucose (blood sugar) and fats from storehouses in the body; these nutrients supply the body with plenty of energy.

This entire process takes only seconds to occur—certainly it took you far longer to read about it than it takes your body to launch the stress response. So now, in the space of seconds, we've got the body and the mind churning on maximum rpms, ready to fight to the death if necessary. What happens next? Once the initial surge of adrenaline subsides, the hypothalamus triggers what's known as the HPA axis. (HPA stands for hypothalamic-pituitary-adrenal.) The HPA axis response is an incredibly sophisticated and complex physiological process, but what you need to know is that the HPA axis is responsible for triggering the adrenal glands to release *cortisol*, a stress hormone you'll be hearing a lot about in this book. Cortisol triggers the continued release of glucose and fats so the body will have ample energy to respond to an imminent threat, and it diverts energy away from low-priority body functions so it can be conserved for lifesaving actions. Cortisol levels remain high—and the entire stress response remains in effect—until our brains perceive that the threat has passed.

Talk about a whole-body response! The stress response is really an amazing process, and it's provided untold benefits to humankind over millennia. But in our day and age, there are few crouching tigers to contend with, and sometimes our brains make mistakes. The "threat" of having to make a spontaneous toast before a large group of colleagues can *feel* as dangerous as a hungry tiger, but in reality the scariest thing in the banquet room is that dry, processed piece of mystery meat lying on your plate. Even more dangerous is the fact that in this day and age, in our stressful society and with too few means to release stress healthfully, cortisol levels often remain stuck on high. This means that our bodies and our minds remain on high alert, constantly revved up, without the opportunity to return to normal levels of rest and relaxation. Yes, short bursts of stress may help us fight that tiger or meet that deadline, but the real problem for us is chronic stress. Even low levels of chronic stress keep the HPA axis revved up and take a toll on our bodies and our minds.

Thus far, we've been looking at the physiological and emotional effects of isolated experiences of stress, but now think of the effect when we're exposed to high stress over a long period of time. For instance, people who are the primary caregivers of loved ones with a serious illness or disability—one of life's most stressful situations—

have been shown to have a 63 percent greater risk of *death* than noncaregiving controls.[15] Caregiving for an ill or disabled spouse has also been specifically associated with increased risk for cardiovascular illness and a 23 percent higher risk of stroke.[16]

Yet despite all these dire research results, remember that the human body is equipped for self-healing. Your body's natural state is to be healthy and highly functioning, not diseased and distressed. Over the course of my career, my patients have included people who've suffered catastrophic cardiac events and who've endured stressful events that would make the hearts of even the most laid-back among us skip more than just a few beats. Even these people have learned to improve and maintain their heart health through lifestyle changes and healthier ways of managing stress.

No matter the state of your current health, you are *already equipped* with the capacity to induce positive emotions that can help protect your heart health. Understanding and learning to use the tools that you already possess will pay great dividends toward improving your overall health—without invasive, costly, and often painful procedures; without medications; and without waiting to treat a heart that is already diseased. What's on our minds really can harm—or heal—our hearts.

The Positive Emotions Prescription: Behavioral Cardiology

Heart disease, while currently our number one killer, is one of our most preventable illnesses. The vast majority of cardiovascular illnesses can be prevented by adopting positive lifestyle changes, and finding ways to reduce or better manage stress should be at the top of the list. Our bodies are designed to deal with short-term stress—not chronic stress. To begin better managing and even preventing stress, take at least 15 minutes each day to reflect on positive thoughts. If you keep a journal, record your positive emotions highlight for the day.

CHAPTER 2

Everybody's Got a Hungry Heart

THE MOOD, FOOD, AND HEART HEALTH CONNECTION

WHAT COMES TO MIND when you think of a "heart-healthy" diet? If you're like a lot of my patients when they first come through the door, it might go something like this: no salt, no sugar, no fat, no fun.

Now it's true that you're not going to be doing yo ur body any favors by eating a diet high in saturated fat and sodium. But instead of focusing on what you *shouldn't* eat, I like to help shift my patients' focus to what they *can* eat and enjoy in support of comprehensive wellness. It turns out there's an abundance of nutritious and delicious foods that promote both emotional health *and* heart health. In this chapter, we're going for a win-win-win: Let's take a look at the latest research on foods that taste great, support healthy cardiovascular function, and elevate mood.

The Mood-Food Connection

You may know more than you think you do about the connection between mood and food. Have you ever been stressed-out and turned to a carb-heavy meal for solace? Down in the dumps and shared your sorrow with Ben and Jerry? On the other end of the spectrum, have you ever felt foggy-brained and sluggish and "medicated" yourself with a double espresso or a hunk of dark chocolate? Emotional eating is familiar to almost all of us, and they don't call it comfort food for nothing.

It turns out that there's a neurological basis for why some of us turn to an ice cream sundae for a little stress relief after a tense day at work. And it all has to do with the neurotransmitter known as serotonin.

Serotonin is one of the brain's major mood neurotransmitters. This powerful chemical that helps brain cells speak to each other is responsible for promoting a host of positive feelings, including calmness, well-being, equanimity, and happiness. In addition to helping to regulate mood, serotonin is also responsible for helping to regulate cardiovascular function, sleep, body temperature, and appetite. It can even positively impact cognitive functions such as memory and the ability to learn new information, and it can help suppress the perception of pain.

With all of these good effects, you may be wondering how you can boost your levels of serotonin. In fact, one of the most common therapies for depression—the class of medications known as SSRIs, or selective serotonin reuptake inhibitors—works in exactly this way, by increasing levels of serotonin. But if you're interested in a drug-free way of boosting your serotonin levels, you have four excellent options—all of which happen to have a positive effect on cardiovascular function, as well. They are (1) exercise, (2) exposure to sunlight, (3) improving your mood through self-directed means, such as meditation or positive thinking, and (4) diet.[1] I'll address all of these throughout the book; in this chapter we'll be focusing on diet.

The way to boost brain serotonin production through diet is to eat foods that trigger the production of tryptophan, which is the precursor to, or building block of, serotonin. And guess which foods do this best? Carbohydrates. So that ice cream sundae you use to self-medicate after work may very well elevate your mood. Carbohydrates trigger the production of insulin, and insulin, in turn, lowers the levels of most amino acids—except for tryptophan, which triggers increased production of serotonin. Simple carbs such as sugar, white rice, and white bread can actually trigger a serotonin increase quickly because they produce a spike in insulin. That's why we experience a feeling of calm after eating a bowl of ice cream. But the effect is temporary, and you're better served for emotional and heart health by eating complex carbohydrates such as barley, beans, kasha, lentils, oats, peas, quinoa, and sweet potatoes. (See Chapter 11 for heart-healthy recipes containing these serotonin-triggering foods.)

Healthy Eating for Mind and Heart

The connection between nutrition, neurology, and cardiology is fascinating, complex, and intricate. But what you need to know now for emotional well-being and heart health is actually straightforward and simple. Let's take a look at specific ways to delight your taste buds with filling, nutritious meals that elevate your mood and promote your heart health. We'll begin with some basic principles of healthy eating.

Eat breakfast. Everything you've heard about breakfast being the most important meal of the day is true. Studies have long shown that eating a low-fat, high-fiber breakfast helps you maintain a healthy body weight, jump-starts your metabolism for the day, reduces your tendency to overeat at the next meal, and improves your concentration (not to mention that it precludes the crankiness that can come from hunger).

Now a new study from the Harvard School of Public Health demonstrates the connection between breakfast and heart health. The study found that men who regularly skipped breakfast had a 27 percent higher risk of coronary heart disease than those who did "break their fast" after a night of sleep. Even after researchers accounted for other risk factors such as smoking, lack of physical activity, high blood pressure, diabetes, high cholesterol, and quality of diet, the link between skipping breakfast and heart disease remained. (The same study, by the way, found that late-night eating was associated with a 55 percent increased risk of coronary heart disease.[2])

Keep dinner light. In our culture, the heaviest meal of the day tends to be dinner, just a few hours before bedtime. If at all possible, try to eat your heaviest meal at midday. Keep dinner light—in the 500-to-700-calorie range. A light dinner means fewer calories, of course, but it makes digestion easier, which prevents your metabolism from being so revved up that it could adversely affect your sleep cycle. When you are sleeping, your other bodily functions should be resting as well. Remember those angry macrophages we learned about in Chapter 1? If your body has to work overtime while you're sleeping, you'll be activating those angry macrophages, which will exacerbate the inflammatory process and accelerate the clogging of your heart arteries. This not only occurs when you are stressed-out and unable to get a good night's sleep, but also when you eat heavily enriched, fatty meals, especially late at night.

I'll be the first to tell you that I was guilty of this bad habit when I was in college. After a night of studying, my friends and I would all splurge on a delicious cheesesteak from the famous "grease trucks" on campus. This was most common after midnight, and then with full guts we'd head off to bed. What I didn't appreciate at the time was that the fat from the greasy cheesesteak would take a good 6 to 8 hours to clear from my bloodstream! If I'd eaten the cheesesteak earlier in the day (and that happened quite frequently as well), then some of the fat would have been cleared more quickly because exertional activities, such as running to class after missing the bus (which also happened with some frequency), rev up the enzyme lipoprotein lipase, which is responsible for processing fat. The more efficiently we can break down our blood fats, the lower our risk of developing metabolic syndrome, diabetes, and heart disease. And this leads us to the next principle: why we should restrict our intake of saturated fat.

Avoid saturated fats and trans fats. What's the common denominator between being stressed-out and eating high amounts of saturated and trans fats? The answer is that when you're stressed, your blood fats (also known as triglycerides) are not processed effectively. At the same time, the release of the fight-or-flight compound epinephrine (adrenaline) directly inhibits the processing of enzymes.[3] Under normal conditions, triglycerides are converted into fatty acids that are used by muscles for energy or stored in fat. My patients are always surprised to discover that the reason their triglyceride level suddenly spiked was because of a recent stressful event.

Keeping the amount of saturated fat that you eat low can also keep your postprandial (after-meal) triglycerides from spiking into dangerously high territory. My research team and I found that you can have a perfectly normal triglyceride level and still be at risk for heart disease if your postprandial levels rise too high. We discovered this effect in our "milk shake study." We asked healthy volunteers to drink a milk shake after they'd completed 1 month of a diet that was either high in saturated fat (40 percent of calories) or low in saturated fat (less than 7 percent of calories). What we found was that even though there was no difference in *fasting* triglyceride levels after the high- and low-fat diets, a significant boost in *postprandial* triglyceride levels occurred after the high-fat phase.[4]

We recently extended these findings in another diet study. Our volunteers consumed three different diets, each lasting for 1 month. They were a high–saturated fat diet (Atkins-like), a Mediterranean diet (South Beach), and a very low-fat diet (Ornish). The most important finding of this study was that there was a direct correlation between the high–saturated fat diet and impairment of the endothelium.[5] The endothelium is our protective blood vessel lining, and impairment of the endothelium causes blood vessels to constrict and increases inflammation, platelet stickiness, and cholesterol plaque buildup.

When putting together a diet containing ideal nutrition, the latest research studies now strongly support that we incorporate several different factors. Such a diet includes foods aimed at maintaining or reducing our cholesterol (see "New Cholesterol Guidelines, Triglycerides, and the Positive Emotions Prescription" on page 22), saturated and trans fats, fasting and postprandial triglycerides (see "Triglyceride Trouble" on page 20), glucose, and blood pressure levels. We also want to select foods that have anti-inflammatory properties in order to keep our macrophages from getting "angry," as well as foods that maintain endothelial health and prevent aging of our blood vessels. It is equally important to assess our caloric needs because they decrease as we age.

Base your caloric intake on your BMR. Instead of basing your daily caloric needs on a one-size-fits-all standard, determine the calories *your* body requires using your basal metabolic rate, or BMR. Your BMR, which is sometimes referred to as your resting metabolic rate, is the amount of energy your body uses when you're completely at rest. It's the energy you need to maintain your vital organs.

Figuring out your BMR is easy with an online calculator or health and wellness app. (You can find one at www.bmrcalculator.org.) Once you do, you can use your BMR to factor in how many calories your body requires each day based upon your level of activity. For example, a 50-year-old male who's 5 feet 10 inches tall and weighs 170 pounds has a BMR of about 1,640 calories a day. If he's moderately active, he'll require about 2,500 calories a day to maintain his weight. A 40-year-old female standing 5 feet 7 inches tall and weighing 120 pounds has a BMR of about 1,250 calories a day and needs to consume approximately 1,940 calories a day to maintain her weight if she is moderately active.

What most people don't know is that as we age, our BMR goes down by about 5 calories per day per year. This means that over a 10- to 20-year period, say from age 30 to 50, if we eat the same amount each day and our activity levels do not change, we'll gain 5 to 10 pounds! (And that's one of the reasons for "middle-age spread.") In other words, as we get older we need to either reduce our food intake or burn more calories; it's simply not good enough to maintain the status quo.

I ask all of my patients how much they weighed and what their waist size was when they were in good health, such as in their early twenties. It's pretty amazing that the answer I usually get from my average 5-foot-10 male patient is somewhere between 140 and 175 pounds, and from my average 5-foot-4 female patient is 110 to 135 pounds. The chart on page 23 lists normal body weight for height based upon Centers for Disease Control and Prevention calculations using the body mass index. Also keep in mind that you will lose about ½ inch in height each decade past age 50.

(continued on page 23)

Triglyceride Trouble

The reason triglycerides are so important to your heart health is that they can predict whether you have other dangerous cholesterol-rich particles in your bloodstream. This is because when triglycerides are processed, the by-products are "remnants," cholesterol-rich particles that are different from low-density lipoprotein (LDL). Under normal conditions, "remnants" are digested by the liver. However, if triglycerides cannot be efficiently processed, remnants will accumulate in your bloodstream. As with LDL, remnants get chewed up by macrophages lining your blood vessels, and these normally mild-mannered macrophages then become overstuffed and angry. As we discussed in Chapter 1, angry macrophages cause inflammation by recruiting additional macrophages to the region. In concert, the macrophage team builds plaque and releases enzymes that can cause the cholesterol plaque to rupture and a blood clot to form. The artery becomes obstructed, resulting in a heart attack or stroke.

We often measure triglyceride levels at the same time that cholesterol is measured. If someone has a high LDL level, also having a high triglyceride level increases the risk of a heart attack more than just having the high LDL by itself.[6]

Several years ago, I was invited to chair the American Heart Association scientific statement on triglycerides and cardiovascular disease.[7] We emphasized the importance of lifestyle choices for treating triglyceride levels above 150 milligrams per deciliter (mg/dL). Heart disease starts to ramp up in one out of every three American adults who has a triglyceride level above 150 mg/dL and even more so in one out of every six with triglycerides above 200 mg/dL.

As triglyceride levels climb to the high range of 200 to 500 mg/dL, the risk of cardiovascular death is about 25 percent higher than in those with triglyceride levels less than 150 mg/dL. Then there are the approximately 1 percent of Americans who have extremely high triglycerides—500 mg/dL or higher. At these levels, the risk of heart disease remains dangerously elevated, and as triglyceride levels approach and surpass 1,000, the risk of pancreatitis increases. The symptoms of pancreatitis include pain in the abdomen that can travel or radiate to the back, along with nausea or vomiting. Pancreatitis is a life-threatening condition that requires immediate treatment. In addition to very high triglycerides, pancreatitis is most commonly caused by the lodging of a gallstone in the bile duct or excessive alcohol consumption in a susceptible individual. Triglycerides can also jump to extremely high levels in patients with type 2 diabetes. In these cases, glucose control becomes the central manner of getting triglycerides under control.

So, what are optimal triglyceride levels? In the American Heart Association statement, we also established an optimal triglyceride level of less than 100. In a study done at Johns Hopkins, affectionately termed the Baltimore Coronary Observational Long Term Study, or COLTS, we first suggested that a healthy triglyceride level might be lower than 100. My colleague Tom Pearson, MD, PhD, executive vice president for research and education at the University of Florida Health Sciences Center in Gainesville, Florida, collected detailed information on heart disease risk factors in 1,000 men and women. Over an 18-year period, we found that having a triglyceride level of less than 100 mg/dL resulted in a 50 percent lower risk of a heart attack or death.[8] If you have a triglyceride level below 100 mg/dL, you are very efficient in clearing fat from your bloodstream. Also, your risk of developing type 2 diabetes and heart disease is low as long as you do not smoke or have other risk factors for heart disease.

Among the lifestyle choices that can lower triglycerides, I'm a big fan of adding omega-3-containing eicosapentaenoic acid (EPA) and/or docosahexaenoic acid (DHA) because they are proven to lower triglycerides. And I've witnessed this firsthand: During my first research project at Hopkins, we found that EPA fed to cells reduced the amount of triglycerides produced.[9]

For my patients with triglyceride levels above 150, I recommend a diet that includes omega-3-enriched fish low in mercury. These include salmon, trout, and sardines. (See Chapter 11 for delicious recipes featuring these and other fish.) For every 1,000 milligrams of EPA and/or DHA, triglyceride levels decrease between 5 and 10 percent. The newest kid on the block, krill oil, has recently emerged as another omega-3 product, but studies testing high-triglyceride groups are needed. Unfortunately, the plant-based omega-3 fats, such as the alpha-linolenic acid (ALA) found in flaxseeds, have much weaker triglyceride-lowering effects than EPA or DHA. And we still don't know whether lowering a high triglyceride level lowers heart attack risk, though studies are in progress. A large study using a purified EPA compound is currently under way to answer that question, and a second study using an EPA/DHA combination is in the planning stages.

I have also witnessed patients who have been able to normalize their high triglyceride levels through lifestyle changes alone. In addition to increasing intake of omega-3 marine fats, these lifestyle changes include weight loss, exercise, and reducing saturated fats, trans fats, and alcohol consumption. The Positive Emotions Prescription recipes in Chapter 11 provide a smorgasbord of healthy foods that will keep your triglyceride levels low. Overall, these measures can result in a 50 percent or greater reduction in triglycerides.

New Cholesterol Guidelines, Triglycerides, and the Positive Emotions Prescription

The new cholesterol guidelines recommend starting statin therapy if you are diabetic, have heart disease, or have high levels of LDL (above 190 mg/dL).[10] They do not address what to do if you have triglycerides in the 150 to 500 mg/dL range, but instead instruct you to follow suggestions made in our American Heart Association Scientific Statement. They include losing weight, exercising, reducing simple carbs, and enriching your intake of marine-based omega-3 fats. My view is that if you have heart disease *and* the combination of high LDL and triglyceride levels, it makes sense to keep both your LDL and triglyceride levels low until new research teaches us otherwise. We found that in 4,000 men and women hospitalized after a heart attack, keeping triglycerides, LDL, and C-reactive protein (CRP) below 150 mg/dL, 70 mg/dL, and 2 mg/L, respectively, reduced the risk of future heart attacks by more than 40 percent![11]

So where do we stand with high-density lipoprotein (HDL), the good cholesterol? We've known that having a low HDL level raised the risk of a heart attack. Well, there is new evidence that suggests the old wisdom may only be partially true. We analyzed more than 3,000 records from the long-standing Framingham Study and found that low HDL did not increase risk of a heart attack if triglycerides and LDL were both below 100 mg/dL.[12] This is welcome news if you were born with a low HDL level and haven't been able to raise it. The treatment of choice for someone with a low HDL level but high triglycerides would start with lifestyle changes to reduce triglycerides.

A question I often get is whether it matters what type of diet we subscribe to. Most diets are based on specific nutrition-based philosophies (low carb, high carb, low cal . . . you get the picture). If the diet is reasonable and palatable, it will usually be effective in the short term, such as weeks to months. The problem is that life happens, and when we're hit with a series of stressful events, comfort foods and old habits often return with a vengeance.

The Positive Emotions Prescription program combines all of the latest research in nutrition, heart health, and emotional health and incorporates daily measures to keep you upbeat so that when stress does hit (and it will), you will be better prepared to navigate through the difficult times without falling off the wagon. Just like it takes a lean horse to win the long race, this program is designed for the long haul.

HEALTHY WEIGHT RANGES[13]

HEIGHT	HEALTHY WEIGHT (POUNDS)	HEIGHT	HEALTHY WEIGHT (POUNDS)
4'10"	89–119	5'10"	129–173
4'11"	92–123	5'11"	133–178
5'0"	95–127	6'0"	137–183
5'1"	98–132	6'1"	140–189
5'2"	101–136	6'2"	144–194
5'3"	105–140	6'3"	148–199
5'4"	108–145	6'4"	152–204
5'5"	112–149	6'5"	156–210
5'6"	115–154	6'6"	160–215
5'7"	118–159	6'7"	164–221
5'8"	122–164	6'8"	168–227
5'9"	125–168		

Knowing whether your weight is healthy based on your height is only one part of the equation. The second is your waist size. This is because belly fat is more "metabolically active," meaning that it promotes more inflammation than fat in other areas of your body. The general consensus is that the risk of diabetes and heart disease increases as waist size exceeds 35 inches in women and 40 inches in men.

However, I have seen too many patients over the years with heart problems whose waist size did not approach these levels. That's why I want to know what relative increase in waist size has occurred since early adulthood. If, for example, my male patient's waist size has grown from 30 to 36 inches during the past several decades, I am concerned—and for good reason. One study of more than 30,000 subjects found that just a 2-inch increase in waist size increased risk of cardiovascular death up to 17 percent over a 10-year follow-up period. A larger study of more than 100,000 men and women found that a 4-inch increase in waist size over 9 years raised risk of death as much as 25 percent, even with normal weight at baseline.[14]

The goal of the 28-Day Positive Emotions Prescription is to get you started toward reducing your waist size to within 2 inches of where it was in early adulthood. This plan is geared to get you back into those clothes that fit comfortably years ago. What I can't guarantee is that they will still be in style (though if you wait long enough, they probably will be).

Be sensible, not ascetic. So many diet plans fail because dieters can't maintain the unrealistic goals they set out with. After the indulgences of the winter holidays, for example, many of us make a New Year's resolution to live on salad and spring water, only to do so for a few days or weeks and then make a mad dash to the nearest fast-food restaurant. The Positive Emotions Prescription is not designed to shock your system by starving you. Rather, the goal is to implement small, practical, and easily manageable steps that enhance positive emotions through diet and other lifestyle changes and minimize the physiological dip in serotonin levels that accompanies major dietary shifts (such as carb restriction) and reduces the likelihood of success.

My recommendation for a healthy, realistic diet that also promotes weight loss is that 15 percent of your total food intake can be "reasonably unhealthy" food. This can be three "reasonably bad" meals (one breakfast, one lunch or brunch, one dinner) spread out over the course of the week, *or* 200 to 300 calories daily. In the Positive Emotions Prescription menus in Chapter 10, I use the phrase *'til your heart's content* to denote these "cheat meals." While a little splurge every now and again is fine, my patients understand that they need to be reasonable or they may get sick. It's better to have smaller portions of your favorite steak.

Along these lines, I asked my patient Wendy, a dedicated red meat eater with a history of pericardial effusion (fluid around the heart sac that was associated with fevers, inflammation, lack of energy, and insomnia) to decrease her red meat consumption of 10 to 14 ounces four or five times a week to 8 ounces once or twice a week. Wendy asked for 12 ounces three times a week. We compromised, and she's decreased her red meat consumption to 10 ounces twice a week. She knows that she has a little more to go and feels that this is now attainable with the positive emotions activities built into her regimen. (Wendy's Positive Emotions Prescription includes watching a comedy three times a week, listening to soothing music, and adding an omega-3 supplement to her diet. She has also recently begun working with a personal trainer.) We also compromised on cooking oils. Wendy used to cook exclusively in butter. She now uses extra-virgin olive oil with a bit of butter for taste. Finally, she previously used ¼ cup of heavy cream in her coffee three times a day, which was loading her diet with saturated fats. Because she does not like the taste of low-fat or skim milk, I recommended that she experiment with hempseed, rice, almond, and soy milk to find what works best for her coffee. These are realistic changes that Wendy has incorporated and that she can *maintain* for the long term. She's already experienced a significant reduction in her blood pressure after 6 years of hypertension. Just as important, she has also driven down inflammation measured by high-sensitivity CRP from an alarming 4.5 to normal levels of less than 1 mg/L. And her sleep habits have improved and her energy level and zest for life are the highest they've been in years.

Be carb smart. The 2010 Dietary Guidelines for Americans recommend that carbohydrates make up 45 to 65 percent of your total daily calories.[15] But what I tell my patients is that *no more than 50 percent of your daily intake should be carbs.* A 1,800-calorie diet would consist of 900 calories from carbs, or 225 total grams (4 calories for each gram of carbs). To put that into perspective, a medium-size plain bagel contains about 56 grams of carbohydrates. That's a quarter of your daily allowance of carbs—from one naked bagel! Cream cheese may be low in carbs, but regular cream cheese contains 35 milligrams of cholesterol per ounce, or 12 percent of the Recommended Dietary Allowance (RDA)—and a walloping 30 percent of your daily recommended intake of saturated fat. Finally, there's the calorie count. Each ounce of a bagel is approximately 70 calories. If the average bagel is 4 ounces, then you're consuming 280 calories—and again, that's if you eat a naked bagel!

All that said, carbohydrates are not public enemy number one. We all need carbohydrates for energy, and as we've seen, carbs improve mood by triggering the release of serotonin. Limiting carbs too much (less than about 130 grams per day) can impair concentration, learning ability, mood, and creativity. Women tend to have lower concentrations of serotonin than men and may be at higher risk of mood-related issues when on a highly carb-restricted diet.[16, 17]

So how do we eat "carb smart"? First, if your diet is too high in carbohydrates—which is the case for most Americans—it's easy to start reducing carbs by 50 grams or 200 calories a day. I recommend first eliminating one or two slices of bread daily. Simply cutting out one slice of bread (at 50 to 60 calories per slice) can result in up to a 5-pound weight loss per year. As you will see in the Positive Emotions Prescription Nutrition Plan in Chapter 10, there is no bread after lunch, except when you use the free, or *'Til your heart's content*, meal.

Second, carbs should be primarily consumed during the day. I recommend to my patients that they avoid "white" carbs (white potatoes, breads, pasta, and rice) after 6 p.m. or within 4 hours of bedtime. White carbs should be replaced with "colorful" carbs, which are found in veggies and fruits and are packed with vitamins, minerals, fiber, and antioxidants that help to keep mild-mannered macrophages from becoming angry. Again, you will not find white carbs in the Positive Emotions recipes.

Ironically, many popular nutrition books still promote a carb snack at night to help promote sleep. But while we are sleeping, human growth hormone (HGH) is released. HGH not only helps to promote growth and repair of tissues, but also helps break down fat, maintain our sleep cycle, and regulate our mood. Insulin suppresses HGH, so when we eat carbs late at night, insulin is released and the benefits of HGH are blunted, resulting in poor mood, poor sleep habits, and weight gain. Conversely, sleep deprivation promotes weight gain due to increased calories eaten, especially late at night.[18]

Read labels. When buying cereal, aim for no more than 5 grams of sugar per serving, optimally with 5 or more grams of fiber. Steer clear of any food products that list partially hydrogenated ingredients, and monitor sodium intake. If you are over 50, have a history of high blood pressure, or have kidney disease, your total sodium intake should be less than 1 teaspoon per day, or about 2,300 milligrams. I tell my medical students that the most deceptive hidden factor on labels is the serving size. Sometimes the serving size is so small that the total number of calories is essentially hidden, or at least misleading. Finally, I also ask them to read the ingredients on the label, and if these science majors don't recognize or cannot pronounce any of the listed ingredients, chances are it is an over-processed product that should be placed back on the shelf.

This is one of the lessons we began teaching more than a decade ago when we were among a handful of medical schools to receive a grant from the National Institutes of Health to educate our medical students about the importance of nutrition for cardiovascular health. With my colleague Steve Havas, MD, we set up a hands-on cooking class where students learned healthy cooking techniques and how to read labels, and to pass this message to their patients when they went into practice.

Employ some tricks of the trade. To help curb your appetite in the evening, I recommend the following: Have an apple or one of the midafternoon snacks listed in our Positive Emotions recipes an hour before dinner, if possible. Drink a full glass of water or water filled with ½ to 1 teaspoon of chia seeds (let it sit for 10 minutes) a half hour before dinner. Then, while eating dinner, make sure to put your fork down between bites to allow time to chew and enjoy your food. Eating slowly also improves digestion and satiety. Floss and brush your teeth about 1 hour after dinner to reduce snacking temptations. And as a heart-health bonus, good dental hygiene also reduces inflammation!

The Positive Emotions Prescription Top 50 Foods and Food Groups

Now that we've got some basics under our belt, let's move on to the fun part: the food! I'm going to give you a list of 50 delicious foods and food groups that dilate blood vessels, reduce plaque buildup, fight infections, and yes, elevate mood. I recommend that one serving of at least five items on this list be consumed each day to maximize heart and emotional health.

But before we begin, here are a couple of tips to help you get the most benefit from these foods and food groups. The highest concentration of antioxidants resides in the skins of fruits and vegetables. Because pesticides can reduce nutrient quality in addition to showering food with toxic chemicals, I recommend buying organic, especially if a fruit or vegetable is thin-skinned or has no coating. If organic produce is unavailable, you can soak fruits and vegetables in warm water for 5 minutes, then soak them in a 3-to-1 solution of white vinegar and water for 1 hour. It takes some time, but this process removes most of the toxic material and is well worth it for your health. If organic produce is unavailable *and* you don't want to be bothered with the vinegar and water bath, a good alternative is to opt for fruits and vegetables that, according to the Environmental Working Group, are less likely to be sprayed with pesticides. This list contains fruits and vegetables that also promote good blood flow: asparagus, avocado, broccoli, cantaloupe, eggplant, grapefruit, kiwi, mango, mushrooms, onions, papaya, peas, pineapple, sweet potato, and watermelon.

Patients also frequently ask me about the value of juicing. If you don't enjoy eating veggies, this would certainly be a good way to get your daily dose of greens. However, until well-conducted research studies prove otherwise, there's actually no evidence that using expensive and heavily promoted high-speed machines that "unlock" nutrients provides additional nutritional value beyond eating fruits and veggies in their natural state. Equally important is that evidence is lacking that taking antioxidant supplements provides value beyond consumption of fruits and veggies. In fact, few if any recent studies have demonstrated benefit. Mother Nature knows best—for the best absorption of nutrients, consume whole foods that have not been tainted with chemicals.

To make it into the Positive Emotions Prescription Top 50, a food had to meet three criteria. First, it must taste delicious. (In some cases the product is only available in powder form, which is used in the recipes found in Chapter 11.)

Second, the food has to possess heart-healthy properties. These include effects on blood levels of cholesterol (LDL and HDL), triglycerides, and glucose. Heart-healthy foods contain soluble fiber and marine-derived omega-3 fatty acids and stabilize blood sugar. They also possess antioxidant compounds, including flavonoids and resveratrol. Foods that reduce blood pressure, such as products enriched with potassium or blood vessel dilators like magnesium, citrulline, and 3-n-butylphthalide, also made the list.

Third, the food must catalyze the release or production of one or more of the "supermood" brain chemicals: endorphins, dopamine, gamma-aminobutyric acid (GABA), serotonin, and norepinephrine. (You'll learn more about the specifics of each of these powerful mood-regulating neurotransmitters throughout the book.) The list also includes foods that supply melatonin, as melatonin helps to regulate sleep, and a good night's sleep works wonders for our mood.[19]

So without further ado, here are 50 foods that are delicious, heart healthy, and mood-elevating.

1. ALCOHOL

Delicious: See Amaretto Amore (page 274).

Heart Healthy: In moderation, consuming alcohol provides a host of heart-protective benefits, including reducing stress, raising HDL, and lowering fibrinogen (a protein involved in blood clotting). It also leads to a 30 percent reduced risk of developing diabetes and an overall 25 to 40 percent decreased risk of heart disease. And it turns out that all varieties of alcohol, not just red wine, offer heart protection. However, the high content of antioxidants, especially resveratrol, found in red wine and dark beer (such as my favorite, Guinness) may give them a slight heart-protective edge.[20]

Moderation is defined as 3 to 7 drinks per week for women and 3 to 14 drinks per week for men. One drink is defined as 4 ounces of table wine, 12 ounces of beer, or a 1-ounce shot of spirits. Drinking higher amounts has been associated with breast cancer in women and with high blood pressure and high triglycerides generally. Drinking larger quantities of alcohol (at least 4 drinks a day) can lead to pancreatitis as well as liver and heart failure.[21]

Mood Elevating: Alcohol releases endorphin-like opioid compounds that are likely to contribute to uplifting mood. Proceed with caution, though: There's a fine line between consuming just enough alcohol to produce an uplifted mood and over-consuming to the point that you experience sensory impairment. My experience is that only a very small amount of alcohol is needed, with the sweet spot for elevating mood at only about half of your favorite drink, if you are a light or moderate drinker.[22]

2. ARTICHOKES

Delicious: See Roasted Jerusalem Artichokes with Herbs (page 269), Green Bean, Artichoke, and Tuna Salad (page 228), Artichoke Frittata (page 222), and Salmon with Asparagus and Artichoke-Mustard Sauce (page 254).

Heart Healthy: Artichokes are number 7 on the USDA list of the top 20 antioxidant-containing foods. Antioxidants help to keep LDL from being engulfed by macrophages and becoming angry, and they maintain the health of our inner blood vessel lining (or endothelium). This leads to improved blood flow, lower risk of cholesterol plaques, and less likelihood of blood clots forming.[23] Artichokes are also an excellent source of magnesium, with a medium artichoke providing 50 milligrams of the 320-milligram RDA for women and 420-milligram RDA for men.[24] Magnesium is one of our most naturally potent blood vessel expanders, and it reduces susceptibility to abnormal heart rhythm.

Mood Elevating: Magnesium has wonderful effects on mood and memory. It can suppress the release of the stress hormone cortisol, and it can prevent the entrance of stress hormones into the brain. Magnesium has also been shown to improve memory in animal studies;[25] research on humans is currently under way.

3. ASPARAGUS

Delicious: See Roasted Asparagus with Shallots (page 265).

Heart Healthy: One of the hallmarks of spring, asparagus is an excellent source of the plant compounds galactolipids, which have powerful anti-inflammatory properties[26] and help to keep our endothelium healthy and our arteries youthful and flexible. Asparagus is also rich in the heart-healthy nutrient potassium. Foods rich in potassium can help lower elevated blood pressure. Asparagus also contains rutin, one of the most powerful natural antioxidants. Rutin inhibits blood clot formation[27] and prevents LDL—the bad cholesterol—from being oxidized, the process that leads to plaque formation and hardening of the arteries.

Mood Elevating: Asparagus is an excellent source of folic acid (or folate). Eating nine spears of asparagus (¾ cup) will provide 50 percent of your daily folic acid requirement and will also help to keep the blues away.

4. AVOCADO

Delicious: See Arugula-Avocado-Almond Salad (page 223) and Avocado Turkey Burger Sprout Wrap (page 229).

Heart Healthy: Avocados are an excellent source of vitamins B_6, C, and K, as well as fiber, folate, and potassium. They also increase the absorption of foods that contain lycopene, the phytochemical that has been found to play a role in preventing prostate cancer, and the absorption of beta-carotene, a main nutrient found in carrots. Despite their relatively high fat content, the majority of the fat in avocados is monounsaturated, and they contain only 2 grams of saturated fat. Importantly, avocados can also lower blood pressure and heart rate.[28] A recent study found that Hass avocado added to a burger offsets the blood vessel constriction that occurs from eating the burger alone and promotes anti-inflammatory effects in healthy individuals.[29]

Mood Elevating: Avocados are a good source of folic acid (three slices, or 1 ounce, contains 50 calories and 6 percent of the RDA for folic acid). Folic acid enhances brain health and improves memory.

5. BEANS

Delicious: See Green Beans with Walnuts and Thyme (page 264), Heartwarming White-Bean Soup (page 240), Stuffed Sweet Potatoes with Beans (page 225), Black Bean Burritos (page 257), and Roasted Green Beans with Garlic and Thyme (page 273).

Heart Healthy: Beans of all varieties are a great source of fiber. These complex carbs not only blunt the spike in glucose that accompanies the ingestion of simple carbs, but they also reduce inflammation. One cup of black beans provides 15 grams of fiber, which is 50 percent of the suggested daily amount. Some beans are also rich in soluble fiber, which lowers LDL cholesterol. They include black beans (2.4 grams), navy beans (2.2 grams), kidney beans (2 grams), pinto beans (1.4 grams), and chickpeas (1.3 grams), all per ½ cup. Adzuki beans are also high in soluble fiber.

The folate in beans lowers homocysteine, a protein that at high levels is toxic to your blood vessel lining (endothelium). Beans are also an excellent source of magnesium and an outstanding source of antioxidants such as anthocyanins and quercetin. Red beans, including kidney beans, have the highest concentration within the bean family. Soaking beans overnight is often suggested to reduce gas production and to optimize the absorption of magnesium.

Mood Elevating: Complex carbs increase tryptophan levels in blood that crosses over into the brain, where the tryptophan is converted to serotonin. Beans (and legumes) are an excellent source of folate to drive dopamine and norepinephrine levels. They are also a good source of selenium. Lima beans and soybeans are also excellent sources of phenylalanine. Chickpeas contain vitamin B_1, which promotes brain and nervous system health, and tryptophan, which can boost your serotonin levels.[30]

6. BEETS

Delicious: See Glazed Beet and Red Grapefruit Salad (page 229), Quinoa Salad (page 232), and Chocolate Chip–Beet Cake (page 281).

Heart Healthy: The red color of beets comes from betanin, a powerful antioxidant that protects the lining of your arteries from free radicals and that may reduce levels of the atherogenic amino acid homocysteine.[31]

Mood Elevating: Beets are a great source of folate and betaine, a derivative of the amino acid glycine that stimulates production of S-adenosylmethionine, or SAMe. (SAMe is a naturally occurring compound in the body that, among many other functions, increases brain levels of serotonin and dopamine. Studies have also suggested that SAMe helps treat depression by boosting serotonin.[32]) The high concentration of uridine and natural nitrates in beets (as well as radishes; see page 53) increases blood flow to the brain, leading to improved mood as well as increased cognition.[33]

7. BERRIES

Delicious: See Blueberry-Cashew Treat (page 275), Strawberry-Pineapple-Kale Smoothie (page 219), Frozen Coconut-Chia-Blueberry Parfait (page 276), Apple-Blueberry Crisp (page 277), and Pistachio-Crusted Tilapia with Strawberry Salsa (page 262).

Heart Healthy: Loaded with B vitamins, vitamin C, antioxidants such as flavonoids and resveratrol, and more than 40 different anthocyanins (pigments that give berries their red, purple, or blue color), berries of all sorts are a treasure trove of healthy compounds. But anthocyanins provide far more than color; they also protect our brain cells and keep cognition and memory intact. Strawberries are loaded with fisetin, a flavonoid that improves long-term memory and reduces diabetes complications. Raspberries contain tiliroside, a flavonoid that inhibits inflammation and free radical activity. They're also a great source of fiber at 8 grams per cup. Blackberries, raspberries, and strawberries contain high amounts of the phenol antioxidant catechin, and blueberries provide an excellent source of the flavonoid myricetin. All of these compounds promote vessel expansion, and a recent study found that consuming strawberries and blueberries three times a week reduced heart attack risk in young and middle-aged women (age range 34 to 61) by more than 30 percent.[34] In addition to antioxidant activity, exotic berries such as acai and goldenberries have also been shown to have cholesterol- and glucose-lowering properties.[35, 36]

Mood Elevating: Recent research has uncovered that strawberries, blueberries, and raspberries contain flavor components that bear similar structures to the mood-stabilizing medication valproic acid.[37]

8. CELERY

Delicious: See Grilled Chicken and Celery Salad à la Marcella (page 233) and Celestial Celery Root and Apple Soup (page 237).

Heart Healthy: Celery is among the most underappreciated yet powerful vegetables for heart health. It has proven blood pressure–lowering properties, and drinking one to two glasses of celery juice daily is commonly recommended to treat hypertension.[38] Alternatively, eating three or four celery ribs each day can lower blood pressure. The active compound believed to be responsible for this effect is 3-n-butylphthalide.

Another compound in celery is the flavonoid luteolin. Also present in thyme, parsley, peppermint, hot chile peppers, green bell peppers, and rosemary, luteolin has been shown to have cardiovascular anti-inflammatory and antioxidant properties that not only reduce the severity of heart attacks,[39] but also improve memory in rodent models.[40]

Mood Elevating: Though not thought of as an aphrodisiac, celery contains the pheromone androsterone, which can enhance both mood and arousal. The compound phthalide has also been suggested to reduce levels of stress hormones and have an overall calming effect.[41]

9. CHERRIES

Delicious: See Butternut Squash with Baby Spinach (page 272).

Heart Healthy: Another great source of anthocyanins and other flavonoids, cherries are not only superb sources of fiber, iron, magnesium, potassium, and vitamins A, B_6, C, and E, but they also have one of the highest antioxidant concentrations of all fruits.[42]

Not all cherries are equal. For example, Rainier cherries have only 25 percent of the antioxidant content of Bing cherries. Cherries should have bright green stems and be consumed within 3 days of picking to have the most potent antioxidant effects. Buy organic cherries or grow your own dwarf varieties, as cherries are among the most pesticide-ridden fruits in the United States.

Mood Elevating: Tart or sour (Montmorency) cherries are high in the sleep-regulating hormone melatonin. Drinking a tart cherry juice concentrate each night for a week improves overall sleep quality. In fact, just 3½ ounces of a tart cherry juice concentrate provides the average amount of melatonin released by your brain's pineal gland. A prior study found that an elderly group who drank a tart cherry juice blend for 2 weeks also experienced a decrease in insomnia. Alternatively, you would need to eat about 11 ounces of tart cherries to get the minimum amount of melatonin release. Unfortunately, the melatonin content of sweet cherries is not well established, so it is unlikely that your "nightcap" with the maraschino cherry will help you fall asleep.[43]

10. CHILE PEPPERS

Delicious: See Roasted Butternut Squash and Black Bean Tacos (page 261) and Gazpacho Soup (page 242).

Heart Healthy: Capsaicin, the active ingredient in chile peppers (a family that includes cayennes, jalapeños, and habaneros), can improve heart health in at least two different ways. First, capsaicin blocks a gene that causes arteries to contract and in doing so induces blood vessel dilation and blood pressure lowering. Second, it has also been shown to lower cholesterol by increasing its excretion.[44]

Mood Elevating: If you're ready to spice it up with capsaicin, you'll be serving yourself a mood-boosting dose of the fat-soluble molecule that gives chile peppers their heat. While your brain releases endorphins that increase blood flow and elevate mood in response to the heat generated by capsaicin, be careful not to eat too much at a sitting, as reports of skyrocketing blood pressure have surfaced.[45] As the saying goes, too much of a good thing is a bad thing. Nevertheless, chiles are rich sources of vitamins C (which increases absorption of iron), B_1, B_2, and E. If you mistakenly get too much heat, counter it with a fatty food such as guacamole to relieve the burning sensation; the fat in the guacamole absorbs the capsaicin.

11. CHOCOLATE

Delicious: See Almond-Chocolate Bark (page 279), Cashew Butter Granola Bars (page 282), Chai Hot Chocolate (page 280), and Chocolate Chip–Beet Cake (page 281).

Heart Healthy: I've never had a patient who hasn't been pleased to hear about the health benefits of chocolate. Chocolate is chock-full of flavonoids such as epicatechin, which improves blood flow to your brain and heart. Dark chocolate contains much, much higher levels of flavonoids—between 90 and 650 milligrams of epicatechin per 3.5 ounces—than milk or white chocolate, which have less than 40 milligrams and zero milligrams, respectively.[46] The European equivalent to the FDA states that eating at least 200 milligrams of cacao flavonoids daily improves endothelial function.

Chocolate is also a rich source of magnesium, which relaxes smooth muscle; hence, premenstrual cramping is often a trigger for chocolate cravings. Chocolate also contains methylxanthines that induce bronchodilation and will open your airways if you have asthma. Take a deep breath after some chocolate, and you'll be amazed at how clear your lungs feel.

Mood Elevating: Chocolate contains the amphetamine-like compound phenylethylamine and the marijuana-like compound anandamide, both found in cacao beans. While both compounds get broken down fairly quickly, leaving only minute quantities available to the brain, at least three flavonoids (kaempferol, genistein, and daidzein) can delay the breakdown of anandamide. Foods highest in kaempferol are capers and kale, while the richest source of genistein and daidzein is soy flour and soybeans (edamame).[47] No wonder I love Trader Joe's dark chocolate–covered edamame!

The amount of cacao polyphenols sticks around longer and thus may play a more prominent role in elevating mood. In a recent study of 72 healthy middle-aged men and women (aged 40 to 65 years), those who consumed the greatest amount of dark chocolate (500 milligrams a day of cacao polyphenols in a drink) over a 30-day period reported that they were more content and relaxed than those receiving the chocolate drink without the polyphenols. Interestingly, more moderate amounts (250 milligrams per day) did not result in any significant benefit.[48] Another study of younger volunteers also found that a high dose of cacao flavonoids (450 milligrams) increased blood flow in the brain region responsible for cognition, while lower doses (150 milligrams) had no effect.[49]

One of the major misconceptions is that the darker the chocolate, the more cacao flavonoids, but the correlation is poor. Although more research is needed to determine the precise amount of dark chocolate that exerts health benefits at the lowest caloric expense, I recommend 2 to 4 teaspoons of cacao powder each day; this amount provides about 125 milligrams of flavonoids at fewer than 20 calories. If you prefer to eat chocolate, then I recommend a daily dose of no more than one-quarter of a 3-ounce bar or a serving size of 150 calories, whichever is lower.

Alternatively, there are now cacao extract supplements such as Mars CocoaVia that can provide 250 to 500 milligrams daily in capsule or powder form. I have tried these and you do get a mental boost, but I recommend starting at 125 milligrams and building up slowly and taking them in the early hours of your day. A dose of 500 milligrams of cacao flavonoids has also been shown to lower systolic blood pressure by up to 3 mm Hg (millimeters of mercury).[50]

12. CINNAMON

Delicious: See Baked Apples with Cinnamon (page 279), Pumpkin Pie Smoothie (page 216), and Apple-Blueberry Crisp (page 277).

Heart Healthy: This aromatic spice helps to regulate glucose by delaying the emptying time of the stomach.[51] It's also been found to lower cholesterol and triglycerides. Cinnamon may also reduce blood pressure by an order of magnitude consistent with taking one blood pressure medication.[52] The health benefits reside in the oil contained in cinnamon bark.

Mood Elevating: Smelling cinnamon can boost memory and alertness, and several drops of cinnamon bark oil taken by steam inhalation has been reported to induce euphoria. In fact, a recent study found that combining the fragrances of peppermint and cinnamon in cars reduced fatigue and increased alertness.[53]

13. COFFEE

Delicious: Consider adding cacao powder and/or cinnamon for a flavor boost (see The 28-Day Positive Emotions Prescription Nutrition Plan, Day 1, on page 185).

Heart Healthy: One cup of coffee contains more antioxidants than a glass of grape juice or a serving of spinach. It also contains phytonutrients that may reduce depression, improve motor control in patients with Parkinson's disease, and reduce its onset.[54]

Drinking as little as 3 cups of coffee daily was found to be associated with a 65 percent reduced risk of Alzheimer's disease, as well.[55] And for every 2 cups of coffee consumed, there is an approximately 12 percent lower risk of developing diabetes.[56] Coffee contains chlorogenic acid, which has been shown to reduce absorption of glucose in the gut[57] and is believed to be a basis for reduced risk of type 2 diabetes. It also reduces LDL and triglyceride levels, as well as susceptibility to LDL oxidation.[58]

Mood Elevating: As previously described for chocolate, coffee also contains methylxanthine. This compound blocks the chemical adenosine. (By the way, that is the reason why you cannot have a cup of coffee prior to a "chemical" stress test when the chemical used is adenosine.) Adenosine normally inhibits the activity of the pleasure chemicals dopamine and glutamate. As a result, these neurotransmitters increase pleasure, attention, and concentration.

I generally recommend 2 cups of coffee daily to my patients, the first in the morning and the second, if needed, 4 to 5 hours later. Keep in mind that the effects of caffeine can last up to 8 to 10 hours, so it is important not to drink it too close to your bedtime. I recently saw a patient who was having a difficult time falling asleep; it turned out that he was having his last cup of coffee at 4 p.m. and wondered why he could not fall asleep at 10 p.m. Once he stopped drinking coffee so late in the day, he experienced more restful sleep.

14. CRUCIFEROUS VEGGIES

Delicious: See Honey- and Maple-Glazed Brussels Sprouts (page 269), Sautéed Kale (page 265), Mediterranean Kale Tart (page 255), and Sesame Chicken Stir-Fry (page 244).

Heart Healthy: Included in this group are arugula, bok choy, broccoli, broccoli rabe, Brussels sprouts, cabbage, cauliflower, collard greens, kale, mustard greens, turnip greens, and watercress. These malodorous veggies contain the isothiocyanate sulforaphane, which reduces inflammation and is an inducer of the powerful antioxidant glutathione. They are also rich sources of potassium, which helps to regulate blood pressure and reduce the aging of your blood vessels. All cruciferous veggies are high in fiber, which tempers postprandial spikes in blood insulin and glucose levels. To lower their cholesterol levels, I often recommend soluble fiber–rich Brussels sprouts (4 grams per cup) and broccoli (2.4 grams per cup) to my patients as part of a comprehensive plan to reduce heart disease.[59]

Mood Elevating: Broccoli and Brussels sprouts are excellent sources of folate, with about 25 percent of the RDA in 1 cup's worth. At this amount, broccoli, Brussels sprouts, cauliflower, and bok choy provide from 50 percent to more than 100 percent of the RDA of vitamin C. When steamed, the absorption of vitamin C is enhanced. This is important for mood regulation because vitamin C is integral to the production of dopamine, norepinephrine, and serotonin. When buying these veggies, try to find those with a dark green or purplish hue to attain the highest content of vitamins and antioxidants.

15. FERMENTED FOODS

Delicious: See Avocado Turkey Burger Sprout Wrap (page 229) and Fish Tacos (page 260).

Heart Healthy: Fermented foods include cabbage (kimchi), sauerkraut, and pickled vegetables. Fermentation helps to optimize the gut microflora. Recent studies by my colleague Stan Hazen, MD, PhD, section head for cardiovascular medicine at the Cleveland Clinic, have shown that after eating animal-derived fatty foods such as eggs, red meat, and dairy products, the gut bacteria break down certain fats (known as phospholipids) into a by-product known as TMAO (or trimethylamine N-oxide). It turns out that TMAO is involved in plaque development, and the higher the TMAO levels, the greater your risk of heart disease. Fermented vegetables generate probiotics that aid in rebalancing normal gut flora and keep TMAO levels under control. Maybe that's why sauerkraut is placed on hot dogs![60]

Mood Elevating: Fermented foods produce the neurotransmitter gamma-aminobutyric acid (GABA) in the gut and increase its brain receptors. GABA mediates the production of endorphins. And let's not forget about fermented drinks. My wife and kids enjoy Kombucha as an after-school and after-work pick-me-up.

16. FIBER (SOLUBLE)

Delicious: See Pumpkin Pie Smoothie (page 216), Deeply Satisfying Kasha Porridge (page 214), Banana-Mango-Ginger Smoothie (page 215), Spinach-Mango Salad with Hempseeds (page 226), and Spinach Salad with Berries and Honey Pecans (page 236).

Heart Healthy: Dietary fiber consists of all the parts of plant foods that can't be digested. These complex carbs include soluble and insoluble fiber, both of which delay the absorption of glucose and are easier on the pancreas with respect to insulin release than are simple carbs. In contrast to insoluble fiber, found in wheat-containing products, soluble fiber also lowers LDL cholesterol.

While a total fiber intake of 20 to 30 grams is recommended, eating 5 to 10 grams of soluble fiber each day should lower both your LDL cholesterol and your risk of heart disease by 10 to 15 percent.[61] By incorporating the foods listed in "The Best Sources of Soluble Fiber" (see page 38), it's rather easy to get this amount into your daily dietary regimen.

Mood Elevating: Soluble fiber enhances the absorption of tryptophan, which in turn bolsters the brain's production of serotonin to improve mood. Keep in mind

THE BEST SOURCES OF SOLUBLE FIBER

PRODUCT	AMOUNT (GRAMS)
Mango (1 small)	3.4
Benefit (3/4 cup cereal)	2.8
Black beans (1/2 cup)	2.4
Navy beans (1/2 cup)	2.2
Grapefruit, fresh (1 medium)	2.2
Pear, fresh, with skin (1 large)	2.2
Oat bran (3/4 cup cooked)	2.0
Kidney beans (1/2 cup)	2.0
Brussels sprouts (1/2 cup)	2.0
Apricots, fresh, with skin (4)	1.8
Orange (1 small)	1.8
Sweet potato, flesh only (1/2 cup)	1.8
Asparagus (1/2 cup)	1.7
Turnip (1/2 cup)	1.7
Barley, pearled, cooked (1 cup)	1.6

that if you have a gluten sensitivity, there is no cross reactivity with soluble-fiber-containing products, except for barley. Oats should not pose a problem, provided that the food-processing plant does not cross-contaminate them with wheat residue.

17. FISH

Delicious: See Rockfish Cakes (page 246), Super-Easy Steelhead Trout Teriyaki (page 253), Roasted Salmon with Orange-Herb Sauce (page 258), Asian Baked Halibut (page 259), Fish Tacos (page 260), Pistachio-Crusted Tilapia with

PRODUCT	AMOUNT (GRAMS)
Oatmeal (1/3 cup)	1.4
Figs, dried (1½)	1.4
Chickpeas, dried (½ cup)	1.3
Green peas (½ cup)	1.3
Broccoli (½ cup)	1.2
Cheerios (1¼ cups cereal)	1.2
Carrots (½ cup)	1.1
Flaxseeds (1 tablespoon)	1.1
Lima beans (½ cup)	1.1
Plums, fresh (2 medium)	1.1
Strawberries (1¼ cups)	1.1
Apple, fresh, with skin (1 small)	1.0
Peach, fresh, with skin (1 medium)	1.0
Prunes, dried (3 medium)	1.0

Adapted from J. W. Anderson, *Plant Fiber in Foods,* 2nd ed. (Lexington, KY: HCF Nutrition Research Foundation Inc., 1990).

Strawberry Salsa (page 262), Flounder in White Wine Sauce (page 245), Baked Rainbow Trout with Dates and Almonds (page 248), Sesame Miso Cod (page 253), and Cedar-Planked Wild Salmon (page 247).

Heart Healthy: An important study several years back revealed why fish is a brain food. Researchers studying our early human ancestors found that as they migrated from inland toward the ocean, their brain size significantly increased. The "brain booster" primarily responsible is the omega-3 DHA. High DHA levels in blood are associated with better memory and a higher level of cognition. Omega-3 intake is also linked to lower risk of depression.

DHA is found in breast milk and, like EPA, the other well-known omega-3, is found in cold-water fish. Brain development is most critical during the first 5 years of life. (As an aside, my wife took fish oil capsules throughout her pregnancies and while breastfeeding; after that, we pierced the capsules and squirted the omega-3s directly into our kids' mouths.) The best sources of marine-derived omega-3s are anchovies, herring, roe, sable, salmon, sardines, trout, tuna, and whitefish.

Speaking of anchovies, these tiny fish are a great source of vitamin D and calcium. King salmon has the highest concentration of nervonic acid, an omega-9 fatty acid. Mackerel is another good source, but it is too high in mercury to recommend. Sardines are also an excellent source of calcium. Fatty fish also increase vitamin D by enhancing calcium absorption. Cold-water fish, as well as shellfish, are an excellent source of A and B vitamins (including B_{12}) and choline. Both fish (sardines) and shellfish (clams and shrimp) are also rich in iodine, which is needed to maintain healthy thyroid function.

Mood Elevating: Clams are an excellent source of iron, which has a direct effect on regulating mood by affecting dopamine and serotonin. Mussels and oysters boast high concentrations of B_{12}, zinc, iodine, magnesium, and selenium, which work cohesively to maintain alertness and serve as mood boosters. Cod is high in the mood-boosting chemicals tryptophan and selenium and contains heart-healthy quantities of the powerful antioxidant glutathione. In addition to being a powerhouse of omega-3 DHA, wild salmon is replete with vitamins B_6 and B_{12}, copper, selenium, and zinc. It is also a good dietary source of vitamin D.

Fish is one of the few foods high in choline, which helps to curb anxiety. Choline also reduces homocysteine levels; too much of this amino acid is toxic to the arteries and blood vessels. Fish is also a good source of zinc. Populations that eat the most fish consistently demonstrate the lowest rates of depression. In fact, people diagnosed with depression have 20 to 30 percent less DHA in their brains.[62]

18. FRUITS (CITRUS)

Delicious: See the smoothie and positive emotion elixir recipes in Chapter 11.

Heart Healthy: Citrus fruits contain flavonoids like hesperetin and naringenin that help improve blood flow. Naringenin is the flavonoid responsible for the bitterness in grapefruit. It also lowers LDL, improves insulin sensitivity, and is being examined to treat diabetic and overweight men and women. Citrus fruits, especially lemons and limes, are loaded with limonoids that keep your heart healthy by lowering LDL and serving as potent antioxidants. This is in addition to the LDL-lowering properties of the soluble fiber (discussed earlier) contained in fruits such as oranges and grapefruits.

Mood Elevating: The aroma of citrus fruits has been shown to have a positive impact on mood.[63] I recommend that my patients eat at least one orange or one grapefruit daily. Half a glass (4 ounces) of your favorite nonconcentrated citrus fruit juice can also pack a decent punch of vitamins and minerals, but larger amounts will add an excess of calories. For example, 4 ounces of orange juice will add only about 55 calories but will still provide 15 percent of your daily potassium requirement.

19. FRUITS (OTHER THAN CITRUS FRUITS AND BERRIES)

Delicious: See the smoothie and positive emotion elixir recipes (pages 215–219 and 283–288).

Heart Healthy: Eating non-citrus fruits daily is another excellent way to maintain if not improve heart health. Bromelain, a heart-protective protein found in pineapples, is a natural blood clot buster.[64] Apples are an excellent source of quercetin, which in supplement form at doses of 150 milligrams per day was found to reduce systolic blood pressure between 3 and 4 mm Hg and reduce plaque-forming, oxidized LDL.[65] Each apple with skin contains about 10 milligrams of quercetin. While I wouldn't recommend eating 15 apples a day, eating apples on a daily basis is associated with reduced risk of heart disease and stroke. In a study of 35,000 women living in Iowa, intake of the apple antioxidants catechin and epicatechin was associated with reduced death from heart disease.[66] Simply eating one apple a day would prevent thousands of heart attacks and strokes each year, based on a recent United Kingdom study.[67]

Apples are a good source of fiber (a small apple has 1 gram of soluble fiber), and a study in older women found that eating one apple daily for 6 months reduced LDL by up to 24 percent.[68] Eating apples on a regular basis may also reduce the risk of stroke.[69] Just don't eat the seeds, because they contain trace amounts of cyanide that if consumed in abundance may be toxic. The same may apply to cherry, peach, and apricot pits.

All fruits contain heart-protective compounds. A healthy intake of fruits that are rich in potassium and magnesium will keep your heart healthy and boost mood. We should aim for between 4,000 and 5,000 milligrams of potassium each day, and for the RDA of magnesium (310 to 320 milligrams for women and 400 to 420 milligrams for men). If your potassium is too low, your physician may prescribe potassium supplements (measured in milliequivalents, mEq). A prescription for 20 mEq corresponds to 782 milligrams. As you can see in the chart below, eating a selection of the fruits listed will help to maintain these important electrolyte chemicals in balance.

FOOD	POTASSIUM (MG)	MAGNESIUM (MG)
Raisins, golden seedless (½ cup)	615	29
Mango (1 whole)	564	34
Dates, Deglet Noor (½ cup)	482	32
Kiwifruit, green (1 serving)	462	25
Banana (1 medium)	422	32
Cantaloupe (1 serving)	358	16
Prune juice (4 ounces)	353	18
Guava (½ cup)	344	18
Watermelon (1 serving)	314	28
Honeydew (1 serving)	306	13
Papaya (1 small)	286	33
Peach (1 medium)	285	14
Orange (1 serving)	256	17
Orange juice (4 ounces)	248	14
Plum (1 serving)	237	11
Strawberries (1 serving)	225	19
Prunes, dried (3)	209	12
Grapefruit, pink/red (1 serving)	206	14
Pear (1 medium)	206	12
Pomegranates (½ cup arils)	205	10
Apple with skin	195	9
Kumquats (5)	186	20
Apple without skin	145	6
Blackberries (½ cup)	117	14
Fig (1 medium)	116	8
Apricot (1 medium)	91	4
Pineapple (1/2 cup)	90	10
Persimmon (1 medium)	78	0
Blueberries (½ cup)	57	4
Cranberries (½ cup)	42	3
Raspberries (10)	29	4

Source: U.S. Department of Agriculture (USDA). http://ndb.nal.usda.gov/ndb/search/list.

Mood Elevating: In addition to magnesium, fruits are also an excellent source of vitamins B_6, B_9 (folate), and C, all of which are instrumental in raising brain levels of serotonin and regulating dopamine release. Guava has the highest content of vitamin C (followed by kiwifruit and mango) at nearly 200 milligrams per ½ cup. Fruits with the highest folate content are mango, papaya, oranges, kiwi, and strawberries, and vitamin B_6-rich fruits are bananas, mangos, raisins, and apricots.

20. GARLIC

Delicious: See Roasted Green Beans with Garlic and Thyme (page 273), Roasted Broccoli (page 272), Curried Cauliflower (page 270), Roasted Jerusalem Artichokes with Herbs (page 269), and Sautéed Spinach with Lemon and Pine Nuts (page 268).

Heart Healthy: Eating one garlic clove daily has been shown to result in a 20 percent lower risk of heart disease.[70] Eating one-half to one clove of garlic per day may lower cholesterol levels by 5 to 10 percent.[71] And ¼ ounce of garlic extract has been shown to reduce blood clotting and systolic blood pressure by more than 5 percent.[72]

On the other hand, garlic supplements have been shown to be less effective. When crushed, garlic releases the chemical allicin, which, when dissolved in an oil (e.g., olive oil), releases the by-product ajoene. Ajoene is the active compound that reduces blood clot formation and inflammation[73] and is believed to be pivotal in contributing to the heart-protective properties of garlic.

Mood Elevating: Garlic relaxes blood vessels due in part to the content of the trace mineral chromium. Chromium increases release of tryptophan, which is the precursor to the mood-enhancing transmitter serotonin.

In addition to chromium, garlic is a good source of vitamins B_6 and C, which regulate dopamine. By reducing oxidative stress and increasing oxygen supply through blood vessel dilation, garlic has also been shown in several Japanese studies to reduce symptoms of fatigue, and it has been used in treating chronic fatigue syndrome.[74] There's nothing like improving your energy level to lift your spirits!

21. GINGER

Delicious: See Banana-Mango-Ginger Smoothie (page 215) and Asian Baked Halibut (page 259).

Heart Healthy: Ginger contains a host of antioxidant compounds that help to lower stress levels.[75] It also contains gingerols that prevent damage caused by free radicals, leading to reduced plaque buildup that can accelerate hardening of the arteries. Ginger supplementation of 1 gram was shown to reduce chronic inflammation.[76] An important anti-inflammatory ingredient is cineole. In addition to ginger, cineole is found in cardamom and rosemary, and recent studies link it to improved cognitive performance and mood (see "Mood Elevating" on the opposite page).

Mood Elevating: Ginger is a good source of magnesium, selenium, and zinc, prime chemicals involved in mood enhancement. It was also shown to reverse the depletion of the mood-enhancing chemicals serotonin and dopamine caused by monosodium glutamate (MSG)—the flavor enhancer used in processed foods.[77]

22. GOJI BERRIES

Delicious: See Red Chakra (Root) Elixir (page 286).

Heart Healthy: Goji berries contain kukoamines, which reduce blood pressure and improve blood flow; some studies suggest that it may also slow aging of the brain. If you take warfarin (coumadin), you should not eat goji berries because of a potential interaction that increases bleeding risk.[78]

Mood Elevating: Goji berries are high in L-glutamine, the precursor of GABA that promotes endorphin release, and L-arginine, the precursor of the blood vessel dilator nitric oxide. Gojis are also a good source of choline, the by-product of the neurotransmitter acetylcholine, which helps to regulate mood. A small handful should have the desired effect.

23. HERBS (BASIL, HIBISCUS, OREGANO, ROSEMARY, AND SAGE)

Delicious: See Pesto Portobello Pizza (page 249), Tuna and Chickpea Salad (page 230), Green Bean, Artichoke, and Tuna Salad (page 228), Honey- and Maple-Glazed Brussels Sprouts (page 269), Flounder in Garlic White Wine Sauce (page 245), Apple-Rosemary Elixir (page 287), Roasted Jerusalem Artichokes with Herbs (page 269), and Mediterranean Kale Tart (page 255).

Heart Healthy: Basil has a high content of heart-healthy flavonoids that inhibit free radical production to keep our cells intact. In rodent and animal models, basil and sage reduced blood pressure.

Hibiscus is rich in the powerful antioxidant flavonoid and associated anthocyanin pigments, and a review of both animal and human studies has found it to effectively lower LDL, triglycerides, and blood pressure.[79] Drinking 3 cups of hibiscus tea each day can lower blood pressure by 8.5 mm Hg compared to a placebo, approximating the benefit seen with a single blood pressure medication.[80, 81]

Oregano is rich in the antioxidants rosmarinic acid and quercetin, which are effective in reducing LDL oxidation and production of free radicals that stimulate growth of cholesterol plaques. In rats, oregano extract has been shown to reduce heart damage after an induced heart attack.[82]

Rosemary also possesses potent antioxidant properties to neutralize destructive free radicals and limit arterial aging.[83]

Mood Elevating: A type of basil referred to as holy basil has been shown to reduce anxiety.[84] In mice, hibiscus extract was found to engender antidepressant effects.[85] Oregano enhances mood by inhibiting the enzyme monoamine oxidase (MAO). MAO is responsible for degrading mood neurotransmitters such as serotonin and dopamine.[86] Healthy volunteers exposed to the aroma of rosemary demonstrated increased arousal, better performance on assigned tasks, and an overall improved mood.[87] Sage inhibits acetylcholinesterase, reducing the breakdown of the mood-uplifting receptor acetylcholine and resulting in improved mood and improved cognitive performance.[88] Sage has also been shown to dramatically improve postmenopausal symptoms, and that should put affected women in a better mood.[89]

24. KALE

Delicious: See Mediterranean Kale Tart (page 255), Strawberry-Pineapple-Kale Smoothie (page 219), and Sautéed Kale (page 265).

Heart Healthy: A leafy green vegetable that has become popular in recent years, kale is an excellent source of calcium, lutein, and the antioxidant vitamins A, C, and E. In addition to containing powerful antioxidants, kale is a good source of the omega-3 ALA that helps to reduce inflammation. Soluble fiber in kale lowers LDL cholesterol, and its magnesium and potassium keep blood pressure levels better regulated.

Mood Elevating: A recent study from the Harvard School of Public Health found that optimism was highly correlated with vitamin A–derived carotenoids.[90] Kale has one of the highest concentrations of vitamin A among vegetables, trailing behind sweet potatoes, carrots, and spinach. At just below 9,000 IU per ½ cup of cooked kale, the RDA for vitamin A (for men, 3,000 IU; for women, 2,310 IU) is easily met. The only caution about eating kale and other greens applies if you are taking warfarin (Coumadin), because the high vitamin K content may counteract warfarin's anticlotting effect.

25. LOTUS ROOT

Delicious: See Roasted Lotus Root (page 266).

Heart Healthy: The lotus root contains proanthocyanidins, chemicals that have anti-inflammatory and antioxidant properties that lower cholesterol and triglycerides and reduce fatty liver in an animal model of obesity and diabetes.[91] Fatty liver not only raises the risk of diabetes and liver failure, but has also been shown to increase the risk of heart disease.[92]

Mood Elevating: Lotus root is a good source of mood-uplifting compounds vitamin B_6 and folate. When roasted, it has a crunchy, sweet, mouthwatering flavor.

26. MACA

Delicious: See Maca Date Shake (page 274) and Pumpkin Pie Smoothie (page 216).

Heart Healthy: Native Peruvians living in the Andes have been shown to have overall good health and reduced levels of inflammation, which is believed to reflect daily consumption of maca, a vegetable akin to the radish.[93] In animal models, maca has antioxidant properties and lowers LDL, triglycerides, and glucose.[94]

Mood Elevating: This Peruvian root has a long history as an aphrodisiac. Reduced libido commonly accompanies depression and, while antidepressants can help, a recent study found that when a group of men and women taking antidepressant medications added 3 grams of maca a day to their diets, their libidos improved.[95] Maca is best used in smoothies and adds maltlike flavor. I recommend that you purchase organic raw maca powder. One teaspoon contains about 5 grams of maca.

27. MUSHROOMS

Delicious: See Pesto Portobello Pizza (page 249) and Grilled Portobello Burgers (page 250).

Heart Healthy: When exposed to sunlight, mushrooms are good sources of vitamin D. And they are great sources of trace minerals like copper, which is essential for collagen production and healthy skin. Recently it was demonstrated that mushrooms possess properties similar to ACE (angiotensin-converting enzyme) inhibitors, medications commonly used to lower blood pressure.[96] Further research is needed to determine the magnitude of this effect. Another recent study found that substitution of mushrooms for red meat (the "Mushroom Diet") resulted in an average weight loss of 7 pounds in overweight subjects over a 1-year period.[97]

Mood Elevating: Of all the available edible mushrooms, one in particular, *Hericium erinaceus,* or Lion's Mane, received a lot of attention recently when a Japanese study found that symptoms of depression and anxiety improved after eating this mushroom daily for 1 month.[98] Lion's Mane mushroom has also been shown to stimulate nerve regeneration and improve cognition. Other mushrooms that may elevate your spirits are shiitakes, due to their favorable content of selenium and magnesium.

28. MUSTARD

Delicious: See Rockfish Cakes (page 246), Salmon with Asparagus and Artichoke-Mustard Sauce (page 254), Orange-Spinach Salad (page 227), and Tuna and Chickpea Salad (page 230).

Heart Healthy: Mustard is one of the heart-healthiest condiments. It is a rich source of magnesium and selenium, which have anti-inflammatory and mood-altering properties. Mustard is also a natural source of vitamin B_3 (aka niacin), which has intrinsic cholesterol-lowering properties. Simply adding 1½ tablespoons of mustard to a meal speeds up your BMR, or basal metabolic rate,[99] which can assist in weight loss. Mustard is also a good source of the omega-9 fat nervonic acid, which helps to preserve myelin sheaths and keep our brains healthy. Another important compound in mustard (as well as wasabi, daikon, and horseradish) is the enzyme myrosinase; this helps to release sulforaphane. Foods high in sulforaphane, such as broccoli, have been shown not only to kill cancer cells, but also to reduce oxidative stress in diabetes. And here's a special tip: Combining cruciferous vegetables with this condiment enhances these antioxidant properties.[100]

Mood Elevating: Both the magnesium and the selenium in mustard are involved in regulating the neurotransmitters dopamine and serotonin. The yellow color in mustard is turmeric, which contains the compound curcumin; curcumin has been shown to have antidepressant effects in rodents (see Turmeric on page 58). A small study of 40 men and women found a trend toward early improvement in symptoms of depression after consuming 500 milligrams of turmeric a day over a 5-week period.[101] When you buy mustard, make sure that it contains turmeric and mustard seed rather than just vinegar and yellow food dye.

29. NUTS

Delicious: See Almond Cookies (page 275), Ultimate Date Cake (page 278), and Almond-Chocolate Bark (page 279).

Heart Healthy: Nuts are a superfood. They're great sources of folate and fiber, and fiber lowers cholesterol and helps to regulate blood glucose levels. Some nuts, like walnuts, are good sources of the omega-3 ALA. Overall, eating nuts reduces risk of heart disease,[102] and there is up to a 35 percent lower risk of heart attacks and sudden cardiac death in those who eat nuts at least twice a week, compared to those who don't. The reasons for these benefits are multifold and include reducing LDL oxidation and uptake by macrophages to form cholesterol plaque and maintaining healthy endothelial function. A healthy endothelium produces cardioprotective chemicals like nitric oxide that offset inflammation and reduce susceptibility to blood clot formation.[103] And despite their high caloric density, nuts can be eaten in programs aimed at weight reduction.[104]

Nuts are potent sources of antioxidants. The following five nuts have high concentrations of antioxidants and are excellent sources of other vitamins and minerals: hazelnuts (L-arginine, copper, manganese); almonds (calcium, magnesium, potassium, phosphorus, vitamin E); pecans (calcium, vitamin A, phosphorus, potassium); walnuts (calcium, L-arginine, magnesium, omega-3 alpha-linolenic acid); and pistachios (vitamins A and E, lutein, L-arginine, magnesium, potassium, phosphorus). Pistachios have been found to better reduce triglycerides (33 percent) and body mass index (0.8 kg/m2) in comparison to a refined carbohydrate snack in obese subjects on a 12-week weight loss program.[105] L-arginine, the precursor of nitric oxide, helps to maintain endothelial function by dilating blood vessels and increasing blood flow.

Mood Elevating: Eating 1 ounce of mixed nuts (almonds, walnuts, and hazelnuts) each day was shown to be associated with an increase in serotonin metabolites.[106] While the study did not measure mood characteristics, a recent study in Spain that evaluated new cases of depression in diabetics found that supplementing their diets with nuts reduced their risk of depression by more than 40 percent.[107]

Nuts are excellent sources of magnesium, selenium, and zinc, all of which are involved in activating the neurotransmitters serotonin, dopamine, and GABA. The Brazil nut is the "queen bee" when it comes to selenium; just two Brazil nuts a day will fulfill your daily selenium needs.

Because nuts are densely caloric, the trick is to eat no more than a handful, which will only set you back 150 to 200 calories. I recommend this portion size to my patients as a midafternoon snack or to eat en route when they're driving home from work (see the 28-Day Positive Emotions Prescription Nutrition Plan on page 182). This serves two purposes: first, to have a healthy snack; and second, to have a filling snack, which can effectively curb appetite so that you don't overeat during dinner.

30. OLIVES

Delicious: See Mediterranean Salmon with Sun-Dried Tomatoes, Capers, and Olives (page 252) and Moroccan Chicken (page 256).

Heart Healthy: Olives serve as the principal component of the oil used in the Mediterranean diet. The principal fat of an olive is oleate (or oleic acid). Switching from a high-carb to a Mediterranean-based diet lowers triglycerides by 10 to 15 percent. Oleate also lowers LDL and reduces its susceptibility to plaque formation by inhibiting LDL oxidation. A recent study in Barcelona found that a Mediterranean diet supplemented with extra-virgin olive oil reduced risk of a first heart attack by 30 percent compared to the control group.[108]

Mood Elevating: A principal by-product of oleate is oleamide, which has a direct effect on regulating serotonin receptors. This finding has translated into real-world experience based on recent studies, including one from Athens that found that the higher the intake of extra-virgin olive oil, the greater the effect over a 6- to 13-year period.[109, 110]

31. ONIONS AND SHALLOTS

Delicious: See Roasted Asparagus with Shallots (page 265), Lightly Sautéed Purslane (page 266), Pistachio-Crusted Tilapia with Strawberry Salsa (page 262), Gingered Carrot Soup (page 241), Stuffed Sweet Potatoes with Beans (page 225), Quinoa Salad (page 232), Celestial Celery Root and Apple Soup (page 237), and Butternut Squash with Baby Spinach (page 272).

Heart Healthy: Onions have anticlotting properties.[111] Just as in garlic, ajoene is released from onions when they're sautéed in oil to produce heart-healthy antioxidant effects. Onions are excellent sources of flavonols (a group of flavonoid compounds that includes apples, broccoli, cacao beans, red wine, and certain teas) and the antioxidant glutathione. Consumption of high amounts of flavonoids has been associated with improved endothelial function, reduced blood pressure and risk of vascular disease, and reduced risk of neurological disorders, including Alzheimer's and dementia.[112] These effects translate into an overall 20 percent lower risk of heart disease.[113]

Shallots are rich sources of flavonoids, with at least five times more than Vidalia onions. These *Allium* compounds are also a potent source of the flavonoid quercetin (see also Fruits on page 41 and Beans on page 30), which is a more powerful natural antioxidant than vitamin E.

Mood Elevating: Onions exhibited antidepressant effects in an animal model of depression.[114] These effects may be attributable to their high chromium content. Chromium has been shown to regulate blood glucose and may blunt some of the midday mood slumps that occur following the glucose spike after lunch. It has also been shown to reduce symptoms associated with some forms of depression.[115, 116] (In addition to onions, tomatoes and oysters are also good sources of chromium.) I recommend that my patients consume at least three onions or shallots each week. The good news is that they can be eaten raw or sautéed without reducing the benefits of quercetin or chromium. To limit eye irritation and tearing, chill onions for 30 to 60 minutes prior to use. Any residual onion-related tears will then be tears of happiness!

32. PERSIMMONS

Delicious: See Persimmon-Mozzarella Panini (page 231).

Heart Healthy: Persimmons are robust in calcium, iron, magnesium, manganese, and potassium. In a recent head-to-head comparison to apples, they were found to contain more fiber and antioxidant capacity.[117] Supplemented persimmon extract has also been shown to reduce insulin resistance, and its catechin and gallocatechin tannins help to preserve the endothelium, dilate blood vessels, and reduce blood pressure. Please make sure that you've selected ripe persimmons because if you eat them when underripe, not only will your mouth become excessively dry as a result of tannin-induced astringency, but you may also experience some stomach irritation.

Mood Elevating: Persimmons are sources of vitamin C (as well as potassium and iodine, which may be useful in regulating moods by reducing oxidative stress and maintaining thyroid health), and the polyphenol tannins contained in the persimmon leaf possess skin-related antiwrinkle effects.[118] If having younger-looking skin doesn't improve your mood, what will?

33. POMEGRANATE

Delicious: See Orange-Spinach Salad (page 227).

Heart Healthy: Pomegranate seeds contain ellagitannins, one of nature's most powerful antioxidants. Drinking one glass (8 ounces) of pomegranate juice once a day for 3 months improved blood flow to the heart in both men and women.[119] Pomegranate juice also reduces plaque formation and blood pressure by acting in a similar way to the heart-protective ACE inhibitors.[120]

Mood Elevating: In a recent study, 60 men and women aged 21 to 64 drank one glass of pomegranate juice a day for 2 weeks. At the end of the study, blood pressure was lowered 4 mm Hg (similar to results from taking a mild blood pressure medicine), with a 24 percent increase in salivary testosterone levels. Mood was also lifted, with corresponding reductions in anxiety and depression.[121]

34. POTATOES

Delicious: See Sweet Potato–Miso Spread (page 267), Stuffed Sweet Potatoes with Beans (page 225), and Baked Sweet Potato Fries (page 263).

Heart Healthy: Sweet potatoes are a great source of the carotenoid beta-carotene, the precursor to vitamin A. In fact, of our top heart-healthy and mood-enhancing foods, sweet potatoes rank first in vitamin A content (21,909 IU for a medium potato), followed by carrots (10,191 IU for one medium carrot), spinach (9,433 IU for ½ cup, cooked), and kale (8,854 IU for ½ cup cooked). While antioxidant supplements (vitamins A, C, and E) have not been shown to be cardioprotective, eating foods enriched with antioxidants of the carotenoid class has been shown to reduce cardiovascular risk.[122]

Potatoes are also high in potassium, and a medium potato contains twice as much vitamin C as a tomato. Kukoamines are chemical compounds found in potatoes; they've recently been discovered to lower blood pressure and may slow the aging of our brains.

Mood Elevating: In general, potatoes are loaded with vitamin B_6 and folate to enhance release of the neurotransmitter serotonin. Potato skin is replete with iodine and enables proper functioning of your thyroid gland, which is vital for maintaining good moods.

35. POULTRY

Delicious: See Sesame Chicken Stir-Fry (page 244), Moroccan Chicken (page 256), and Avocado Turkey Burger Sprout Wrap (page 229).

Heart Healthy: Poultry is an excellent source of animal protein that is rich in vitamins B_6 and B_{12}, selenium, zinc, and the antioxidant vitamins A and E.

Mood Elevating: Chicken and turkey are excellent sources of tryptophan, which is an important chemical for the mood-regulating neurotransmitters serotonin, norepinephrine, and dopamine.

Although tryptophan can be partially converted to melatonin and help to regulate sleep, this is less likely to occur when poultry is consumed with other foods. The fatigue we experience on "Turkey Day" is more likely the result of the fat-rich meal many of us indulge in.

36. PUMPKIN

Delicious: See Butternut Squash with Baby Spinach (page 272), Roasted Butternut Squash and Black Bean Tacos (page 261), Pumpkin Pie Smoothie (page 216), Mouthwatering Watermelon Salad (page 234), and Apple-Blueberry Crisp (page 277).

Heart Healthy: Pumpkin is an excellent source of vitamins A and C, potassium, iron, and fiber. In clinical trials, pumpkin extract improved blood glucose levels in diabetics and exerted antioxidant effects. One of the antioxidant compounds isolated from pumpkin, D-chiro-inositol, is believed to play a role in limiting destruction of the pancreatic beta cells that produce insulin. If these findings can be reproduced in humans, it will be a new way to treat men and women at risk for or in the early stages of diabetes.[123]

Animal studies have found pumpkin seeds to have cholesterol-, blood pressure–, and weight-reducing properties. We await further confirmation of these effects in men and women.[124,125]

Mood Elevating: Pumpkin seeds are packed with the L-tryptophan that our brain uses to make the neurotransmitter serotonin to improve mood. Pumpkin seeds also represent our top heart-healthy, mood-regulating source of magnesium (156 milligrams in 1 ounce), and their high zinc content helps activate the neurotransmitters serotonin (via conversion of tryptophan) and GABA.

37. PURSLANE

Delicious: See Lightly Sautéed Purslane (page 266).

Heart Healthy: Purslane is a weed that has an underappreciated role in promoting cardiovascular health even though it actually has the ability to block important proteins that cause vascular inflammation.[126, 127] Purslane reduces LDL and triglycerides while raising the good cholesterol, HDL.[128] Purslane also contains a high amount of plant omega-3 ALA (up to 475 milligrams per ½-cup serving). That compares favorably to walnuts (700 milligrams per tablespoon) but is lower than flaxseeds (2,200 milligrams per tablespoon).[129, 130] A review of studies evaluating dietary sources of plant-based omega-3s found that consumption of plant-based omega-3 alpha-linolenic acid was associated with a relatively modest 10 percent reduced risk of heart attack and stroke deaths.[131]

Mood Elevating: The omega-3s in purslane are involved in controlling the mood-regulating neurotransmitters dopamine and serotonin. Purslane is also a rich source of vitamin A (1,065 IU), which is associated with lifting mood. Like tart cherries, purslane is also a good source of natural melatonin and may help to produce a good night's sleep. As a weed, purslane can be easily grown in your yard, or it may be purchased at your local farmers' market.

38. QUINOA

Delicious: See Warm Beet Quinoa Salad (page 232).

Heart Healthy: This gluten-free grain is an excellent source of fiber (3 grams total, with 1.1 grams of soluble fiber per ¼-cup serving) and can modestly reduce LDL. Quinoa is also an excellent source of the antioxidant flavonoids kaempferol and quercetin, which reduce LDL oxidation and plaque formation.

Mood Elevating: Quinoa is an energy-boosting food that is high in magnesium, manganese, zinc, and vitamin B_6, nutrients that activate mood-boosting neurotransmitters (serotonin and GABA) and reduce aging of our body tissues.

39. RADISHES

Delicious: See Arugula-Avocado-Almond Salad (page 223).

Heart Healthy: Radishes belong to the brassica family of vegetables, which includes broccoli and cabbage. Their peppery taste is due to glucosinolates that block cancer cell formation. Radishes may improve blood flow to the brain in part because they contain natural (not processed) nitrates, which stimulate production of nitric oxide.[132]

Mood Elevating: Radishes are a good source of folic acid, vitamin C, and beta-carotene and may uplift mood by stimulating the release of dopamine and norepinephrine.

40. ROSEMARY

Delicious: See Heartwarming White Bean Soup (page 240) and Grilled Portobello Burgers (page 250).

Heart Healthy: Another antioxidant powerhouse, this herb contains cineole, which increases blood flow to the heart and the brain. Cineole has also been shown to act as a bronchodilator and reduce symptoms of shortness of breath.

Mood Elevating: Recent studies suggest that rosemary oil improved mental alertness, cognitive performance, contentedness, and overall mood by between 5 and 10 percent when various word recall and memory tasks were tested.[133, 134]

41. SAFFRON

Delicious: See Saffron Split Pea Soup (page 238).

Heart Healthy: In a rabbit model, the addition of saffron's carotenoid antioxidant crocetin to a high-fat diet for 8 weeks resulted in reduced cholesterol plaques compared to a high-fat diet alone. Saffron's powerful antioxidants (crocin, lycopene, and beta-carotene) are believed to contribute to this effect. Saffron is also an excellent source of vitamin B_2 (riboflavin), which has been linked to lower blood pressure and reduced homocysteine levels. Saffron may also be the most highly concentrated source of manganese, which reduces free radical buildup, cell damage, and aging. For a serving size of only ½ teaspoon (2.5 grams), saffron provides 0.71 milligram of manganese, representing 30 percent or more of the RDA (for men, 2.3 milligrams; for women, 1.8 milligrams). The only other top heart-healthy and mood-enriching food sources higher in manganese per serving are chickpeas (0.85 milligram per ½ cup cooked), spinach (0.83 milligram per ½ cup cooked), pineapple (0.77 milligram per ½ cup), pumpkin seeds (0.74 milligram per 1 ounce), and edamame (0.71 milligram per ½ cup cooked).[135, 136]

Mood Elevating: Saffron may be the world's most expensive spice, but recent studies are proving that it's well worth its price. Saffron improved cognitive function in patients with early-stage Alzheimer's disease over 4 months.[137] Saffron has also been shown to improve symptoms of PMS[138] and to improve the symptoms of mild to moderate depression as effectively as common medications used to treat depression. Although the amount of saffron used in these trials was higher than the RDA and in capsule form (30 milligrams of the crocus petal), the results do support the use of saffron as a potential mood-altering compound.[139, 140]

The biggest concern when purchasing saffron is ensuring its authenticity. One recommendation is to purchase a product that has been graded by the International Organization for Standardization, or ISO. The deeper the color, the better the quality of the saffron. Aim for an ISO of 190 or greater. Note: Saffron stimulates the uterus, and even though this generally occurs at higher doses than are commonly used in foods, I would recommend that you either avoid it during pregnancy or discuss its use with your obstetrician first.

42. SEAWEED

Delicious: See Miso Soup (page 243).

Heart Healthy: Seaweed contains antioxidants. Of specific interest was the recent discovery that seaweed possesses chemicals that are similar to ACE inhibitors, medications that lower blood pressure and dilate arteries. Various types of seaweed include nori, used for sushi rolls, which is high in omega-3 fatty acids; hijiki used for miso soup; and wakame, the dark green seaweed often used in miso soup and which is high in magnesium and folate.[141] In fact, wakame is now offered daily at our university café. Its primary pigment, fucoxanthin, prevents diabetes and diet-induced obesity in mice.[142]

Mood Elevating: Seaweed is a great source of iodine, which helps to regulate your thyroid, but perhaps even more importantly, it's among the richest natural sources of selenium. In fact, several studies have now shown that selenium supplementation improves mood, while low levels in the blood have been linked to depressed states.[143, 144] Seaweed contains vitamins (A, B_{12}, and C) and magnesium, which is involved in the production of mood-regulating neurotransmitters. Not only can you find seaweed in Asian supermarkets and health food stores, but it is also readily available from national retail outlets including Trader Joe's and Costco.

43. SEEDS

Delicious: See Frozen Coconut-Chia-Blueberry Parfait (page 276), Spinach-Mango Salad with Hempseeds (page 226), Sesame Bars (page 276), and Cashew Butter Granola Bars (page 282).

Heart Healthy: Seeds can be lignin-rich, with antioxidant and cholesterol-lowering properties (sesame seeds, flaxseeds), and high in omega-3 ALA and soluble fiber, which lower LDL. They also regulate glucose (chia seeds, flaxseeds, sesame seeds), reduce platelet aggregation and blood clot formation (hempseeds), and lower triglyceride levels in diabetics (sesame seeds).[145–147]

Mood Elevating: Seeds are packed with nutrients that activate mood-uplifting neurotransmitters. They include L-arginine (hempseeds, pumpkin seeds), magnesium (flaxseeds, pumpkin seeds, sesame seeds, sunflower seeds), folate (flaxseeds, sesame seeds, sunflower seeds), vitamin B_6 (chia seeds, flaxseeds, sesame seeds, sunflower seeds), and zinc (chia, pumpkin, sesame, and sunflower seeds).

44. SPINACH

Delicious: See Sautéed Spinach with Lemon and Pine Nuts (page 268), Butternut Squash with Baby Spinach (page 272), Orange-Spinach Salad (page 227), and Spinach Salad with Berries and Honey Pecans (page 236).

Heart Healthy: Spinach is one of the richest vegetable sources of magnesium, vitamin B_6, and folate, all of which lower levels of homocysteine, the amino acid linked to increased risk of heart attack and stroke.

Mood Elevating: Spinach is among the most powerful mood-boosting foods because its leaves are lined with folate (262 micrograms per cup) and antioxidants. Spinach also contains oxalic acid, which interferes with calcium absorption but is easily neutralized by cooking. Keep in mind that the darker the leaf, the higher the calcium content. Spinach is a top source of betaine, tryptophan, and magnesium, with an impressive 78 milligrams in each ½ cup to help combat anxiety and fatigue and improve concentration.

45. SPIRULINA

Delicious: See Almond-Chocolate Bark (page 279) and Green Chakra (Heart) Elixir (page 284).

Heart Healthy: This protein-enriched algae has been consumed for centuries in Mexico and Central Africa. At doses as little as 1 gram daily for 2 months, spirulina has been shown to reduce cholesterol and triglycerides, as well as improve glucose levels in diabetics. Spirulina also has powerful antioxidant and anti-inflammatory properties.

Mood Elevating: Spirulina's reported mood-elevating properties may reflect its high concentrations of vitamin B_{12} and omega-3s.[148] While spirulina has a good safety record, you should only purchase it from a vendor with an unblemished record of excellent quality control due to reports of contamination with mercury and other toxins.

46. TEA

Delicious: See various dessert teas recommended throughout the 28-Day Positive Emotions Prescription Nutrition Plan in Chapter 10.

Heart Healthy: The cardiovascular benefits of drinking tea are numerous. First, all teas contain a class of antioxidants known as polyphenols. While the polyphenols in green and black tea differ, they both have similar heart health properties. Drinking 3 cups of your favorite tea each day reduces cardiovascular risk (heart attack and stroke) by 20 percent. These benefits are due to reduced platelet clumping and inhibited LDL oxidation. It has been suggested that drinking 5 cups of tea each day can effectively detoxify the free radicals that accumulate in response to life's stressors and promote atherosclerosis. Through detoxification, tea can slow aging of our cells and heart vessels.[149] Other antioxidants in teas include catechins, which can cause your metabolism to burn an extra 100 calories per day. In effect, drinking several cups of green tea daily was associated with an approximate 3-pound weight loss over a 3-month period.[150] Recent studies found that drinking up to 3 cups of black tea on a daily basis reduced triglycerides by 30 percent because the tea blocks enzymes in the stomach that digest fat. The same appears to hold true for green tea.

Hibiscus tea can also reduce blood pressure if consumed on a daily basis and acts similarly to the popular class of medications known as ACE inhibitors.[151]

Mood Elevating: Tea consumption improves alertness and arousal, and a recent review found that drinking 2 to 3 cups over 1½ hours improved mood and conferred a greater ability to focus on the tasks at hand. Caffeine and the amino acid threonine are believed to be the factors responsible for these benefits. Other teas such as the green tea matcha (or maccha) were shown to increase concentration and improve mood.[152]

47. TOMATO

Delicious: See Mediterranean Salmon with Sun-Dried Tomatoes, Capers, and Olives (page 252), Sun-Dried Tomato Dip (page 267), and Gazpacho Soup (page 242).

Heart Healthy: Lycopene is the primary dietary carotenoid antioxidant in tomato-based products. The lycopene content of 1 cup of tomato juice or tomato-based soup using ½ cup of tomato sauce varies between 11 and 17 milligrams. Contrast that with ½ cup of watermelon (3.4 milligrams), half a grapefruit (1.8 milligrams), and ½ cup uncooked tomato (2.3 milligrams), though lycopene content is two to three times higher in organic tomatoes.[153] At least seven servings of tomato-based products each week was shown to be associated with reduced risk of heart disease in women; the findings were less consistent in men.[154] Tomatoes may also prevent blood from clotting, as the yellow liquid surrounding tomato seeds inhibits platelet activity in a manner similar to aspirin. However, you need to consume six or more tomatoes to attain this effect.[155] Still, I recommend that my patients pack tomatoes on a long trip that may restrict movement, as they may be at increased risk of a deep venous thrombosis (DVT) or blood clot in their leg. Tomatoes also dilate blood vessels due to their high content of magnesium and chromium. Chromium has also been shown to reduce food cravings.[156]

Mood Elevating: Eating tomatoes twice each week was recently shown to be associated with reduced self-reported depression compared to consuming less than one tomato each week in a group of nearly 1,000 men and women over age 70. In fact, eating a tomato or tomato-based product at least once each day was associated with more than a 50 percent lower reported rate of depressive symptoms compared to consumption at or below once weekly.[157] Whether this may have been the result of the powerful antioxidant effect of lycopene is unknown. I recommend that my patients eat at least one raw tomato each day, in addition to their apple.

48. TURMERIC

Delicious: See Moroccan Chicken (page 256), Sunshine Gold Elixir (page 286), and Apple-Rosemary Elixir (page 287).

Heart Healthy: As the primary spice in curry, turmeric's biological benefits reside in curcumin, a primary antioxidant and anti-inflammatory compound found in turmeric root.[158] Curcumin has also been shown to reduce complications in diabetics. Their high concentrations of glucose result in changes in proteins that produce advanced glycation end products (AGEs). AGEs rev up oxidative damage and, in doing so, convert mild-mannered macrophages into angry macrophages, resulting in endothelial damage and premature vascular disease. Curcumin protects our endothelium against oxidative stress, thereby slowing down cellular aging.[159]

Indeed, turmeric is a dietary staple for Okinawans, who experience healthy aging and longevity.[160]

While studies have demonstrated that curcumin improves glucose control in diabetic rats, there have been no large human trials evaluating turmeric's effect on heart attack and stroke risk. Still, the small-scale human studies are encouraging. Curcumin lowers the anti-inflammatory marker CRP and improves vascular function in women after menopause.[161, 162] At a dose of 45 milligrams per day, it was shown to lower LDL after a heart attack.[163] Exciting preliminary studies also support a potential role for curcumin in treating heart failure.[164] In addition, curcumin was recently shown to slow the vascular eye changes that occur in diabetics and is currently being evaluated as a treatment for a host of other inflammatory and degenerative eye diseases.[165, 166]

Mood Elevating: In addition to the small trial of turmeric to treat depression described on page 47, another recent trial in 60 men and women diagnosed with major depression found that the administration of curcumin at 1,000 milligrams a day for 6 weeks was safe and well tolerated and that it performed similar to Prozac (20 milligrams) with respect to improved mood.[167]

49. VANILLA

Delicious: See Peach and Blueberry Cobbler (page 221), Ginger-Date Smoothie (page 215), Amaretto Amore (page 274), Chocolate Chip–Beet Cake (page 281), and Cashew Butter Granola Bars (page 282).

Heart Healthy: Native to Central America, the vanilla bean possesses natural potent antioxidant properties that can reduce free radical formation and cellular aging.[168] The vanilla bean also contains magnesium, manganese, and zinc, although the quantity of each is modest. Despite a lack of clinical data, I believe that the potential benefit based on the aforementioned characteristics makes vanilla a worthy candidate for inclusion as a top nutrient source.

Mood Elevating: When it comes to enhancing mood, vanilla stands out. Vanilla extract is effective aromatherapy, with a soothing and mood-elevating effect. This was demonstrated in a clinical trial in which smelling a vanilla mist reduced anxiety for cancer patients preparing to undergo MRI scanning, which commonly induces claustrophobia.[169] I recommend vanilla-scented candles to my patients. Vanilla in powder, extract, or (scraped) bean tastes great in frozen banana smoothies and other desserts.

50. WATERMELONS

Delicious: See Mouthwatering Watermelon Salad (page 234) and Watermelon-Mint Elixir (page 288).

Heart Healthy: Watermelons contain high amounts of citrulline, an amino acid that relaxes blood vessels in much the same way that Viagra dilates them. Like tomatoes, watermelon contains lycopene (though in lower quantities) and so provides its antioxidant, heart-protective properties. The edible rind of watermelon contains lots of citrulline. Citrulline is converted to arginine, the precursor of the vasodilator and endothelial protector nitric oxide, and citrulline enrichment reduces blood pressure.[170] In fact, eating just three slices of watermelon a day may prevent a person with prehypertension (systolic blood pressure of 120 to 139 or diastolic blood pressure of 80 to 89 mm Hg) from developing full-blown hypertension. This may be due in part to watermelon's arginine-mediated diuretic effect.[171]

Mood Elevating: Although no scientific studies have specifically addressed watermelon intake's effect on mood, there is good reason to believe it does have mood-enhancing properties. This is based on its high content of vitamin A, previously shown to be associated with optimism and uplifted mood (see Kale on page 24), and lycopene, which has also been shown to reduce symptoms of depression (see Tomato on page 57). The high citrulline content that drives L-arginine– and nitric oxide–mediated vasodilation may also play a role in improved mood, but this will require further study.

Eight Trending Positive Emotions Foods

In addition to the Top 50 Foods, here are eight foods that are just beginning to make it into the public eye. Take a look at these for the latest trends in superfood heart and emotional health.

1. DRAGON FRUIT

Dragon fruit, or red pitaya, is native to Mexico and Central and South America. It has a pleasant, mood-uplifting taste resembling that of kiwifruit, with hints of pear. This fruit is an excellent source of antioxidants and in animal studies has been shown to improve glucose control and blood pressure and reduce stiffness and aging of arteries.[172]

The USDA has only permitted dragon fruit to be imported within the past decade, and therefore you will have the most success finding it at your local Asian market. Do not eat the skin, but rather spoon out the flesh and cut it into cubes. Try it in a salad or on its own.

2. GUARANA

Also known as Brazilian cocoa, guarana seeds are rich in caffeine and antioxidant tannins. Guarana extract at a dose as low as 37.5 milligrams daily is associated with improved mood and alertness.[173]

With respect to heart disease prevention, guarana reduces oxidation of LDL and platelet clumping—both of which raise heart attack risk.[174, 175] Compared to those who don't, elderly folks living in the Amazon who eat guarana tend to have a healthier metabolic profile, including lower blood pressure and cholesterol as well as reduced waistlines in men.[176]

While these studies neither prove that guarana use reduces heart attacks or strokes nor exclude the potential benefit of the caffeine content, they do represent a starting point to support additional research into and testing of this compound. You only need a very small amount (such as one drop of purified liquid extract) to get about 50 milligrams of guarana to boost mood. I would not recommend more than 50 milligrams if you also drink caffeinated beverages.

3. INDIAN GOOSEBERRY (AMLA)

Lots of exciting studies have recently come to light supporting Indian gooseberry as a mood-elevating food with a host of cardioprotective features. While cholesterol- and triglyceride-lowering effects have been shown after eating gooseberries raw or in powder form, the concentrated extract was recently shown to possess powerful anti-inflammatory properties.[177, 178] Healthy volunteers taking 500 milligrams of purified extract for 2 weeks showed significant reduction in artery stiffness.[179, 180]

The same extract given to diabetics, a group with a higher tendency to form clots, was also shown to result in reduced platelet clumping over a 10-day period.[181] Perhaps the most impressive finding was that Indian gooseberries placed first among 20 Ayurvedic remedies for their potent antioxidant properties, which, coupled with their inhibition of an enzyme implicated in dementia, may lead to their playing a future role in treating Alzheimer's disease.[182]

Indian gooseberries may be available at your local Asian market. They have a very sour taste, though they'll taste sweeter if you have a sip of cold water with them. I would recommend starting with just one berry a day. Many enjoy using ½ to 1 teaspoon of the organic powder form in smoothies. You may also consider obtaining it in frozen form in Asian markets or purchasing it in bottled (pickled) or powder form.

4. LUCUMA

This subtropical Peruvian fruit is also known as Incan Gold because of its rich flesh color and deliciously sweet maple flavor. Lucuma is a rich source of the mood-uplifting chemicals magnesium and zinc, and in recent years, it has also been shown to exhibit antioxidant, antidiabetic, and antihypertensive properties.[183]

The easiest way to obtain lucuma is in powder form from your local health food store or from an online outlet such as Navitas Naturals (navitasnaturals.com). Powdered lucuma can be added to smoothies or used to make the popular Peruvian lucuma-flavored ice cream. The typical serving size is 1 tablespoon (10 to 15 grams).

5. MAQUI BERRY (CHILEAN WINEBERRY)

With a taste like blackberries, the delicious and mood-uplifting Chilean maqui berry is superhigh in the purple pigment antioxidant anthocyanin.[184] Like other powerful antioxidants, maqui berries reduce oxidation of LDL, thereby keeping angry macrophages at bay and reducing foam cells, the precursor of cholesterol plaques we discussed in Chapter 1. They also protect us against the oxidative damage we face each day caused by stress and pollutants in our environment.[185] Maqui berries also have anti-inflammatory properties and antidiabetic effects; they improve insulin sensitivity so that glucose can be more readily taken up by our muscles.[186]

Unless you are visiting Chile, the best way to get maqui berries is in freeze-dried organic powder form from an online retailer such as Navitas Naturals. The serving size is about 1 gram daily.

6. MUCUNA BEAN

Also known as velvet beans, this Indian herbal aphrodisiac contains L-dopa, the precursor of dopamine, and has been used to treat depression as well as combat symptoms associated with Parkinson's disease.[187]

In animal models, the mucuna bean has also been shown to lower cholesterol and triglycerides and to possess both glucose-lowering and anti-inflammatory properties.[188, 189]

Organic velvet bean farms are sprouting up here in the United States, and the beans can now be purchased online whole or in powder form. While the taste of velvet beans is delicious, the amount to consume for positive emotional benefits and heart health has yet to be established. Raw velvet beans can be toxic, however, so the beans should be thoroughly soaked and cooked before eating. (The downside of cooking, though, is that it reduces L-dopa content.) Using 5 grams daily of a purified roasted powder reduces some symptoms of Parkinson's disease. If you are healthy and trying mucuna bean powder for the first time, I would recommend much smaller doses, such as 2 or 3 grams. Side effects such as vomiting or mind-altering effects would not be expected at low doses, but they have been reported at a dose of 30 grams per day.[190]

7. REISHI MUSHROOM

Also known as the lingzhi or supernatural mushroom, reishi mushrooms have been used in traditional Chinese medicine for millennia. They have a host of cardioprotective effects that include lowering blood pressure, cholesterol, glucose, and blood clot formation.[191]

In a recent study, 25 women being treated for breast cancer who were assigned to take reishi mushroom powder at a dose of 3 grams a day for a month showed increased physical well-being and reduced fatigue when compared to another group of women with breast cancer who did not receive the powder.[192]

These mushrooms may be found and purchased in fresh, dry, or powder form at your local Asian market. Adding about 1 gram of the powder to smoothies, coffee, or tea may provide you with a modest boost in mood and energy. I add it, along with a teaspoon of cacao powder, to my coffee on superbusy mornings.

8. SEA BUCKTHORN BERRY

These delicious but tart little orange-mango-tasting berries are packed with vitamin C (10 to 15 times more than in oranges) and antioxidant flavonoids like quercetin. The sweet, aromatic scent has mood-uplifting effects. Originally found in the Himalayan regions, sea buckthorn shrubs have now been cultivated in cooler North American climates, including certain parts of Canada and the United States.

A Finnish study of 110 overweight women found that replacement of part of the normal diet with 3½ ounces of these berries for 1 month was associated with lowering of cholesterol and triglycerides.[193] This study adds to prior studies showing mild weight reduction and reduced inflammation. Similar results were obtained with bilberries.[194]

If you do not live in a climate conducive to finding these berries at your farmers' market, they can be purchased in powder form online. Make sure to choose a reputable manufacturer who has a record of only selling products free of mercury, cadmium, and other toxins.

The Positive Emotions Prescription: Nutrition

Choose a minimum of five foods each day from the Top 50 Foods list and incorporate them into your diet for positive emotional health, cardiovascular wellness, and happy taste buds.

CHAPTER 3

Laughing Matters

THE BEST MEDICINE YOU'LL EVER TAKE

ONE OF MY FAVORITE MOMENTS as a physician occurs when, with a very somber look, I inform my patients that there's one thing they *absolutely must do* in order to make a successful recovery after a cardiac event. They're all ears as they brace themselves for a stern lecture on cholesterol or blood pressure or losing weight. So imagine their looks of astonishment when their cardiologist tells them that one of the best things they can do for their hearts is to go home and laugh until they cry.

"Dr. Miller," one new patient said, incredulous, "I'm scheduled for triple-bypass surgery *tomorrow*. What have I got to laugh about?"

"John, instead of *about*, think about *for*," I said. "You've got your entire life to laugh *for*."

After I explained a little about the mind-body connection and how laughter directly affects the cardiovascular system, John began gesturing frantically.

"What is it?" I asked. "What do you need?"

"I need you to get out of the way of that TV," he said. "*The Office* is on in 2 minutes and I need all the help I can get!"

I can't claim that Steve Carell can be given *all* the credit for John's return to health, but I can tell you that this 48-year-old who underwent triple-bypass surgery after suffering his *second* heart attack—his first was at 42—beautifully tolerated surgery and went on to make a full recovery with the help of the Positive Emotions Prescription. In addition to exercise and a *mostly* heart-healthy diet—he indulges in occasional ice cream splurges with his wife—John went all out in making a dedicated practice of laughing on a daily basis through watching movies, reading humorous books, and taking part in his grandchildren's playful antics.

John's heart surgery occurred more than 7 years ago. Since then, he's kept up his heart-healthy habits, and he still includes daily laughter in his overall health plan. He reports that he and his wife are having the most fun they've had in years.

All of John's positive lifestyle choices are working in concert to give him the healthy, active life he deserves. But laughter's role in his recovery and in his ability to maintain his cardiovascular health for years is not to be underestimated. In fact, I think laughter is so important for everyone—whether we have healthy hearts or, like John, we've already experienced heart disease—that I literally prescribe a daily dose of laughter to all of my patients, and I recommend it highly for everyone.

So what's so healthful about laughter? Is it more than a feel-good panacea? Does it really have a measurable impact on our cardiovascular health? And if so, can laughter actually help *prevent* cardiovascular disease before it even begins? Can it help promote all-around health for all of us, regardless of our level of cardiovascular health?

The answer to the last four questions is an unequivocal *yes*. To answer the first question, let's take a closer look at the amazing neurochemical and physiological processes that occur when we enjoy one of life's most pleasurable and beneficial experiences: deep, mirthful laughter that leaves us relaxed and happy and wiping our eyes.

Laughter Really Can Save Your Life

Over the course of my career, I've been involved in a number of research studies, but none has received as much attention as the clinical trials involving the effect of laughter on cardiovascular health. The idea to study the effect of laughter and other positive emotions on the cardiovascular system first came about after studies found that mental stress causes blood vessels to constrict, as we discussed in Chapter 1. This unhealthy response, called *vasoconstriction*, is responsible for reducing blood flow and raising blood pressure. Any reduction in blood flow to your heart can raise your risk of having a heart attack, and high blood pressure has long been known to be a major risk factor for cardiovascular events such as heart attack and stroke.

In one of those early studies on vasoconstriction, my team and I assembled a group of 300 people to study their humor responses. Half of these people had already suffered a heart attack or had undergone coronary artery bypass surgery. The other 150 were healthy, age-matched participants with no history of heart disease. We asked participants to answer two questionnaires.[1] The first presented them with a series of questions and multiple-choice answers to determine how much or how little they laughed in certain situations. They were to rank their responses on a scale of 1 to 5, with 1 being little to no laughter and 5 being enthusiastic laughter. Here are two examples of typical questions:

If you were eating in a restaurant with some friends and the waiter accidentally spilled a drink on you . . .

1. I would not have been particularly amused.
2. I would have been amused, but wouldn't have shown it outwardly.
3. I would have smiled.
4. I would have laughed.
5. I would have laughed heartily.

You thought you recognized a friend in a crowded room. You attracted the person's attention and hurried over to him or her, but when you got there you discovered you had made a mistake and the person was a total stranger. . . .

1. I would not have been particularly amused.
2. I would have been amused, but wouldn't have shown it outwardly.
3. I would have smiled.
4. I would have laughed.
5. I would have laughed heartily.

The second questionnaire asked for a simple "true or false" response and was used to measure a participant's level of anger or hostility. Typical prompts on this second questionnaire included, "I often wonder what hidden reasons another person may have for doing something nice for me," or "I am likely not to talk to people until they speak to me."

What we found across the board was that the people with heart disease were less likely to recognize humor or to use it to get out of uncomfortable situations. Specifically, they were *40 percent less likely to respond with laughter* compared to the patients the same age with healthy hearts.[2] Subjects with heart disease generally laughed less, even in positive situations, and they displayed more anger and hostility.

So, while the people with healthy hearts would've laughed off or even made a crowd-pleasing joke about having water spilled on them in a restaurant, the people with heart disease would certainly *not* have been amused, and some would've reacted with outright hostility. (We did not test to see if spilled water resulted in lower tipping.)

While the conclusions of this study aren't meant to suggest that laughter-prone people will never develop heart disease, nor that all hostile people will develop heart disease, the results were striking enough that they warrant serious consideration for the health and wellness of all of us. (Those of us in the field of behavioral cardiology are already dreaming of a time when routine medical forms assess patients' tendencies toward anger and hostility and their ability to laugh.) And the results were certainly striking enough that we wanted to do further research. If stress and a lack of laughter cause vasoconstriction, could positive emotions and laughter cause the opposite effect, vasodilation, or the expansion of blood vessels?

The question was far from academic. Expanded blood vessels allow free blood flow throughout the cardiovascular system, and as we've seen, vasoconstriction increases the risk of heart attack and stroke by impeding or cutting off blood flow. The most common cause of acute myocardial infarction—heart attack—is the blockage of a coronary artery, usually because a blood clot forms over built-up plaque on blood vessel walls. Without a steady supply of oxygenated blood, the heart muscle will become severely compromised or even die from lack of oxygen, resulting in the person's death. Our team reasoned that if something as easily accessible as laughter could directly contribute to vasodilation, we'd have a powerful—and certainly pleasurable—new line of defense in maintaining cardiovascular health.

My colleagues and I designed a study to find out the potential link between positive emotions and laughter and the ensuing beneficial effects on the vasculature. We asked 20 healthy men and women to watch clips of two movies on different days. One, the violent opening battle scene in *Saving Private Ryan*, would be sure to evoke a stress response; the other clip was a funny scene from *Kingpin*, *There's Something about Mary*, or *Shallow Hal*. Because intense laughter is about 30 times more likely to occur in the presence of others, rather than when we're alone,[3] we invited each volunteer to bring along a few friends when viewing the comedies. We tested the volunteers' vasodilation before and after viewing each of the movie clips by constricting and releasing the brachial artery (located in the upper arm) with a blood pressure cuff and then measuring the blood vessels' function with an ultrasound.

The results? We found remarkable differences in blood vessel functioning depending on which movie the participants watched. Fourteen of the 20 subjects who watched the stressful drama experienced significant blood flow reduction due to vasoconstriction within 1 to 2 minutes of viewing the clip. On the other hand, 19 of the 20 subjects experienced vasodilation and increased blood flow after laughing at the funny movie clip—and again it happened quickly, within 1 to 2 minutes.[4] We were able to conclude that stress has a direct and immediate constricting effect on the blood vessels, while laughter has a direct and immediate dilating effect on the blood vessels. The results couldn't have been any more impressive.

Ultimately we did over 300 measurements on the subjects' blood vessels, and we found an overall 30 to 50 percent difference in blood vessel diameter between the laughter (vasodilation) and mental stress (vasoconstriction) phases. That means that blood vessels were narrowing by 30 to 50 percent during the stress-inducing movie clip—and imagine a 50 percent reduction in blood vessel diameter if your arteries are already compromised due to plaque buildup! What's more, vessel dilation *increased* by 22 percent after laughing. Remarkably, that 22 percent increase is an improvement equivalent to the effect of a 15- to 30-minute workout or the use of a statin to reduce cholesterol. Let me state that another way: After just 15 minutes of laughing, volunteers experienced the same vascular benefit they'd experience from spending 15 to 30 minutes in the gym or from taking a daily statin medication to lower their cholesterol.

With study results so exciting they bordered on too good to be true, the news spread quickly, leading to further investigations and refinements.

One study performed by researchers in Texas reproduced our results demonstrating blood vessel expansion in response to laughter. The added dimension in this study was that researchers monitored the vascular response for a longer period of time. They found that blood vessel expansion *persisted for nearly 24 hours*. In other words, the healthful vascular effects from watching a movie that produces laughter sufficient to bring tears to your eyes can last for the remainder of the day! These results suggest that if you have a good laugh in the morning, your blood vessels remain actively dilated and protected throughout the day, even as stress rears its head. (Morning comedy clubs, anyone?) Regardless of the time of day you laugh, the good news is that within minutes, a good laugh can reverse the vasoconstriction that occurs with stress, and these heart-healthy effects can last for hours.

News of these studies circled the globe, and members of the Associated Press asked my colleagues and me to show them whether it's possible that laughter can improve stress-induced vasoconstriction. To do this, we brought in my patient John. You'll recall that he had heart disease at a young age, and after undergoing triple-bypass surgery and following the Positive Emotions Prescription, he maintained excellent cardiovascular health well into his seventies. With cameras rolling, we first had John watch the opening scene of *Saving Private Ryan*. Although he had not participated in any of our previous studies, he had seen this movie several times in the past. Despite his being familiar with the opening segment, John's arteries constricted within minutes. With those constricted vessels, we then showed him some of the funniest scenes from *Kingpin*, which he had never seen, and with all of us in the room laughing in unison, his blood vessels dilated right in front of us. This astonishing demonstration prompted worldwide interest in the possibility that laughter can counteract the blood vessel constriction that sudden stress causes, *even if you already have heart disease*. Further confirmation requires ongoing research studies in hundreds of patients—scientific work that is now going forward. Yet, even at the outset, it is thrilling to inform the public of the possibility of drug-free dilation of the blood vessels, using laughter as the only medicine.

Meanwhile, the surprises didn't stop there. John not only reversed the stress-induced vasoconstriction within minutes of hearty laughter, but amazingly, his responses were as good as the responses in younger volunteers we had previously studied. John's remarkable results led us to ask another serious question: Can laughter possibly reduce the effects of aging on human blood vessels? Medical textbooks have been teaching us that arteries naturally stiffen and narrow over time, regardless of a patient's lifestyle. But in my patient John, the results suggest that progressive hardening of the arteries is *not* an inevitable consequence of aging. Will our next discovery show that laughter is one of the most natural and effective ways to mitigate the aging process of the vasculature?

Research is under way, and John's results as well as some preliminary studies in Germany are producing exciting results. German researchers showed funny movies to volunteers and then measured arterial compliance, which is a measure of arterial stiffness using pulse wave velocity. Pulse wave velocity is the speed of the blood pressure wave created as blood travels through the aorta, our main artery. Pulse wave velocity helps us to assess the flexibility or elasticity of our arteries. Young, healthy arteries are very elastic and more easily able to adapt to changes in vascular tone, an important component of cardiovascular health. If we have risk factors for heart disease, our blood vessels age and the arteries develop reduced vascular tone and increased stiffness.

After research subjects watched funny movies, arterial stiffness was reduced, which means that vascular tone was improved.[5] We can expect that prolonged improvement in an individual's vascular tone would reduce aging of the arteries, improving overall vascular heath. I have recently incorporated pulse wave velocity in my cardiology practice: I now routinely test the degree of arterial stiffness in my patients. To date, some of my patients (especially those who laugh easily and regularly) exhibit arterial ages that are 10 to 20 years below their chronological age. Studies are now using pulse wave velocity to assess how certain therapies can influence heart disease along with the aging of blood vessels. In the near future, the public will be hearing more about this exciting new way to determine the age of your arteries.

By now you may be wondering exactly how and why laughter has such a profound effect on cardiovascular health. The answers lead us into the fascinating realm of neuroscience and the powerful neurochemicals responsible for these effects on our cardiovascular systems. As you read on, you'll begin to understand more of the intricate interconnection between the mind and the body, and you'll see that the benefits of laughter extend far beyond cardiovascular health. You'll also see why, no matter your current level of health, you have every reason in the world to treat yourself to a daily dose of laughter.

The Science behind Nature's Best Medicine

If the mention of neuroscience and neurochemicals is already raising your blood pressure, set your mind (and heart) at ease. You don't need a PhD or a peer-reviewed research study to demonstrate the clear connection between the mind and the body. Think about the last time you experienced fear—an intense negative emotion that is inherently stressful. Let's say you're cruising down the road at 55 miles per hour when, without warning, a car pulls out in front of you. You hit the brakes and, in a peal of burning rubber, you narrowly avoid a collision. What happens to your body? As adrenaline and the stress hormone cortisol pour into your bloodstream, your heart and breathing rates increase, your blood pressure surges, your pupils dilate, and glucose feeds your muscles, readying them for quick action. You may even feel nausea as your digestive system quickly goes on lockdown. That's a very simple and familiar example of the mind-body connection at work.

Of course, the delicate interconnectedness of the mind and the body works just as powerfully with positive experiences. In the midst of pleasurable occurrences—sex, the familiar runner's high produced by an intense workout, hearty laughter—we just as readily experience the "symptoms" of pleasure. We experience a boost of energy and a sense of well-being. We feel more relaxed, and pain diminishes.

Now let's consider the pleasurable experience of laughter specifically. What happens on a neurochemical level when we laugh? It had long been suspected that laughter, like other pleasurable experiences, triggers the release of endorphins simply because we feel so refreshed and relaxed after a good laugh. Recently, a study conducted by Dr. Robin Dunbar, an evolutionary psychologist at Oxford, was able to provide conclusive evidence that a hearty laugh that induces tears indeed triggers the release of endorphins.[6] Endorphins (natural opioids) are painkilling compounds that foster a sense of well-being, relaxation, and even euphoria. Endorphins are released during times of heightened physical stimulation such as deep laughter, exercise, orgasm, and pain. With our systems flooded by these natural "feel good" chemicals, it's no wonder that laughing until our sides hurt makes us feel so good.

But how is it that laughter triggers the expansion of blood vessels? The answers lie in the interplay between endorphins, the celebrated neurochemical nitric oxide, and the inner lining of our blood vessels, known as the endothelium. The endothelium serves as a conduit for the transfer of blood cells, lipids, and various nutrients to neighboring tissues. Healthy endothelial cells secrete vasoactive chemicals—most notably, for our discussion, nitric oxide. This superstar neurochemical (its discoverers were awarded the Nobel Prize and it was named "Molecule of the Year" in 1992) produces a treasure trove of heart-healthy benefits. Here are just a few things for which we can thank nitric oxide, all of which lower our risk of heart attack and stroke.

- It triggers blood vessel dilation.
- It increases blood flow.
- It reduces vascular inflammation.
- It reduces the buildup of cholesterol plaque.
- It decreases platelet aggregation and platelet stickiness, which reduces the risk of blood clots.
- It reduces leukocyte (white blood cell) adhesion to the endothelium, which reduces the risk of blood clots and plaque buildup on arterial walls.
- It dilates the bronchial tubes (which is why you feel you can breathe easier after laughing).

(And as a vasodilator, we also have nitric oxide to thank for the efficacy of Viagra. But that's a subject for another book.)

So here's the beautiful and powerful sequence that's already built into our bodies and that we are all capable of accessing for heart health: Deep belly laughter triggers the release of endorphins, endorphins activate opiate receptors in the endothelium that signal it to produce nitric oxide (see Figure 3.1), and nitric oxide in turn produces the cornucopia of heart-healthy benefits mentioned above.

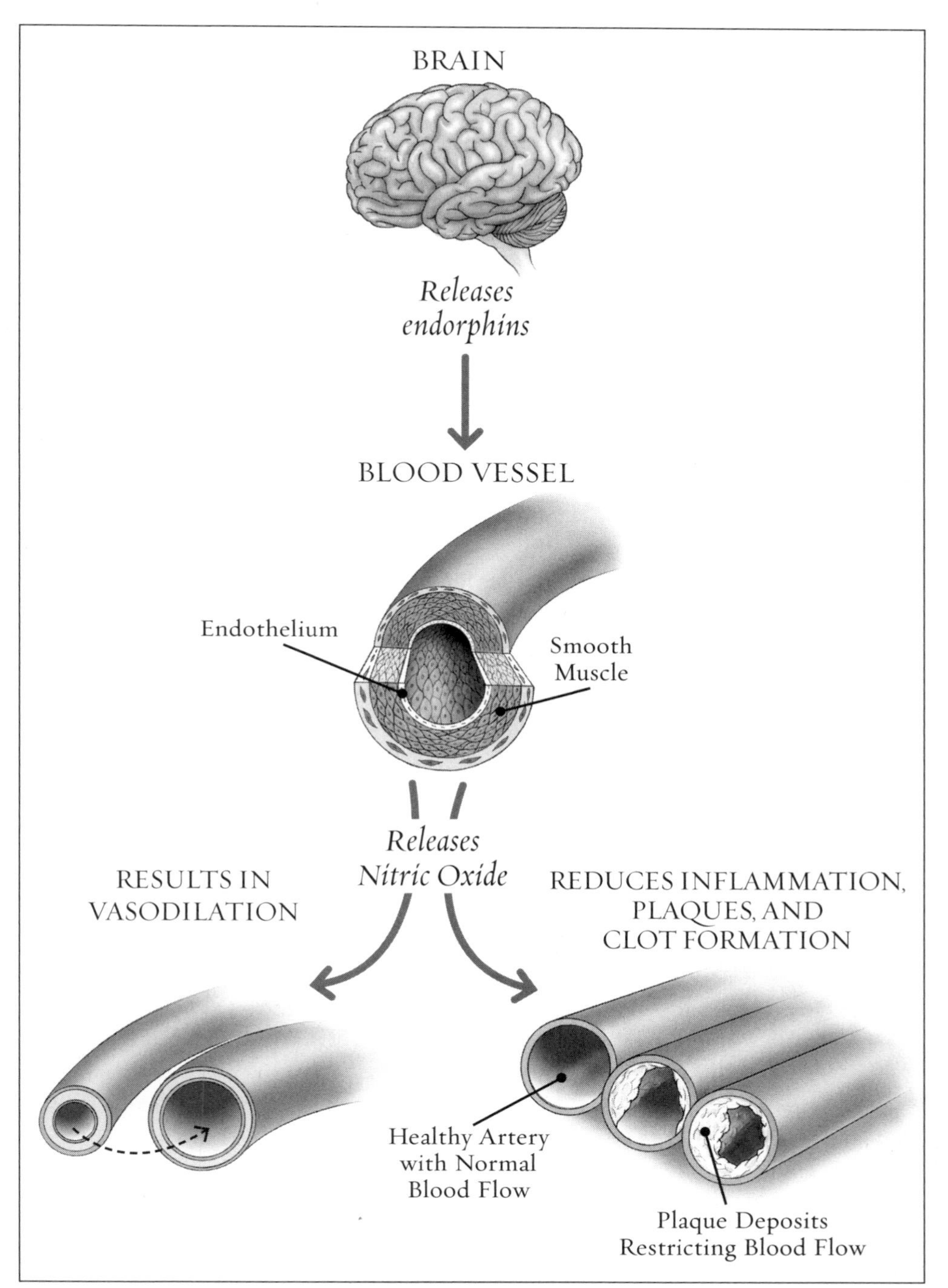
BRAIN
Releases endorphins
BLOOD VESSEL
Endothelium
Smooth Muscle
Releases Nitric Oxide
RESULTS IN VASODILATION
REDUCES INFLAMMATION, PLAQUES, AND CLOT FORMATION
Healthy Artery with Normal Blood Flow
Plaque Deposits Restricting Blood Flow

Figure 3.1

You could say that your brain chemicals "cross talk" with your heart chemicals, resulting in a mind-to-heart connection. It's a beautiful process that highlights the mind-body connection, and more specifically, the interrelationship between emotions and the vasculature. Our studies were the first to show a direct connection between positive emotions and blood vessel expansion, strongly supporting the release of nitric oxide, and thus the host of healthy cardiovascular responses nitric oxide confers.[7] You really can laugh your way to health and well-being.

The Many Health Benefits of Laughter

Thus far we've concentrated on the cardiovascular benefits of laughter, but what about other health benefits? There's plenty of good news ahead. Because your mind and body work together in an intricate and elegant dance, the advantage that one organ system receives applies holistically. Laughter, for example, has been shown to improve sleep, and people who get adequate sleep experience lower stress, improved memory and focus, and decreased effects of heart-damaging insomnia.

Let's take a look at some of the best benefits of laughter, beginning with further cardiovascular benefits and moving on to healthy effects on weight control, sleep, memory, and social connection.

Laughter Counteracts Hardening of the Arteries

For years, medical schools taught that regardless of lifestyle, human blood vessels progressively stiffen and narrow over the course of a life span, aging until one suffers a debilitating or fatal cardiac event. This stiffening or hardening of the arteries—commonly known as arteriosclerosis or atherosclerosis—was assumed to be a natural consequence of aging, as plaques containing cholesterol built up in the arteries, narrowing the arteries and making them stiffer. The narrow, stiff arteries impede blood flow and produce angina over time, and in the worst-case scenario, pieces of plaque can break off and create a full blockage, resulting in heart attack or stroke.

The *results* of arteriosclerosis are undisputed. But as we've seen, research studies are overturning the outdated explanation of "naturally" deteriorating blood vessels. In reality, one of the main causes of arteriosclerosis actually has a great deal more to do with our old enemy, stress—that ubiquitous and underappreciated risk factor.

When you experience even momentary stress, your blood vessels constrict and become less efficient and less able to conduct healthy blood flow throughout your body and to your heart muscle. Vessels are also less able to release protective chemicals such as nitric oxide, and over prolonged periods of stress, your vessels become increasingly rigid. I tell my patients that just like too much sun exposure without adequate protection can cause wrinkles and aging of the skin, the inability to effectively handle daily stressors will advance aging of your blood vessels. This occurs because *your blood vessels mimic your experience of feeling angry or upset.* Far more than passive tubes that afford simple circulatory passage, your blood vessels are dynamic organs that actually mirror your mood.

Here is the new scientific truth you need to know: Hardening of your arteries is *not* a natural or inevitable process of aging, and you *can* intervene. We now know that experiencing positive emotions directly affects vascular health and that through the power of laughter, you can reduce the deterioration of your blood vessels. In effect, experiencing positive emotions that include laughter may help to maintain the youthfulness of your blood vessels in much the same way that sunscreen protects your skin—but without the chemicals, of course!

Laughter Affects Your Blood Pressure

Here's a thought that could raise your blood pressure: For each 20-point increase in your systolic blood pressure (the peak pressure or "top number") or 10-point increase in your diastolic blood pressure (the minimum pressure or "bottom number"), your risk for a heart attack and stroke *doubles.* Most of us can rattle off a short list of factors that contribute to high blood pressure: high sodium intake, smoking, obesity, and lack of exercise. But the single most overlooked reason for hypertension is *stress.*

But if stress can cause your blood pressure to rise, can laughter that reduces stress also reduce your blood pressure? Our study with the movie clips certainly made that case, but further research was needed, and subsequent studies confirmed our results. A study in Japan examined 90 men and women ages 40 to 74. Researchers assigned one group to engage in hour-long laughter or music therapy sessions every other week. The other group received no therapy. After 3 months, the group who had engaged in laughter therapy saw a drop of 5 to 7 mm Hg in systolic blood pressure, lowering the likelihood of blood vessel stiffness.[8]

In a 200-person study conducted in India and presented at the annual meeting of the American Society of Hypertension in 2008, 100 healthy adult men and women participated in seven sessions of laughter yoga over 3 weeks. At the end of the 3 weeks, laughter yoga participants had lower systolic and diastolic blood pressure, lower levels of cortisol (a stress hormone), and less perceived stress than the control group.[9] They experienced a similar reduction in systolic blood pressure (approximately 5 to 7 mm Hg) as the Japanese study found.[10] It's important to note that the Indian study's subjects' average blood pressure before and after the laughter phase (128/82 mm Hg versus 121/79 mm Hg) was not in the hypertensive range, and it would be important to repeat these studies in men and women with high blood pressure.

Still, these results are remarkable, as you could expect a similar reduction in blood pressure if you took a blood pressure medication, followed a low-salt diet (less than 1 teaspoon of sodium per day), or lost 10 pounds.

There's also a question of duration: How long does the positive effect on blood pressure last? Though laughter always causes an initial, momentary increase in blood pressure, especially if we're laughing boisterously, pressure stabilizes over a 30- to 60-minute period. Even though blood pressure differences appear to normalize within an hour, researchers in Japan and at the University of Texas found that patients who watched just 30 minutes of a comedy continued to have increased blood vessel dilation the next day. In other words, a short period of laughter could sustain this heart-healthy effect for up to 24 hours![11]

The bottom line of all of these studies is that, incredibly, the vasodilation caused by laughter was found to be as effective at lowering blood pressure as a daily dose of blood pressure medication. This is bad news for the pharmaceutical companies, but great news for us. We now have a readily accessible, pleasurable, cost-effective, and drug-free way to lower blood pressure: daily doses of mirthful laughter. Now I'm not recommending that you throw away your blood pressure medications if you have a history of hypertension! What I'm suggesting is that once you engage in the Positive Emotions Prescription and reduce your systolic blood pressure by 5 to 7 mm Hg, your physician may be able to reduce the dosage or even eliminate one of your blood pressure medications.

If the entire US population achieved a drop in blood pressure of just 5 mm Hg, the risk of heart attacks or strokes would be cut by 5 to 15 percent. Translation? Even with a conservative estimate, that's as many as 30,000 lives saved per year. These results alone are enough for me to prescribe laughter to all of my patients and to enthusiastically recommend it for everyone. But if you're still not convinced, read on.

Laughter Burns Calories

Laughter is great exercise. Researcher Maciej Buchowski and colleagues at Vanderbilt University evaluated the amount of energy expended when 45 men and women ages 18 to 34 watched video scenes of famous comedians. They found that laughing for 10 to 15 minutes can burn up to 40 calories.[12] The reason appears to be the increased work of numerous muscles in the face, throat, and abdomen that are used during hearty laughter.

There's also evidence that laughter can reduce binge-eating. Following a laughter therapy program allowed author Katie Namrevo to lose 35 pounds, diminish her stress-induced cravings, and gain more energy to pursue aerobic activities. She describes her experience in her 2004 book *Laugh It Off! Weight Loss for the Fun of It.* Mary Dallman, PhD, professor of physiology, and her colleagues at the University of California, San Francisco, have proposed that under chronic stressful conditions, people are subconsciously drawn to comfort foods. These foods, which are characteristically high in fat and carbs, in turn suppress the activity of the stress hormone cortisol.[13] Laughter terminates this vicious cycle. The result is that regular engagement in laughter as part of the Positive Emotions Prescription may result in significant changes in body weight that can reduce the likelihood of insulin resistance, diabetes, and heart disease.

Laughter Improves Your Sleep

When you become sleep deprived (or sleep less than 6 hours each night for adults), the levels of your stress hormones increase. It was once thought that high levels of the stress hormone cortisol produced insomnia, but a 2003 study suggested that the opposite is true: Chronic insomnia—which is often caused by chronic stress!—produces higher levels of cortisol.[14] Thus we're caught (again) in a vicious cycle, and sadly, it doesn't stop there. The familiar grouchiness or even hostility that results from prolonged insomnia can rev up your desire for comfort foods, and ingesting those simple carbs for a quick hit of stress relief inevitably leads to weight gain. Weight gain can lead to sleep apnea, which disrupts your sleep and leaves you fatigued and irritable and at higher risk for hypertension, heart attack, stroke, and diabetes. As we've seen, everything works together. When one part of the body is suffering, the whole body suffers.

The good news is that the same principle applies to health and wellness: Improving one aspect of health improves the whole body. And once again, laughter can come to the rescue. In a Korean study of 109 men and women over age 65, researchers found that just four laughter therapy sessions over a 1-month period were associated with more restful sleep as well as reduced feelings of depression.[15] Insomnia is so common that nearly one out of every two people complains of poor sleep habits!

But the sad reality is that not only does insomnia adversely affect our productivity and emotional state, it also increases our risk of depression, hypertension, metabolic syndrome, and heart disease.

My medical advice? Before bedtime you should turn off the stressful news and look for comedy or lighthearted reading.

Laughter Improves Your Memory

Here's a fascinating fact: The right frontal lobe of the brain processes information related to memory and is also associated with the ability to appreciate humor. One can say that humor and memory work hand in hand, as studies have shown that people remember things that are perceived as humorous. Advertising agencies know this quite well, which is why they strive to outdo each other during the Super Bowl with comical TV commercials that will stick in viewers' memories. (If you want a good laugh, just Google "Funniest Banned Commercials 2013"—viewer discretion advised.) Researchers have long known that memory is enhanced through humor. A recent Japanese study presented 177 college students with cartoons labeled as "high humor" (elephant giving an ant a friendly pat on the back), "low humor" (elephant stepping on an ant), and "nonhumorous" (a spot between a line and a square with some patterns). The students were given a 30-page booklet that contained 30 different images (10 of each humor category) and were asked to rate each picture over a 10-second period. After completing this task, each student was asked to sketch the pictures that he or she could recall. Not surprisingly, memory recall was highest for the high-humor cartoons and lowest for the nonhumorous cartoons.[16]

And when researchers in Germany were studying changes in cerebral connectivity according to different types of laughter—the reflexlike laughter that comes from tickling versus the more complex social laughter that comes from joy—they stumbled upon a fascinating discovery involving memory. When subjects listened to auditory laughter sequences resulting from tickling, different portions of the brain were activated than when joyful laughter sounds were produced. Interestingly, the portion of the brain activated in joyful laughter, the lingual gyrus, plays an important role in visual memory, and if that part of the brain has been damaged, memory is greatly impaired.[17]

Because the brain processes that control humor and memory are closely linked, you can rely on humor as an aid to improve your memory. Humor helps your mind create visual images that become useful as a creative strategy for memory enhancement. When you recount incidents that occurred long ago, you likely find that vividly funny details jump readily to mind. My own experience in a summer job showcases this benefit of memory working in concert with humor. As a young waiter in a busy restaurant, I silently pictured my customers wearing their orders (chicken-à-la-red-polka-dot-dress, steak-on-blue-tie-with-stripes-and-onions). Useful visualizations allowed me to rely on humor to recall and keep track of large tables of diners. Numerous studies have concluded that humorous material tends to be recalled more readily than nonhumorous material, and memory books encourage readers to use humor as an aid in recalling lists of information. Some of my most effective teachers were also dynamic and funny.

Laughter Helps You Form Connections

During prehistoric times, when our language was in its infancy, it is likely that laughter became an important and adaptive socialization skill. In fact, communication through laughter may have been an early test of survival of the fittest because early humans who did not engage in group laughter were likely to be alienated and left to fend for themselves. Even today, laughter is an important and early socialization skill.

Before human language develops, babies laugh as a response to physical stimuli. Soon, the infant begins to use laughter to communicate with adults and other children. As a toddler, the baby laughs to express playfulness. And as a growing child and then as an adult, the individual laughs as self-expression and as an important communication skill. Laughter becomes essential for participation in groups and for achieving social acceptance. It not only relaxes us, it also signals others that they can relax around us. Laughing is a highly effective form of communication and it facilitates connection.

Laughter is also a key ingredient in successful relationships, yet people often underestimate its importance. Research by my colleague Robert Provine, PhD, professor of psychology at the University of Maryland, Baltimore County, has shown laughter's important role in mating. On average, females laugh more than twice as much as males, while males are more likely to try to be amusing. The female's laughter serves as a primary barometer in strong relationships, and the earliest hint of a problem in the relationship is when a woman no longer finds her partner funny.[18] According to independent findings of psychologists Dr. John Gottman and Dr. Michelle Golland, the most important predictor of divorce is the absence of laughter in a marriage.[19] Partners who recognize this important clue at an early stage can increase the likelihood of resolving underlying conflicts before any disharmony spins out of control. Doing so may save the relationship while also protecting the heart health of both partners—divorce is widely known to be one of the most stressful experiences people can endure.

It is absolutely clear that laughing with others—in love, in the workplace, or in any social situation—reduces tension while improving morale, cooperation, and cardiovascular health. So schedule time with your funniest friends, or reach out and reconnect with fun-loving friends with whom you've lost touch. Strong bonds are formed and strengthened when people laugh together, and laughter is always a more enriching experience when it's shared with others.

Tips for Getting Your Daily Dose of Laughter

It would seem that there's virtually no downside to laughter. Laughing promotes whole-body health, it relieves stress, it enhances memory, it facilitates social connection, and it's simply fun. Yet for some of us, laughter doesn't occur on a daily basis. While the average 5-year-old laughs as many as 300 times a day, the average adult laughs a paltry four times a day.[20] Our lives are busy and often stressful, and not all of us have the built-in advantage of living with a funny person or having a close friend or colleague who's particularly funny. This means that most of us are going to have to be quite intentional in seeking out our daily dose of laughter. We all have it in us to laugh heartily every day, and there are some simple, easy measures we can take to increase the likelihood that we will experience episodes of hearty laughter. To lighten up each day, you can make small changes that relieve tension, release you from inhibitions, and foster positive emotions that become a platform for laughter. Here are a few tips I prescribe to my patients to help them find and create more laughter in their lives.

Link to Laughter

With our computers, smartphones, tablets, and handheld devices, we can access information at the speed of lightning. This includes tens of thousands of Web sites that allow us instant access to humor. Keep links to humor bookmarked, and then the moment you find yourself in need of a laugh—that is, in need of stress relief, an energy boost, and a heart-healthy dose of endorphins and nitric oxide—click away. It could be anything from a hilarious clip on YouTube to episodes of your favorite comedies to comedy Web sites like The Onion or CollegeHumor to the latest funny videos on Reddit—whatever tickles your particular funny bone.

There's also the entire world of apps to explore. Developers have designed dozens of apps to elicit laughter, and with everything from recordings of laughing babies to storehouses of jokes accessed with a tap of a finger to one-line "zinger" generators, there's something out there that will appeal to every sense of humor. Perhaps not surprisingly, one of the most notable laughter apps was designed by a former cardiac patient. While lying in his hospital bed recovering from a heart attack, Fred Burger began wondering how he could access instant, genuine laughter that would lift his spirits and get his mind off his troubles. His first solution (well before the dawn of apps) was to create a video of people engaged in deep, mirthful belly laughter, which easily prompted contagious laughter in the viewer. Then, in 2011, his company released an app called "The Gift of Laughter," featuring 50 people laughing; the clips can be viewed one at a time or on a continuous loop.[21] To find "The Gift of Laughter" and other laughter apps, search your app store or Google "laughter apps."

If you prefer more old-fashioned forms of humor—and don't mind doing an Internet search to find some—check out the American Film Institute's 100 Funniest Movies at www.afi.com/100years/laughs.aspx, or this list of 100-plus funniest TV shows: http://nowthatsnifty.blogspot.com/2011/03/100-greatest-american-sitcoms-of-all.html. Or check out this list of 290 comic novels: www.goodreads.com/list/show/5447.Funniest_Novels_of_All_Time.

With the Internet opening up entire worlds of humor, we have 24-hour instant access to laughter. With just a few clicks or the tap of a finger, you can link to the healthful benefits of laughter and begin positively impacting your health from wherever you are.

Participate in Laughter Yoga and Laughter Clubs

If you're feeling adventurous and don't mind looking a little silly for a half hour, laughter yoga and laughter clubs are a great option for getting the deep belly laughter that keeps your heart healthy. The difference between the two is mainly semantic: Both laughter yoga and laughter clubs bring people together to engage in deep-breathing and laughter exercises that promote rollicking, cathartic, spontaneous, and genuine laughter.

Indian family physician Dr. Madan Kataria popularized laughter yoga beginning in the mid-1990s; since then, more than 6,000 laughter yoga clubs have sprung up in at least 65 countries. At a typical laughter yoga session, participants first warm up with a clapping and chanting exercise; the chant of "HO, HO, HA HA HA!" promotes diaphragmatic breathing and gets energy levels up. The laughter leader or teacher then leads participants through a series of exercises that reduce inhibitions and get the giggles going. "Milkshake Laughter," in which you pretend to pour milk from one cup to another while chanting "aeeee," then downing the milk in one gulp, and "Balloon Laughter," in which you pretend to blow up a balloon, throw it on the ground, and then burst into laughter when you pop the balloon with your feet, are just two examples of laughter exercises that look as outlandish as they sound. In laughter yoga, that's the point. Participants approach the sessions with an open, childlike playfulness and maintain eye contact with each other throughout. As you can imagine, laughter that is at first forced quickly becomes genuine. Contagious laughter sweeps the room, and participants are overcome with knee-slapping, eye-watering belly laughter.

After a session of laughter yoga, practitioners widely report feeling more relaxed and connected with others, an overall sense of well-being and optimism (there's those endorphins again), relief from depression, a reduction in pain and/or a higher pain tolerance, and greater energy. With all of these benefits and more, it's well worth it to spend 30 or 40 minutes looking a little silly—or a lot! One of the best ways to increase laughter in your life is to take yourself less seriously, and laughter yoga is excellent for this.

Several years ago, Dr. Kataria invited me down to Miami to lecture and participate in a laughter yoga session with his certified trainers. I was impressed by how much the trainers enjoyed participating in the session and had no doubt that endorphins were being released throughout the seminar hall!

Research on laughter yoga remains sparse yet promising. A study in India found that laughter yoga reduced blood pressure between 5 and 10 mm Hg, results similar to those from taking one prescription medication to lower blood pressure.[22] A study in Iran found that symptoms of depression decreased in depressed elderly women who were assigned either to laughter yoga or to exercise, compared to a control group.[23] And studies using laughter therapy in the elderly have confirmed that the therapy reduces insomnia, as well as anxiety and depression.[24, 25]

Laughter clubs of any sort can meet anywhere groups of people can convene. Group laughter sessions have been practiced in schools, nursing homes, rehabilitation centers, hospitals, public parks, prisons, and workplaces. It's become a global phenomenon—there's even a World Laughter Day that's celebrated the first Sunday of every May—so chances are you can find a laughter club in your area.

And if you can't, start one! There are many training programs available; Dr. Kataria's Web site (www.laughteryoga.org) and the American School of Laughter Yoga's (www.laughteryogaamerica.com) are good places to start.

Old Wisdom, New Knowledge

Laughter is a far more powerful ally in the quest for health than many (even those in the medical community) realize. The latest research in the field of behavioral cardiology demonstrates a clear link between laughter and cardiovascular health, and we certainly know that laughter quickly and effectively counteracts the harmful effects of stress. Those of us in the field of behavioral cardiology look forward to more long-term studies of patients who have laughed their way to heart health versus control sets of patients who rarely laugh. That said, the evidence we do have is altogether persuasive enough that it belongs—today—in the hands of every person who is recovering from heart disease or who wishes to preserve his or her healthy heart. Laughter, with its ability to quickly trigger vasodilation, zap stress in its tracks, bring us closer to others, and bring a little more fun and happiness into our lives, couldn't be a better line of defense in the fight against heart disease. So eat your veggies, get some exercise, don't smoke, and treat yourself to nature's best medicine: a daily dose of robust laughter.

The Positive Emotions Prescription: Laughter

Every day, aim for at least one good belly laugh that brings tears to your eyes. In other words, laugh until you cry!

CHAPTER 4

With a Song in Your Heart

THE HEALING POWER OF MUSIC

RECORDED HISTORY OFFERS countless tales of how music can soothe the savage beast (or breast, to cite the original quote), assuage madness, offer balm to the grieving, increase joy or incite euphoria, and even, in the mythical tale of Orpheus and Eurydice, cheat death. Music has the power to alter our mood, boost our energy, and create connection between people. And medical science is now proving what people have known for hundreds of years: that music is deeply healing. It may indeed be, to use the words of renowned neurologist and best-selling author Oliver Sacks, our "profoundest nonchemical medication."

The diversity of symptoms and syndromes for which music has proved beneficial is truly astonishing. It's been shown to ameliorate the symptoms of anxiety, depression, and PTSD; boost the immune system; improve memory; help retrain aphasic patients to speak and help those on the autism spectrum to express themselves; open airways for asthma sufferers; treat nausea; decrease the perception of pain; improve sleep; help recovering addicts maintain sobriety; ease chronic or acute pain; improve motor skills; promote the sucking instinct in premature infants; treat symptoms of neurological disorders such as schizophrenia, Alzheimer's, and Parkinson's; improve the quality of life for residents of nursing homes; speed recovery from surgery and injury; decrease violence in correctional facilities; and enhance cognitive functioning. This is just a *partial* list, but it gives you some idea of the depth and breadth of music's healing power.

Of course, in this book we're going to focus on the role that music plays in supporting the health of your cardiovascular system. Because of the universal love of music and the ease with which we can avail ourselves of this "treatment," music is arguably the most enjoyable aspect of the Positive Emotions Prescription. In a perfect world, I could convince all of my patients to fall in love with exercise and to find mung beans utterly irresistible, but that's about as realistic as yours truly singing at the Super Bowl halftime show. But on the other hand, I've never met a person who didn't like some type of music. An effective, quick-acting dose of heart health and emotional wellness is literally as simple as clicking Play.

Hearts and Happiness in Tune

The newest research from the field of behavioral cardiology has measured changes in blood pressure, heart rate, and heart rate variability in response to different kinds of music. For a study conducted at my lab, we asked 10 healthy, nonsmoking volunteers to select music that in the past evoked joy for them ("joyful music") and music that provoked feelings of anxiety or stress ("anxious music"). (Biochemically speaking, the joyful music would stimulate the release of endorphins and dopamine, and the anxious music would stimulate the release of the stress hormone cortisol.) We asked that volunteers not listen to their musical selections for a minimum of 2 weeks prior to the study in order to minimize emotional desensitization. For one phase of the study participants would listen to joyful music, for a second phase they'd listen to anxious music, and for a third phase they'd listen to recordings of relaxing sounds such as ocean waves and other calming sounds. A fourth phase of the study had volunteers view comical video clips in order to induce laughter, similar to what we had originally done years earlier, as described in Chapter 3.

Volunteers completed each phase over the course of 4 to 6 weeks. On the mornings of testing, they spent 15 to 20 minutes listening to joyful music, anxious music, or the relaxation tape, or watching the funny video. After each session, we assessed endothelial function by measuring the blood flow and dilation of the brachial artery, just as we'd done in the clinical trials on the effects of laughter.

The results were impressive. Subjects experienced a 26 percent increase in blood vessel dilation after listening to joyful music, a 19 percent increase in response to the funny video, and an 11 percent increase after the relaxation tape. In contrast, the anxious music produced a 6 percent *decrease* in blood vessel dilation.[1] It's also worth noting that these results occurred quite quickly. Subjects experienced blood vessel dilation within minutes of hearing the joyful music or the relaxing sounds, and also within minutes of laughing at the funny video. Likewise, blood vessels constricted within minutes of hearing the anxious music, and the effect generally lasted for at least 2 hours.

Among this particular group of study participants, country music happened to be the most commonly selected "joyful music" and heavy metal the most commonly selected "anxious music." Currently, however, there is no evidence that one particular genre of music is best for heart health. As musical tastes are highly particular, what one individual finds soothing or joyful could be boring or irritating to another. Musical taste aside, it's clear that music of *any* genre has a physiological effect not only on heart rate, blood pressure, and breathing rate, but also on the lining of our blood vessels. The endothelium, that barometer of emotions, dilates to the music the listener finds joyful and constricts during music that provokes the stress response. Our research and that of others demonstrate that listening to the music that *you* most enjoy leads to the release of nitric oxide—the heart-protective chemical that reduces inflammation, plaque acceleration, and blood clot formation. You now have scientific evidence to support your taste in music, even if your spouse finds it insufferable or your kids think it's lame.

A recent study from Serbia reproduced our results in test subjects with heart disease. Men and women were divided into three groups. One group was placed in an exercise program for 3 weeks. A second group did the same 3-week exercise program, but they also listened to their favorite musical selections for 30 minutes every day. The third group only listened to their favorite music, without participating in the exercise program. At study completion, blood vessel dilation improved by 39 percent in the group that combined music, and exercise, 29 percent in the group that listened to music only, and just 19 percent in the group that did the exercise program alone.[2]

Multiple studies have demonstrated the heart-healing power of music. In one study, researchers found that listening to music 25 minutes daily for 4 weeks resulted in a 12 mm Hg reduction in systolic blood pressure (the top number) and a 5 mm Hg decrease in diastolic blood pressure (the bottom number). Results like these are equivalent to taking a strong blood pressure medication![3]

In another study, researchers studied the effect of music on patients admitted to the hospital for a heart attack. They found that listening to 20 minutes of classical music during the first 72 hours following a heart attack led to immediate reductions in heart rate and respiratory rate. These heart-healthy benefits lasted at least an hour in each test subject, and overall anxiety levels were reduced as well.[4]

A study evaluating postoperative heart surgery patients found that listening to

20 minutes of music resulted in significant reductions in pain and anxiety levels.[5] Similarly, a study that monitored hospitalized patients who were confined to bed rest after cardiac surgery found that listening to music daily for a 30-minute period significantly lowered blood pressure, respiratory rate, and overall anxiety levels.[6]

The calming effect of music is so powerful, in fact, that one study found that listening to relaxing music before cardiac surgery was more effective at reducing stress than the sedative medication Versed (midazolam). The same study demonstrated that the group that listened to music after surgery fared better than patients who received midazolam. Because of the potential adverse effects of the medication, music turns out to be the preferred method for assuaging anxiety and bringing relaxation.[7]

Another study of patients who'd undergone open-heart surgery found that listening to soothing music while recovering releases the neurochemical oxytocin, which is among the most powerful chemicals producing positive emotions.[8] Oxytocin facilitates social bonding and is released during cuddling and hugging. Unfortunately, after heart surgery, hugging won't be easy to do for at least 4 to 6 weeks. In its place, the next best thing to release oxytocin is to listen to music!

The reason music has such a profound effect on us psychologically and physiologically remains somewhat mysterious. Evidence-based research is still needed in this area, and there are some exciting studies currently under way, such as a research project called "The Body's Musical Score" taking place in Gothenburg, Sweden, and work being done by researchers at McGill University in Montreal. But here's a little about what we do know.

One theory explaining music's effect on us is that music acts directly on the body's autonomic nervous system, which is located in the lower brain stem. The autonomic nervous system is responsible for involuntary actions such as heart rate, blood pressure, digestion, perspiration, sexual arousal, and respiration. In other words, it would seem that an appreciation of music is one of our most fundamental impulses, "wired in," if you will, to the same areas of the brain that regulate such basic functions as our heartbeat and our breathing. The McGill University researchers described it this way: Music "initiates reflexive brainstem responses" such as "heart rate, pulse, blood pressure, body temperature, skin conductance, and muscle tension."[9]

Further evidence has found that music's *tempo* affects all of these involuntary functions. Specifically, slow music induces a slower heart rate, a slower respiration rate, and lower blood pressure, whereas fast rhythms have the opposite effect. Perhaps not surprisingly, musicians are more attuned to these effects.[10] It's also been shown that loud music raises heart rate and blood pressure, whereas soft and soothing music set at a low volume lowers heart rate and blood pressure.[11] It's truly as if we're wired to be in sync with music.

The Importance of Heart Rate Variability

One of the more fascinating links between music and cardiovascular health involves one of the known markers of a healthy heart, *heart rate variability*. Heart rate variability is one of the many involuntary responses controlled by the autonomic nervous system. Heart rate variability, or HRV, is the variation in intervals between heartbeats. Along with a low resting heart rate (less than 60 beats per minute), HRV is one of the primary indicators of a healthy heart. In healthy hearts, the beat-to-beat intervals can vary quickly and extensively. Healthy hearts can respond and adjust appropriately to stress. You could say that a person with good heart rate variability has a nimble and flexible heart.

If you're an athlete or have ever given special attention to your breathing, such as by practicing meditation or yoga, you may have already noticed heart rate variability. If your heart rate increases readily during aerobic exercise and decreases in response to slow, deep breathing, that's good HRV.

In contrast, in cases of stress, lack of sleep, or heart ailments such as a heart attack, the fight-or-flight response takes over and the sympathetic nervous system control limits heart rate variability. Decreased HRV is associated with increased risk of cardiac death. This is especially the case if you've experienced a heart attack already, in which case having poor heart rate variability raises your risk of another heart attack, heart-related arrhythmia, and sudden cardiac death. If you've already experienced one or more heart attacks, poor HRV has been shown to increase cardiac death fourfold![12]

Think of reduced heart rate variability as a rigid system that cannot adjust or adapt to sudden changes that affect your environment. Your heart, in other words, has lost that ability to respond with alacrity to whatever comes your way. Someone who has good heart rate variability, or as cardiologists often refer to it, good parasympathetic tone, can more easily adapt to changes in his or her world. In a way, good HRV means that your heart is flexible and can adapt more readily to stress-induced changes that come your way. Consequently, your heart can respond more appropriately to a range of emotions, with less risk of harm occurring when emotional extremes arise. Listening to music that you find soothing and relaxing is an excellent way to improve heart rate variability.[13]

Training your heart to improve heart rate variability is important because without it, your risk of having a first heart attack may be increased. Fortunately, we have excellent means at our disposal to improve HRV. They include improving positive emotions through effectively managing stress (see Chapter 1), improving poor sleep habits, engaging in regular exercise (see Chapter 5), and, equally important, listening to relaxing music.[14]

Music and Inflammation

By improving parasympathetic tone, listening to soothing music may also have anti-inflammatory effects. This is because a key inflammation protein, interleukin-6 (IL-6) is inhibited by vagal or parasympathetic stimulation. If interleukin-6 is activated by fat cells, it sends a signal to the liver to release CRP, or C-reactive protein, the well-known marker of inflammation that we discussed in Chapter 1.

At least two studies have now demonstrated that music reduces IL-6. In the first study, 87 elderly patients with cardiovascular disease were assigned to music therapy for 45 minutes each week over a 10-week period. Researchers found that this group had significantly lower levels of IL-6 compared to the control group. This was associated with reduced episodes of congestive heart failure, a condition characterized by high sympathetic tone that soothing music appears to counter.[15]

The second study examined the effect of opera and classical music in transplanted hearts of mice. Following a heart transplant, mice were assigned to listen to continuous music from Verdi's *La Traviata,* selections from Mozart, the Irish singer Enya, or single monotones. The longest-surviving mice were those randomized to either Verdi or Mozart, with blood samples revealing reduced levels of inflammation, better immune function, and lower rates of organ rejection. Investigators also confirmed that another group of deaf mice exposed to the various music selections did not demonstrate benefit from the Verdi and Mozart selections (just to show that it wasn't dumb luck and that mice, in fact, have good musical taste).[16]

Music and Hospital Recovery Time

A number of studies have now shown that music therapy may shorten postoperative recovery time and hospital stay. One study was conducted in a Florida community hospital with 60 men and women ages 65 and over who were admitted for coronary artery bypass surgery or valve replacement. The evening prior to surgery, patients assigned to music therapy selected their music from a collection of available CDs. Music was then played continuously throughout their surgeries and during recovery in the surgical intensive care unit (ICU). The results were significant. In addition to the expected effect of reducing anxiety, the patients who listened to music were also able to have their breathing tubes removed several hours earlier than the control group (6.5 hours on average following surgery, compared to 10 hours). As any patient who has ever had to have a breathing tube inserted will tell you, the quicker you can get that thing out, the more comfortable you will be and the quicker your overall recovery![17]

Another study provided a choice of multiple music channels for patients undergoing coronary artery bypass surgery to enjoy. The postoperative time spent in the surgical ICU for those assigned to music was reduced from nearly 28 hours to 22 hours. At first glance, this may not seem like a much shorter period of time, but if you are a patient, the quicker you can be moved out of the ICU to a quieter and more private area, the closer you are to recovery, hospital discharge, and rehabilitation.[18]

My recommendation is that if you need to have surgery, you should discuss with your surgeon the possibility of bringing in a selection of music that soothes and relaxes you. Music can be played during surgery if the surgeon allows it, and certainly after surgery as a means to speed up your recovery.

Music and the Frisson Effect

How do you know whether you've attained the health benefits of music? Just like tears are the physiological response to laughter, the *frisson effect* represents the physiological response to music. Frisson is the sudden sensation of "chills down the spine" that occurs when listening to music we thoroughly enjoy.

What causes the frisson effect? Recently, scientists at McGill University used brain scans to demonstrate that listening to pleasurable music released the neurotransmitter dopamine. The more joyful the music, the more the brain scans lit up. As we discussed, dopamine is a primary chemical that is an integral component of the brain's reward structure, meaning that when dopamine is released, pleasure sensations are released from the brain down the spinal cord and throughout the body. That's why the sensation is literally described as "chills down the spine." In addition to being triggered by joyful music, dopamine is also released in response to other pleasurable activities, such as eating delicious foods and using certain illicit drugs.[19]

To maximize the frisson effect, I suggest to my patients that they find musical selections they truly enjoy and, if at all possible, haven't listened to in quite a while. They should select music that's associated with good times in their lives and that will elicit good memories. For example, you may be able to remember a specific song you listened to when you had a memorable relationship, or maybe there was a song that you and a friend spontaneously sang in unison when it came on the radio. When I was a medical student, I remember driving down to Florida with an old girlfriend, listening to Steve Winwood's *Arc of a Diver*. Years later, after not having heard that CD in the meantime, the first bars of "While You See a Chance" came on the radio. It immediately brought back so many great memories and triggered the frisson response. The same thing happened with Van Morrison. My college roommate, Leo, had all of Van's music on eight-track tapes (you can get a great deal on eBay!) and played them constantly. Leo and I got to see Van Morrison play live while at Rutgers. Soon after my wife, Lisa, and I began dating, she bought me the CD *The Best of Van Morrison*, which blew me away because not only had I not heard some of his great songs, such as "Wild Night," in years, but I'd never mentioned anything about Van Morrison to her! Her gift of music gave me a double dose of the frisson effect.

It only takes seconds to achieve the frisson effect, and improvement to the health of your endothelium follows just moments later. This is a particularly great way to combat stress if you have to drive to work and hit a lot of traffic en route. In addition to the traditional ways of purchasing CDs, downloading songs to your musical device, or subscribing to satellite radio, many local libraries have CDs that can be checked out for free (or for a nominal charge). My recommendation is to check out one or two CDs a week and listen to 5 to 15 minutes of your favorite songs each day. Or better yet, dust off your old CDs or visit your attic and grab some of those old vinyl LPs that are now back in style. But don't overdo it, because overplaying the same song more than a few times will diminish the frisson effect.

Singing Your Way to Health

If listening to music lowers blood pressure and heart rate, what about the direct physiological effects that occur from singing? Believe it or not, there isn't a whole lot of research in this area. However, there is a recent case report of a woman undergoing surgery who had spiking high blood pressure that could not be effectively controlled with blood pressure medications. The 76-year-old woman was scheduled to have her knee replaced due to arthritis, but despite a regular regimen of blood pressure medications *and* an additional dose of nifedipine and Lasix prior to surgery, her blood pressure remained dangerously high at 240/120 mm Hg. After hours with no improvement, the patient asked if she could sing. It was her habit to sing when she was worried and to cheer herself up or calm herself down. After singing just two songs (she was a devout Seventh Day Adventist and sang sacred music), her pressure dropped to 180/90. As she continued to sing, her blood pressure continued to drop, until it was low enough to permit surgery. Her knee replacement was performed without complications, and she had no problems with blood pressure after surgery.[20]

Personally, I need look no further for the healing power of singing than my patient Doug, who describes himself as "genetically cursed" when it comes to heart disease. His youngest brother was born with a congenital heart defect, his father and oldest brother died from heart disease, and a brother who is younger than he has already had a double bypass. Doug also describes himself as a "chronic worrier" and has an extremely stressful job in television. After a catheterization test revealed an 80 percent blockage in a coronary artery, he gave serious attention to getting in shape and managing his stress level. His primary form of stress management? Music.

During his 35-minute commute to work, Doug sings constantly. He's sung since he was young, but after the blockage was discovered he said he "just stepped up the singing, because it's a great release and such a stress reliever." In the last few minutes of his commute, he tunes in to "elevator music" to bring an extra dose of calm. Finally, any time he finds himself particularly stressed out, he turns to music. "I go away and hide somewhere and put in the earbuds and listen to soft orchestral music," he said. "I'm an obsessive person, and I take my blood pressure a lot. I disengage and let the music play, and then I literally watch my blood pressure drop before my eyes." Doug is doing well and the only medication he takes is a very low dose of a beta-blocker. He maintains his heart health and emotional wellness through music, exercise, and diet.

Studies evaluating singing's effect on the heart found that singing in a choir leads to synchronization of heart rate and heart rate variability among choir members. This suggests that subconsciously, closer social bonds are being formed and raises the possibility that singing in unison is even more beneficial for your heart than singing alone. I have heard from both patients and colleagues that being part of a choir, whether at church, school, or as part of a musical production, produces a sense of euphoria and a frisson response similar to if not greater than that achieved by listening to music. But you don't have to sing in a choir or even go outside your home to get this benefit. Simply singing in the shower or performing karaoke along with Guitar Hero, or Singtrix to songs you enjoy should provide a nice frisson effect.[21, 22]

And once again, you have scientific evidence to support your taste in music. If your partner is flummoxed by your enthusiasm for yodeling or your neighbor doesn't exactly approve of your attempts at arias, kindly inform him or her it's doctor's orders. A nice pair of noise-canceling headphones also helps.

The Positive Emotions Prescription: Music

To boost positive emotions and heart health, listen to music, sing, or even play an instrument for 20 minutes at least four times each week.

CHAPTER 5

Lighthearted and Light on Your Feet

YOUR EMOTIONAL HEALTH AND PHYSICAL ACTIVITY

LOOKING FOR A QUICK, effective, drug-free, and inexpensive way to give yourself a dose of heart-protective happiness? Look no further than your next workout.

Both medical science and conventional wisdom have long supported the association between physical activity and improved mood. If you've ever sought relief from a stressful day at work by taking a stroll around the block or remedied a case of the blues with a walk in nature, you may be following deeply intuitive wisdom to boost your mood by putting your body to work. Your muscles are made to move and to keep your body *and* your mind well.

Exercise for Body and Mind

Exactly how exercise improves mood isn't entirely understood, but we know that the powerful "supermood" brain chemicals endorphins, dopamine, GABA, serotonin, and norepinephrine are involved. *Endorphins* trigger positive feelings, and like their chemical cousin morphine, diminish our perception of pain. They're partially responsible for the fabled "runner's high" or sense of euphoria that some athletes experience as a result of an intense workout. *Dopamine* is a neurotransmitter that's involved in the reward centers of the brain. Pleasurable activities such as eating and having sex stimulate the production of dopamine, and exercise has been found to do so as well. Dopamine can also blunt the brain's response to stress and increase our pain threshold. *GABA* is an amino acid that acts as a neurotransmitter and produces a feeling of calm and tranquility. *Serotonin*, as we've seen, is the neurotransmitter that wears many physiological hats, as it regulates sleep, mood, appetite, memory, and cardiovascular function. The popular selective serotonin reuptake inhibitor (SSRI) antidepressants (such as Zoloft, Prozac, and Lexapro) work by boosting levels of serotonin. Finally, *norepinephrine* is a hormone and a neurotransmitter that plays a major role in heart function. It's released during exercise, and decreased levels of norepinephrine have been found in people suffering from depression. Considered together, these powerful brain chemicals, all of which are triggered by exercise, constitute a positive mood cocktail that supports cardiovascular health as well as emotional wellness.

Though we don't know exactly *how* exercise enhances mood, we do know a little more about *why*. In addition to the feeling of well-being or even euphoria that exercise can trigger, exercise is a well-known stress reducer. My patient Scott, whom I've been treating for nearly 20 years, puts it simply: "If I don't exercise, I feel the stress." After recovering from surgery to place a multilayer stent, Scott got serious about improving his diet, exercising, and experiencing positive emotions. He dropped nearly 30 pounds, exercises 4 or 5 days a week, and laughs with his wife on a regular basis. Now 45, and with two sons who keep him on his toes, he's healthier than he was at 25.

Some researchers have suggested that the rise in body temperature that comes from exercise has a calming effect on the mind. Exercising on a regular basis can improve sleep, while poor sleep habits adversely affect both metabolism and mood.[1] Exercise has also been shown to alleviate symptoms of both anxiety and depression. In fact, some studies have revealed that exercise is just as effective at treating depression as taking an antidepressant and that exercise's effect lasts longer than that of antidepressants.[2] Performed in a group or with a partner, exercise can get you interacting with others, so you'll reap the benefits of social interaction as well. Exercising can boost your self-esteem by giving you the confidence to reach your goals and by improving your appearance as you become more fit. And it can provide a healthy distraction by taking your mind off of your worries or negative thoughts.

Yet another interesting theory suggests that exercise gives your body practice runs at dealing with stress. During exercise, the body's physiological systems communicate more closely than usual—the cardiovascular system communicates with the muscular system, which communicates with the digestive and renal systems, which communicate with the brain centers that deal with the stress response, and so on. The more sedentary we are, the less practice our bodies get in dealing with stress and the less efficient they are in communicating.[3]

Finally, some of the latest research is revealing that exercise can protect your heart and improve your mood by activating your stores of brown fat. Now, if you're one of the many people who didn't know there was any other kind of fat than the kind you don't want on your belly, you're in for a treat. Researchers are beginning to discover that fat has more positive functions in the body than we'd assumed. Brown fat, for instance, which is found in higher proportions in lean people than in overweight people, releases energy and generates heat, and it burns calories when stimulated. And guess where those calories come from? White fat, which is the fat we think of when we're lamenting our spare tires or our cellulite. Brown fat gets its color because, unlike our more plentiful white fat, it's chock-full of iron-rich mitochondria—our cells' main energy suppliers.

If fully activated, even small amounts of brown fat can burn 300 to 500 calories a day! That's enough to lose a pound a week.[4] Unfortunately, as we age, our stores of white fat increase and our stores of brown fat decrease.

Brown fat is correlated with reduced body fat percentage as well as body mass index, and efforts are under way to devise strategies aimed at stimulating "brown-like" fat in order to treat and even prevent obesity.[5] A major step in this direction follows the recent discovery by scientists at Harvard University that we actually have a *third* type of fat, referred to as beige fat. In contrast to brown fat, located in specific regions that include the nape of the neck, collarbone, and the upper and spinal regions of the back, beige fat is based in white fat regions and, if stimulated by exposure to cold or hormones like irisin, which is secreted during exercise, can be converted to calorie-burning brown fat.[6]

THE MOOD-ENHANCING EFFECTS OF BURNING FAT

Amazingly, all of the known ways to convert white or beige fat to brown fat or increase brown fat activity also enhance mood. The first is to exercise, as recent studies suggest that aerobic conditioning may lead to the "browning" of white fat. How much exercise, as well as the intensity required to produce this effect, are not entirely clear, and further research is clearly needed to sort this out.[7] Until then, I recommend the activities discussed on pages 106–112, such as brisk walking for 30 minutes a day or 150 minutes each week, because they release endorphins, burn calories, lower triglycerides, and improve overall heart health.

A second way is to ingest spices that activate a family of protein receptors known as TRPs (transient receptor potentials). Studies of capsaicin, found in chile peppers, demonstrated that taking 9 milligrams of purified capsinoid capsules (the amount found in about nine chile peppers) daily for up to 6 weeks activated brown fat regions and transformed inactive white fat regions (beige fat) to energy-burning brown fat. [8, 9]

At the University of Maryland School of Medicine, my colleague Dr. Soren Snitker has shown that taking as little as 6 milligrams of capsinoid capsules daily for 6 weeks reduced waist size by 1.2 inches.[10] Finally, another study, from UCLA, found that a dose of 9 milligrams of the capsaicin compound dihydrocapsiate (DCT) resulted in an extra 80 calories burned each day in obese subjects on a very low-energy (800-calorie) diet. Because low-calorie diets reduce basal metabolic rate (see Chapter 2), the amount of calories burned due to brown fat activation is actually quite impressive.[11]

While it is still premature to recommend capsinoid supplements based on these short-term studies and because our bodies do become sensitized to the effects of capsaicin over time, it's best to switch it up with other spices and herbs that also activate TRPs. They include piperine (the pungent spice of pepper and gingerols, and similar to the shogaol found in ginger), allyl isothiocyanate (found in mustard seeds, horseradish, and wasabi—Japanese horseradish), and menthol (the cooling, flavorful compound in mint).[12]

I recommend and incorporate these compounds into the Positive Emotions Prescription Plan in Chapter 10 not only because they activate brown fat, but also because they enhance positive emotions through the activation of endorphins and serotonin.

The third way to increase brown fat activity is through cold exposure. One study placed volunteers in a thermal suit cooled down to 64 degrees for 3 hours, which resulted in 250 calories burned. The writers of the accompanying editorial ironically quipped that activating brown fat is akin to "being on fire"![13] But if you don't have a thermal suit handy, taking a cold shower may be particularly good because it increases brown fat and also releases the supermood chemicals endorphins and norepinephrine. A temperature as low as 73°F is safe, and a shower lasting as little as 2 minutes can produce this heart-healthy and mood-enhancing effect.[14] Now how cool is that?

THE DIRECT CARDIOVASCULAR BENEFITS OF EXERCISE

Whatever the how and why, it's clear that exercise protects your heart by improving your cardiovascular health and by elevating your mood. Before we move on to the types of exercise that work best for emotional and physical health, let's briefly look at some of the many ways exercise supports and improves your cardiovascular system.

Exercise increases your breathing and heart rates and, by doing so, enables your heart muscle to become stronger. Cardiovascular fitness increases the efficiency with which your muscles extract oxygen. Over time, your heart becomes a more efficient pump and, as a result, does not have to work as hard during normal activities or exercise.

With improved cardiovascular function, your heart rate also slows down at rest. The average resting heart rate is between 60 and 100 beats per minute, and athletic training can reduce that by 10 to 20 beats per minute. (You can test your heart rate by placing your index and middle fingers on the pulse point of your wrist and measuring the number of pulse beats over 1 minute.)

A lower resting heart rate has long been known to be an indicator of fitness. Well-conditioned hearts, as are commonly found in athletes, have slow pulse rates (50 to 60 beats per minute) that can run as low as the 40s during sleep. A slow heart rate allows for more oxygen to be delivered to the coronary arteries. This process occurs during the heart cycle's relaxation phase (known as diastole) and is one of the reasons that medicines like beta-blockers, which slow the heart rate, can be effective in treating angina.

In addition, a well-conditioned heart is also more adaptable to stressful changes in the environment, such as what might occur during moments of anger and hostility and in situations over which you have no control. Adaptable hearts have excellent heart rate variability and are more successful in "riding the crests" and blunting significant rises in blood pressure and heart rate that might otherwise occur in less-well-conditioned hearts.

Conversely, higher resting heart rates are associated with increased risk for heart disease. In the Framingham Heart Study, men with a resting heart rate greater than 88 beats per minute had a four times greater risk for sudden cardiac death compared to those with resting rates below 65 beats per minute.[15] And a 2010 study from Scandinavia found that for each 10-beat increase in a resting heart rate, the risk of death from a heart attack increased by 18 percent in women under 70 years of age and 10 to 11 percent in men across age groups.[16]

So is there such a thing as a "happiness" muscle? You bet! There are lots of them, in fact. All 600-plus of your skeletal muscles (the muscles that actually move bone) as well as your heart—arguably the most important muscle—are directly involved in emotional wellness. They're *all* happiness muscles, because physical exertion is one of the best ways to trigger the release of the supermood neurotransmitters dopamine, endorphins, norepinephrine, GABA, and serotonin. Exercising to the point of muscle fatigue is the best way to trigger these extraordinary mood boosters, but take heart: Lower-intensity workouts such as taking a walk can also stimulate serotonin and improve mood.[17]

FINDING YOUR EXERCISE SWEET SPOT

If you're over age 50 or you have health concerns, it's always best to check with your doctor before starting an exercise program; below I'll mention a couple of specific tests to consider. But generally speaking, even those with sedentary lifestyles should be able to begin adding increased physical activity to their lives. Remember, too, that *any* exercise is better than none, and that includes any activity that gets your heart pumping and your body burning calories. Yard work, gardening, and cleaning house are all physical activities that count as exercise.

How Much Exercise Do You Really Need?

Now, if the last time you've seen the inside of a gym was at your high school prom, don't let the words *workout* or *exercise program* intimidate you. Research has shown that just a single aerobic activity lasting 30 minutes and done at a moderate pace improved mood in people suffering from depression.[18] Other studies confirm that brisk walking (walking the equivalent of a 15- to 20-minute mile or 3 to 4 miles per hour on a treadmill) for at least 30 minutes 5 or more days a week is a powerful tool for improving mood, reducing depression, and also lowering risk of heart disease by 20 to 30 percent.[19] While the best results for your emotional and physical health will come from a *regular* exercise program, any exercise you can add to your day can confer heart-healthy benefits and boost your mood.

So how much exercise is necessary to maintain good heart health and emotional wellness? Turns out that all you need is moderate activity lasting 2½ hours (150 minutes) each week or intensive activity for 1¼ hours (75 minutes) weekly.

With respect to cardiac health, research has shown that there's a U-shaped curve when it comes to exercise. At either intensity extreme, too little or too much, the risk of death increases.

First, let's consider the problem of too little physical activity. If you're sedentary, or if you're getting fewer than 2½ hours a week of activity that elevates your heart rate, you're not getting enough exercise for your body or your mind. In those who are sedentary, body weight, blood pressure, cholesterol, glucose, and insulin levels tend to be less well controlled. Consequently, there is an increased risk of heart disease and certain cancers, particularly of the colon and breast.[20]

In our culture, which increasingly calls for jobs that require many hours of sitting in front of a computer, it seems we have to go out of our way to add physical activity into our daily routines. But making an effort to get up and add some exercise to your day is nonnegotiable. Sitting for extended periods of time is bad for both your heart and your mood. A recent large study out of Australia found that sitting for more than 4 hours each day was associated with chronic diseases such as diabetes.[21] In a large study of middle-aged women, researchers found that sitting for 16 hours a day raised the risk of a heart attack by nearly 70 percent compared to that for women who sat less than 4 hours daily. Similarly, watching TV for more than 4 hours a day was associated with doubling the risk of heart attack and death from heart disease compared to watching less than 2 hours a day.[22] Yet another recent study of middle-aged women found that test subjects who sat for more than 7 hours daily doubled their risk of depression compared to active women who sat for less than 4 hours each day.[23]

We all know why inactivity is bad for our bodies, but why is it bad for our emotional health? In addition to reduced release of those supermood chemicals like endorphins and serotonin, periods of inactivity may also be associated with reduced blood flow to regions of the brain involving emotions, such as the amygdala and the brain-adrenal axis that protects against the release of stress hormones.[24] And sitting still—staying in one place—may increase the likelihood of dwelling on negative thoughts or problems. Exercise is a wonderful distraction from our cares and concerns.

Now, let's consider the other extreme: overactivity. Inactivity is the far more prevalent problem in our culture, but it *is* possible to overdo it and cause problems for your heart. At my lab, we discovered how overactivity damaged the heart in one of our patients, a middle-aged male who had jogged at a fast pace for an hour every day for 30 years. One day, he went for a free screening test that measured the amount of calcium in his heart arteries. A normal exam would reveal a calcium score of zero, and a high reading is above 100. Yet, despite being in excellent shape—with normal cholesterol, blood pressure, glucose, and body weight—this patient had a calcium score of 1,200! When we examined him further, it turned out that while his resting blood pressure was perfectly normal (110/70 mm Hg), when he exercised his systolic pressure went through the roof, with readings above 220 mm Hg.[25]

The condition for which he had absolutely no symptoms (such as headache or blurriness of vision) is called "exercise-induced hypertension," and it is undoubtedly much more common than we appreciate. As the resting blood pressure is perfectly normal during any routine exam, the only way to identify this condition in the absence of symptoms during exercise is to measure blood pressure during physical activity. Under normal stress test conditions, the systolic blood pressure should not exceed 200 mm Hg, and the diastolic pressure should not exceed 100 mm Hg.[26]

If you are spending 30 to 60 minutes a day keeping your blood pressure this elevated, it is not healthy for your endothelium and can lead to accelerated plaque formation, as evidenced in our patient.[27]

Exercise-induced hypertension has now been shown to predict heart attacks, stroke, and increased risk of death. Overall, there is an increased risk of developing full-blown hypertension, as well as doubling cardiovascular death rates. For each 10-mm Hg rise in systolic pressure during exercise, there is a 4 percent increased risk of cardiovascular events that is independent of other heart disease risk factors. Exercise-induced hypertension would not be expected to occur with moderate activities such as brisk walking, light jogging, and swimming, but rather with more intensive or competitive-based aerobic activities. For this reason, *I recommend that my patients have a baseline stress test prior to embarking on an intensive aerobic training program, such as training for a marathon.*[28] This is different from having a stress test to rule out blockages in the coronary arteries that may be suggested by symptoms of angina (chest pressure or tightness) or "anginal equivalence" (such as shortness of breath and abdominal discomfort) that occur during exertional activities and progress over time.

Another tool that we use in our practice is testing for *arterial stiffness or excessive aging of the artery* (see Chapter 3 for how this test has been used to study the benefits of laughter). By placing a small transducer over the radial artery pulse on the front of the wrist, pulse wave speed is measured and calibrated in the aorta, the main artery of the body. A good pulse wave reading shows that the aorta is elastic and distensible, whereas poor readings indicate stiffness and advanced aging. Some of my patients can have an arterial age that is 10 to 20 years younger or older than their actual age. Even though risk factors such as cigarette smoking, hypertension, high cholesterol, and diabetes advance the age of your arteries, stress management also plays an important role. Some patients have been baffled to find that despite good control of their risk factors, their arterial age is a decade or more older than their actual age. The most common unifying element is that these folks have not managed their stress well. This can be due to having poor sleep habits, eating too much junk food, being constantly on the go with insufficient downtime, bickering with loved ones or coworkers . . . you know the drill. The good news is that engaging in the Positive Emotions Prescription Plan can help to reverse this process and improve the age of your arteries.

Because of the severity of our patient's exercise-induced hypertension, he was treated with blood pressure medication to lower the risk of further damage to his endothelium, and he has done quite well. He continues to exercise, with adequate warmup and cooldown periods. Now in his midsixties, he remains free of cardiovascular disease despite a super-high calcium score.

By the way—and contrary to popular belief—there is very little evidence that calcium buildup recedes. The upside of this buildup, however, is that calcium also increases stability of the plaque, making it less vulnerable to rupture. Then again, we also have to take into account noncalcified plaque, or the soft deposits of plaque that accumulate on artery walls. And herein lies the danger: A very high calcium score (above 1,000) strongly suggests the presence of noncalcified areas that may be more prone to rupture and to cause a heart attack if risk factors are not under good control. And once again, optimizing management of stress is as critically important as our traditional risk factors.

Other studies have identified additional damage to the heart resulting from overexertion. German investigators found that their marathoners had an excessive amount of calcium in their coronary arteries, similar to what our patient had demonstrated. Another study in the United States also found high levels of coronary calcium in runners who had completed 25 or more marathons. High-intensity activities have also been associated with an up to fivefold increased risk of atrial fibrillation.[29,30] Marathoners can also exhibit premature aging of their blood vessels due to chronic stress and excessive wear and tear on their endothelium.[31]

Just to be clear, the kind of overactivity I'm talking about does not include moderate activities like brisk walking and noncompetitive swimming. To better define differences between moderate and more intense activities, let's turn our attention to metabolic requirements (see "Exercise and MET" on page 104).

(continued on page 106)

EXERCISE AND MET

The Metabolic Equivalent of Task, or MET, represents a simple way to express the amount of energy used during physical activity as a function of your resting metabolic rate. One MET represents activity during rest, with higher levels associated with greater intensity of the activity. Listed below are moderate activities (those assigned METs ranging from 3 to 6) and intense activities (defined as greater than 6 METS).[32]

MODERATE ACTIVITIES (METS IN PARENTHESES)

Ballroom dancing, slow (3.0)

Bicycling, <10 miles per hour, to work or for pleasure (4.0)

Bicycling, stationary, 100 watts, light effort (5.5)

Bowling (3.0)

Calisthenics, home exercise, light or moderate effort, general (3.5)

Caribbean dancing (3.5)

Carpentry, home remodeling, moderate effort (4.0)

Carrying a 1- to 15-pound load up stairs (5.0)

Chopping wood, moderate effort (4.5)

Elder care, care of disabled adult, bathing, dressing (4.0)

Fishing, general (3.5)

Frisbee playing, general (3.0)

Golf, general (4.8)

Horseback riding, general (5.5)

Household tasks, moderate effort (3.5)

Hunting, general (5.0)

Mowing lawn, general (5.5)

Painting (4.5)

Pilates, general (3.0)

Raking lawn (4.0)

Table tennis (Ping-Pong) (4.0)

Tai chi and pilates (3.0)

Walking 3 to 4 miles per hour on flat ground (3.5– 5.0)

Water aerobics (5.3)

Yard work, moderate (4.0)

Yoga, power (4.0)

INTENSE ACTIVITIES

Bicycling 10 to 12 miles per hour (6.8)

Calisthenics (pushups, pullups, jumping jacks), vigorous effort (8.0)

Carrying a 16- to 24-pound load upstairs (6.0)

Jogging, general (7.0)

Jumping rope (10.0)

Running, 4 miles per hour (15 minutes/mile) (6.0)

Running, 5 miles per hour (12 minutes/mile) (8.3)

Running, 6 miles per hour (10 minutes/mile) (9.8)

Running, 6.7 miles per hour (9 minutes/mile) (10.5)

Running, 7.5 miles per hour (8 minutes/mile) (11.5)

Shoveling snow, by hand (6.0)

Skating, roller (7.0)

Skiing, general (7.0)

Skipping rope (12.0)

Soccer, casual (7.9)

Swimming, leisurely (6.0)

Tennis, doubles (6.0)

Tennis, singles (8.0)

Both the moderate and intense activities listed in "Exercise and MET" do *not* produce the METs seen when training for marathons or other events for elite athletes. In these instances, the MET range is often closer to 15 to 20. It is under these conditions, done year-in and year-out, that calcification of the coronary arteries has been reported, as well as changes in the architecture of the heart muscle due to chronic dilation that may lead to scarring; at its extreme, this condition can result in an abnormal heart rhythm and sudden cardiac death.

The bottom line is that unless you are training over a relatively short time frame (measured in months, rather than many years), I do not recommend daily intense activities but rather advocate for more moderate exercise that generates the health benefits without prematurely aging your heart and blood vessels. *Improved mood will occur whether you perform moderate or intense activity, provided that the duration is at least 30 minutes and that your muscles are fatigued.* Moderate activities are also easier on your joints and less likely to cause the rapid changes in heart rate and blood pressure that occur with intense activity. This represents the sweet spot in my activity recommendations because it is attainable for most people on a daily basis, improves mood, and is good for your heart with little, if any, downside.

What Kinds of Exercise Are Best?

First things first: Whatever exercise you choose, don't underestimate the importance of an adequate warmup and cooldown period. For traditional aerobic workouts such as running, walking, weight lifting, or swimming, I always recommend 5- to 10-minute warmup and cooldown periods for my patients. In addition to preventing the potential muscle strain that may be more common in deconditioned and older individuals, warmup periods allow for adjustments to blood vessel dilation, blood pressure, and body temperature. The 5- to 10-minute cooldown period not only allows for equilibration of these factors, but also could prevent complications that might otherwise arise if there is an underlying heart condition.

A classic example is someone with a significant narrowing of the aortic valve that has gone undetected due to lack of symptoms. If during aerobic exercise a person with significant aortic stenosis stops exercising suddenly, there can be inadequate blood flow to the brain and body, resulting in a fainting episode or, in rare cases, sudden death. I advise all of my patients over the age of 50—regardless of their health status—to include adequate warmup and cooldown periods to reduce their risk of heart-related issues such as an abnormal heart rhythm, because as we age, our hearts become more temperamental regarding sudden changes in activity levels.

But what about types of exercise? I'm often asked if specific kinds of exercise are best for cardiovascular health and for improving mood. I think the best barometer for exercise is any activity that you like well enough that you'll engage in it with regularity. The most benefits can be gained with *regular* exercise, practiced five times a week. That said, here are some exercises I routinely recommend to my patients, as they're doable for most people and they count as that moderate level of activity we're aiming for.

Brisk walking (3 to 4 miles per hour on flat ground, or 15 to 20 minutes per mile) is one of the best ways to get some moderate activity and has been shown to reduce the risk of a heart attack.[33] Not only is the "brisk" pace cardioprotective, but another surprise is that walking at a slower pace (2½ miles per hour or less, or 24 minutes per mile) actually *increases* overall risk. A pace slower than 2½ miles per hour was associated with a 44 percent increased risk of death, heart attacks, and stroke and a fivefold increased risk of dementia despite walking the recommended 150 minutes per week![34] Of course, one of this study's shortcomings was that many of the older folks destined for cardiovascular events or dementia had already developed symptoms that limited their motor skills. In other words, the poor motor skills weren't the main reason for their increased risk of events. Ongoing studies are under way to investigate this surprising result.

Walking appears to offer benefits similar to running when it comes to reducing major heart disease risk factors. For example, a good friend of mine, Paul Thompson, MD, a 1972 US Olympic finalist and director of cardiology at the Hartford Hospital, along with his colleague Paul Williams, MD, evaluated the records of 33,000 runners and approximately 16,000 walkers over a 6-year period. Not surprisingly, both running and walking reduced the risk of hypertension, high cholesterol, and diabetes. The risk of developing heart disease was also reduced in walkers (9.3 percent) and in runners (4.5 percent),[35] those these differences were not significant.

Dancing is another great activity and one of the best ways to stay in shape and elevate mood. Its benefits include:

- An uplifted mood from endorphin release, social interaction, and exercise
- Increased blood flow through dilation of the endothelium
- Improved learning and focus through coordinated activities of new moves with yourself and a partner
- Reduced risk of dementia

In a study of septuagenarians followed over an average of 5 years, dancing was associated with a reduced decline of memory. (Playing board games, reading, and playing a musical instrument also had a positive effect on memory.)[36] Social dancing is also associated with better balance and reduced likelihood of falling, which can pose greater danger in the elderly.[37] Hip fracture in the elderly is one of the most ominous predictors of death, with more than one in four dying within a year after such a fracture.[38]

Even men and women with a history of heart failure (meaning the heart's pumping function has decreased to less than 40 percent of normal) can benefit from dancing. In a group assigned to alternating slow and fast waltzing lasting 21 minutes, three times a week, for 2 months, not only was waltzing safe, but it also dilated blood vessels and improved overall fitness and mood. These results were comparable to those from another group assigned to a supervised aerobic program, but I bet that the dancers had more fun because of the added emotional component of participating with partners.[39]

Swimming is one of the best aerobic activities you can do for several reasons. First, no other exercise utilizes more muscles than the various strokes employed in swimming. Because swimming is a resistance exercise, it tones muscles as well as strengthens muscles and bones. Swimming also cushions the body and reduces aches associated with degenerative arthritis.[40]

Swimming tends to produce less bronchoconstriction than other aerobic activities such as running, and is usually better tolerated in those who experience exercise-induced asthma.[41] Doing this activity for just 30 minutes at an easy pace burns 200 calories, and as a regular activity, swimming reduces the risk of death by 50 percent compared to a sedentary lifestyle.[42] It also provides a great platform to release endorphins. Interestingly, in one study, women tended to experience less tension and anxiety after swimming than their male counterparts. As with running and brisk walking, you get the most bang for your buck with endorphin release if your duration is at least 30 minutes and your muscles are fatigued after the swim.[43]

If you can't or don't like to swim, try walking in the water. You can start waist deep and progress to chest immersion or, alternatively, use the water flotation aqua belt. In deep water, you can burn 500 to 600 calories in an hour. (Now, if you can walk *on* water, you won't burn any calories. But then again, you shouldn't need to.)

Cycling, like swimming and other aerobic activities, dilates blood vessels to release nitric oxide. However, in contrast to laughing or listening to joyful music, the dilation occurs as a result of an increase in sheer stress of blood flow against the blood vessel wall. Cycling can burn 250 to 350 calories an hour, which can lead to a 5- to 10-pound weight loss over a year. It also protects against heart disease.

What about Weight Training?

Weight training releases endorphins and can also be protective for your heart, but there is a trick to best accomplishing both. Lifting heavy weights promotes endorphin release, but it also changes the architecture of the heart muscle, causing it to develop hypertrophy (enlargement), and raises blood pressure. The rise in blood pressure can be significant during a workout, with systolic and diastolic levels increasing by 50 percent or more, depending on the intensity of the workout. Long-term hypertension can also occur with high-intensity weight programs.

Using lighter weights with sufficient repetitions and a minimal rest between sets is sufficient to release endorphins, provided again that you experience muscle fatigue. If the exercises are not challenging, it is unlikely that you will derive benefit with regard to positive emotions.[44]

For upper arm and chest workouts, I recommend that my patients work up to three sets of 10 repetitions each, with a 1-minute rest period between sets. For leg exercises, build up to three sets of 15 repetitions per set. I recommend alternating days of weight training with aerobic activity, for four to six total sessions each week.

Weight training has also been shown to reduce the risk of diabetes in women. A study of nearly 100,000 women aged 36 to 81 (the Harvard Nurse's Health Study) found that combining 150 minutes a week of aerobic exercise with 60 minutes a week of strength training translated into a 67 percent reduced likelihood of developing diabetes over an 8-year period.

Similarly, in middle-aged men who participated in weight-training and aerobic activities for at least 150 minutes each week, there was a 41 percent reduction in risk of diabetes compared to nonexercisers over an 18-year follow-up period.[45, 46]

This adds to the growing literature on combining weight training with aerobic activity to decrease risk factors for heart disease, on top of increasing endorphin release. The seminal study in this regard was the Harvard Health Professionals' Follow-Up Study, which found that weight training for at least 30 minutes each week resulted in a 23 percent lower risk of a heart attack or death from heart disease. In addition, brisk walking (3 to 3.9 miles per hour) for 30 minutes per day reduced risk by another 18 percent.[47] Practiced within these parameters, the combination of aerobic activity and weight training is an important part of the Positive Emotions Prescription for great heart health.

Cycling for at least 30 minutes each day reduces heart disease risk by 20 percent, and other studies suggest up to a 50 percent reduced risk of heart disease from cycling 20 miles each week. Once again, cycling represents a great activity to release endorphins. All you need to do is bike for at least 30 minutes and ensure that your legs (and arms, if you do resistance biking) get a good workout. Arm cycling can burn 400 calories over a 30-minute span.[48] Overall, both upper arm and lower leg exercises are effective for releasing endorphins.[49]

More Exercise Ideas

As we saw from the MET table, there are far more ways to burn calories and get our blood flowing than just traditional exercises like running, walking, swimming, and cycling. Here are a few more techniques some of my patients have used to burn calories and add physical activity to their routines.

Playing active video games like Nintendo's Wii Fit can be a fun way to burn calories, lose weight, and feel great. In a 2013 study, women in the postpartum period were assigned to either Wii Fit Plus for 40 days or to no activity. After the study period, the Wii Fit group had burned an average of 200 extra calories each day and lost 5 pounds![50] When using video games as an exercise tool, the most important factor is to choose a game that you enjoy. Like most things in life, the more enjoyable the activity, the greater the likelihood that you will keep it up and reap the benefits.[51]

Rebounding is another way to improve mood and support heart health. Bouncing on a mini trampoline can increase heart rate to moderate- and high-intensity levels (55 to 90 percent of maximal heart rate for age) and burn about the same amount of calories (approximately 5 to 10 calories per minute) as jogging on a treadmill at 5 to 6 miles per hour. Rebounding has a low impact on your joints and is a great option for people who have painful feet while wearing shoes during exercise, since it can be done barefoot. I recommend one of the newer mini trampoline models that are bungee cord rather than spring loaded, such as Bellicon (www.bellicon-usa.com) or JumpSport (www.jumpsport.com), because they provide a gentler, lower-impact bounce that's easier on your joints. The American College of Sports Medicine recommends target exercise expenditure between 150 and 400 kilocalories each day to optimize heart and overall health. This is likely to be met by 30 minutes of brisk walking or 15 minutes of rebounding, both of which are guaranteed to elevate your mood.[52]

Being NEAT is another great way to add more movement and burn more calories. NEAT stands for *nonexercise activity thermogenesis* and is our ability to burn fat in the absence of formalized activity. Virtually anything that you do throughout the day, excluding exercise or being a couch potato, counts as NEAT.

One of the very best-kept secrets as to why thin people stay thin (and a secret that even thin people themselves may not realize) is that they are super NEAT achievers. Many thin people never sit still, even when they are supposedly relaxing. The next time you're able, notice the behavior of your thin colleagues or friends when they're at rest. Do you recall that guy at the office whose foot is tapping all day long, or the woman who's always jiggling her crossed leg? That's super NEAT behavior. Thin people also tend to sit about *2½ hours less each day* than obese men and women. Not only does having a high NEAT score keep someone moving and therefore burning calories, but it also improves his or her mood by keeping those super-mood chemicals revved.[53]

It has been suggested that adapting to a NEAT lifestyle can burn about 350 additional calories each day.[54] Over the course of a year, conversion to a NEAT lifestyle can lead to a 30- to 40-pound weight reduction! To rev up your NEAT profile, I recommend the following:

- Try to walk up one or two additional flights of stairs in addition to those in your residence at least once daily. For example, if your job is located on the tenth floor, get off the elevator on the eighth or ninth floor and walk the rest of the way up. As your strength and endurance improve, add more flights.
- When you're out shopping, park at the far end of the lot. Not only will you improve your NEAT profile, but you'll also be less stressed because your auto will be less likely to be hit by the rushed, type A drivers in some of these densely populated parking lots.
- Chop, slice, and dice your veggies rather than purchasing them already prepared. Every extra bit of movement counts.
- Fidget throughout the day. I tell my patients who have desk jobs never to sit still. Fidgeting, also known as incidental or spontaneous physical activity, in itself can burn anywhere from 100 to 800 calories each day![55] Specifically, I recommend that my patients stay in motion throughout the day by quietly tapping their feet or drumming their fingers. Burning as little as 100 calories daily through fidgeting can translate into a 10-pound weight loss over the course of a year.[56]

- In addition to moving their extremities, people with desk jobs should make a habit of standing and walking around the room or hallway every 15 to 20 minutes to improve their circulation and burn some calories.

Finally, don't underestimate the power of *doing what you love*. My patient Woody, for example, is an avid sailboat racer. This isn't one of the traditional exercises that so often make Top 10 lists, but it does provide a workout as well as an enormous mood boost. "Ocean racing is a real rush for me," he said. "It can be stressful physically and mentally, but it feels euphoric afterwards." In other words, Woody is getting the same endorphin high that we traditionally think of as reserved for runners. I met Woody 20 years ago, just a few months after he had a quadruple bypass, and he has had no cardiac issues since. He's a classic type A personality who never sits still for long, and he credits sailboat racing as his secret for stress relief and overall health and wellness.

The Positive Emotions Prescription: Exercise

You don't need to be an athlete to generate benefits for your cardiovascular system, as well as your mood. Moderate-intensity activities will yield heart-healthy dividends and provide a quick boost to your mood, as well as a more substantive increase in positive mood over time. To reap the benefits for both your heart and your mind, participate in an aerobic activity for 30 minutes a day or 150 minutes each week, and maximize NEAT by moving every 15 to 20 minutes during the day.

CHAPTER 6

Having a Heart-to-Heart

POSITIVE EMOTIONS AND YOUR PERSONAL LIFE

AS IF WE NEEDED ANY additional reason to desire meaningful personal relationships, there is now a vast body of research that demonstrates that love and friendship contribute significantly and directly to heart health. Let's look at some of the latest studies and explore why healthy relationships are important for your heart and how you and your loved ones can influence and optimize each other's cardiovascular health.

Your Relationship Status and Your Heart Health

Research has long shown that married people are less likely to suffer from cardiovascular illness than those who are single. In one of the most recent studies, researchers in Finland studied more than 15,300 patients ages 35 to 99 with acute cardiac syndrome (ACS). Regardless of gender or age, those who were single were two to three times more likely to die of a heart attack than married people. The study concluded quite simply that living alone or being unmarried "increases the risk of having a heart attack and worsens its prognosis both in men and women regardless of age."[1]

Married people also fare better in the aftermath of cardiac surgery. In the 3 months following surgery, unmarried people were 233 percent more likely to die than their married counterparts, and they were 71 percent more likely to die in the following 5 years.[2] Another study showed that married men who received bypass surgery were 2.5 times more likely than single men of similar ages to be alive 15 years after surgery.[3]

Interestingly, the connection between marriage and heart health is different for males and females. For men, being married has long been associated with better health overall. Married men also enjoy improved heart health and better recovery rates after a heart attack or heart bypass surgery. The Framingham Offspring Study followed nearly 3,700 men over 10 years and found that married men had a 46 percent lower rate of death than unmarried men—and this was true even after taking into account traditional cardiovascular risk factors such as smoking, hypertension, high cholesterol, and diabetes.[4]

When women are happy in their spousal relationship, their risk of heart disease is reduced fourfold. However, an unhappy marriage offers no heart health benefit compared to single women,[5] and women fare worse than men when it comes to the effects of marital discord. In one Swedish study of 30- to 65-year-old women who'd been previously diagnosed with coronary heart disease, those who were experiencing stress in their marital relationships (or in their relationship with a cohabitating male partner) were nearly three times as likely to experience recurrent coronary events. In this study, "recurrent coronary events" were defined as acute myocardial infarction (heart attack), revascularization procedures, and even cardiac death. The researchers adjusted for a host of additional risk factors, including age, diabetes, hypertension, smoking, and elevated cholesterol and triglycerides. The study also compared women's work-related stress to marital stress and found that, as opposed to men, work stress was *not* a predictor of recurrent coronary events for women.[6] Generally speaking, in other words, work-related stress compromises men's heart health, while marital-related stress compromises women's heart health. It seems that for women, not just *being married,* but being in a nurturing, supportive marriage is necessary. It's not the institution of marriage that confers health benefits, but the quality of the relationship.

In fact, research shows that regardless of gender, being in a stressful, strife-filled relationship is far worse for your health than being single. (If you've been considering a shotgun marriage to protect your health, you can cancel those drive-thru wedding plans.) By now this should be no surprise because of what we know about the unhealthy effects of stress on the entire body. Relationships in which there is frequent discord or especially hostile arguments prove to be the most harmful to our health—and this is true for marital relationships as well as relationships between friends and family. A study of more than 9,000 British workers found that experiencing negative aspects in close relationships of any sort was associated with a 34 percent increased risk of heart disease.[7]

In the Framingham Offspring Study discussed above, the researchers also looked at how married men and women behaved during times of conflict and what effect their behavior had on their heart health. Researchers concluded that women who "self-silenced" during an argument were four times as likely to die compared to women who spoke up and argued back![8] Now, no one is advocating shouting matches, but these results do speak to the harm that bottling up your negative emotions can have on your physical health. Couples need to find effective styles of communicating *and* listening to each other, even in the midst of volatile, high-tension situations.

The Heartbreak Effect

Now, what about one of life's most stressful situations, divorce? As you may surmise, divorce is terrible for your health. A recent paper from the *Journal of Men's Health* concluded that divorced and unmarried men have mortality rates up to 250 percent higher than unmarried men. The causes of death for divorced men are the familiar culprits of cardiovascular disease, hypertension, and stroke. The paper also reported that divorced men suffer from higher rates of a host of ailments, including everything from the common cold to cancer. Even more chillingly, divorced men's suicide rates are 39 percent higher than married men's.[9]

Neither are women immune to the physical toll of divorce. A study from the Population Research Center found that divorced middle-aged women are 60 percent more likely to have cardiovascular disease than women who remain married. What's more, these negative cardiovascular effects tend to stick around long after the divorce is finalized.[10]

A 2006 study of almost 9,500 people between the ages of 51 and 61 found that both men and women who experienced divorce or the death of a spouse had a higher rate of cardiovascular disease than their continuously married counterparts. How much higher? Approximately "10.7% of remarried women, 11.6% of divorced women, and 10.8% of widows report having cardiovascular disease compared to 8.7% of continuously married women." For men, the odds were worse: "About 16.4% of remarried men, 17.7% of divorced men, and 16.5% of widowers report having cardiovascular disease compared to 13.5% of continuously married men."[11] Interestingly, another study based on the same data found that the continuously married and the *never* married have better cardiovascular health than those who have been through a divorce or who have lost a spouse. And people with multiple marital losses suffer the worst health outcomes.[12] Research has shown that in the first 24 hours after losing a spouse, the risk of a heart attack in the surviving spouse increases by more than twentyfold. Even after 1 month, the risk remains four times higher compared to those who have not lost a spouse.[13]

Given that losing a spouse or partner through divorce or death is one of the most stressful events a person can experience, it's no wonder that so many negative health effects come from losing a loved one. There's even the relatively rare but substantially documented phenomenon known as "broken heart syndrome." Also known as stress-induced cardiomyopathy or Takotsubo cardiomyopathy, this condition occurs under extremely stressful conditions where there is a sudden outpouring of stress hormones that causes the heart essentially to shut down. The causes of broken heart syndrome can vary, but because losing a loved one (especially unexpectedly) is such a stressful event, there is a strong correlation between the death of a spouse or partner and this aptly named heart condition. Postmenopausal women tend to be most vulnerable to broken heart syndrome because of changes in estrogen levels that may raise susceptibility to abnormal function of the heart's left ventricle.[14]

Broken heart syndrome can closely mimic a heart attack. The main difference is that the coronary arteries are usually free of major blockage. When a patient is identified with broken heart syndrome, she is treated with the traditional medications used to treat heart failure. Fortunately, because the shocked heart muscle is only temporarily damaged, there is usually rapid improvement in days, with complete recovery and very low likelihood of recurrence.[15] It's one of the most dramatic examples of the direct, immediate—and sometimes deadly—impact of our emotional health on our heart health.

Cardiac Rx: Healthy Relationships

Thus far, we've focused mainly on the role that romantic partnerships play in heart health. But if you're single, there's no need to think you need to run out and get married in order to keep your heart healthy. Research has shown that supportive, close relationships with friends and family members also have a wonderfully beneficial effect on your heart, as well as your entire body.

A study of 13,301 Finnish men and women found that the more social connections a person had, the lower the risk of heart disease.[16] Another study of more than 32,000 male health professionals ages 42 to 77 found that socially isolated men had nearly twice the risk of dying from heart disease and a 2.2 times greater risk of having a stroke or dying from accidents and suicides. Social isolation was defined as being unmarried, having fewer than six friends or family members, and being without membership in a religious group or community organization. Socially isolated men were also two times more likely to die of stroke.[17] Echoing these results, a 15-year study of middle-aged and older men (aged 50 when the study began) also found that men at the lowest levels of social integration had a 60 percent increased risk of heart disease compared to men who were more socially attached.[18]

Women are by no means protected against cardiovascular disease if they are exposed to poor social and work relationships. For example, women who have poor social networks with few friends and family members and who do not volunteer or belong to a club or church are at a nearly threefold higher risk of stroke compared to women with good social networks.[19] Similarly, women with few social networks are more likely to smoke and are also associated with having a greater risk of diabetes and hypertension and having more than twice the overall risk of death compared to women with a more robust social network.[20]

A recent review of studies published over a 15-year period (from 1995 to 2009) found that women tend to fare better than men in dealing with work-related stress and hostility, and this may reflect women's tendency to have a better social network in place.[21]

So why are women better able to handle the stress of negative social relationships than men—and what can we learn from this? For one thing, men tend to exhibit the fight-or-flight response when reacting to stressful social relationships—they are more likely to become combative or to isolate themselves when a relationship becomes stressful. In contrast, women tend to be less combative and more likely to seek additional emotional support through their social networks and to work toward an amicable solution. Researchers also found that when estrogen signaling was activated in male rats, they were much more responsive to their surroundings under stressful conditions and responded in a manner similar to the female rats. Conversely, when scientists blocked estrogen signaling in the brains of female rats, the rats reacted to stress in a similar manner to the way the male rats had before estrogen activation.[22]

There's even some evidence that women's brains may be more wired for connectivity than men's. Women may have stronger emotional connections due to more neuronal connections between the brain's left and right hemispheres, as recently demonstrated in a study of nearly 1,000 men and women. These neuronal connections may strengthen a woman's ability to process and integrate social and emotional memories and to exhibit superior social cognition skills. On the other hand, the neural circuitry in men's brains is more tightly aligned from the front to the back of the brain, thereby facilitating better motor coordination and spatial resolution. Although there is certainly no excuse for men to forget important dates in a relationship, there may be a physiological basis for it.[23] (Please note that this study was not conducted at my lab.)

Lessons from Long Relationships

Let's turn for a moment from the clinical research and examine the more anecdotal evidence. When it comes to the realm of the human heart in the literal and the figurative sense, we can learn a great deal from those who've maintained long-lasting relationships, whether that's a marriage or partnership, an enduring friendship, or close ties with family members. As many of my patients have been married for 25 years and longer, I've asked them what they believe to be their secret to a successful marriage. David, a retired professor at the University of Maryland School of Dentistry who suffered a heart attack nearly 20 years ago but has done well ever since, has been married for over 50 years. He attributes his successful marriage *and* his continuing physical health to having a very supportive wife. "My wife is smarter than me," he said with a grin. "She's always been a hardworking and caring person." She is as invested in his health as he is.

I'm always impressed when spouses accompany patients to their follow-up appointments. In the vast majority of these cases, the patient is male and his spouse tends to be especially concerned about his prognosis and whether or to what extent additional testing or treatments may be needed. I also asked David how his wife and he interact when conflict arises. "She doesn't get vicious during arguments," he said. "And during an argument, I walk out and cool off." Now in his late seventies, David remains very active with his grandchildren and loves to canoe when he is back at his hometown in southern Ontario.

Another patient, Geraldine, is in her early seventies and has been married for more than 40 years. Like David's wife, Geraldine's husband has never missed one of her appointments. Years ago, Geraldine was diagnosed with a debilitating medical condition that required a liver transplant—yet you'd never know by looking at

Geraldine that she's ever been ill. She maintains a great attitude about life and attributes her long-standing marriage to "enjoying each other's company and sharing a great sense of humor." Geraldine and her husband are very active in their church and are convinced that their faith has played a major role in stabilizing her medical condition. The social interaction they enjoy through church functions and gatherings supports her health, as well. Both she and her husband enjoy nature. They live in the woods and spend time outside listening to the sounds of birds in their area, and they relax to soft, soothing music. Because of the care Geraldine and her husband put into their physical *and* emotional health, Geraldine's prognosis looks great, despite significant health challenges in the past.

One of my most unusual cases is 33-year-old Jason, who at age 9 was the youngest person in the world to be diagnosed with a rare condition known as familial lecithin-cholesterol acyltransferase (LCAT) deficiency.[24] LCAT (pronounced "ell-cat") is an enzyme that transfers cholesterol into HDL in order to enable its transport to the liver, adrenal gland, and reproductive organs for processing. When a genetic defect occurs in the LCAT gene, cholesterol cannot be effectively transferred into HDL. As a result, HDL particles are broken down quickly and HDL levels in blood are low. (Normal HDL levels in men and women average at least 45 and 55 mg/dL, respectively.)

When a faulty LCAT gene is passed on from one parent, this results in a partial LCAT deficiency. In these situations, HDL levels are usually about 10 to 15 mg/dL lower than average. Many people with partial LCAT deficiency don't know it unless they've been tested, because aside from the low HDL, most will lead normal, healthy lives. The problem occurs if a faulty LCAT gene is passed on from both parents. In these cases of complete LCAT deficiency, HDL levels are usually less than 10 mg/dL and abnormal lipids accumulate in certain body tissues such as the kidneys, corneas, and red blood cells. As the disease progresses, patients are at high risk for renal failure, and at the age of 29, that's exactly what happened to Jason.

A kidney transplant was necessary, and as Jason is, in his words, "very blessed to have lots of great friends and family," he received many offers of the gift of a kidney. But as genetics would have it, his wife turned out to be the perfect match, so they both readied themselves for the transplant.

But during the pre-op procedure the medical team discovered nodules in Jason's lungs, and after a wedge resection, he was diagnosed with the fungal infection histoplasmosis. The transplant had to be put off for 6 months in order to treat the histoplasmosis, and in the meantime Jason went on dialysis. Finally, he received his wife's kidney in April 2011, and the surgery went splendidly.

The next step for Jason's long-range recovery was a partial liver transplant. The hope was that healthy liver tissue could begin producing LCAT. With liver transplants, however, the tissue comes from a live donor, and the sickest patients receive transplants first. At that rate, Jason would never have made it up the list, and again, his extraordinarily supportive family and friends intervened. "I had people jumping in line to donate," he said, "but again, my wife not so much volunteered as insisted." The medical team was hesitant because of his wife's weakened state due to the donation of her kidney, but, as Jason said, "She wasn't taking no for an answer." Amazingly, during the pre-op procedure, doctors discovered that she had an extra vein going to her liver, which gave her increased blood supply. Because she was such a perfect match and because of the extra blood supply—and yes, because of her extraordinary commitment to her husband's health—Jason received his wife's liver tissue.

Today, both are doing well, and Jason credits his wife and the "incredible support" from his friends and family with helping him recover from three major surgeries and with his continuing health. "All throughout my ordeals," he said, "even when I was at my sickest, my closest family and friends were absolutely relentless with the joking and making me laugh. I wouldn't trade it for the world—not even right after the lung resection, when it really *hurt* to laugh!" His is an amazing story of the incredible power of a strong support network.

Personally, the most sage advice I ever received on relationships came years ago from our office manager at the time, Kate McWilliams. She told me that the one piece of relationship advice she'd been taught and found most effective was to refrain from saying anything she might later regret. Holding your tongue in the midst of an argument can be difficult, but like my patient David, you *can* learn to give yourself a time-out to gather your composure and give thought to what you're going to say and the effect it will have. The old adage about "sticks and stones" becomes less applicable as we get older and words become more emotionally meaningful—and impactful.

Now of course I'm not a psychologist or a relationships expert, but through personal experience as well as what I've observed from my patients in long-term relationships, I've learned some lessons about what keeps a relationship going for the long haul. In addition, the lessons I learned from the failure of my first marriage have enabled me to find a better path toward a more sound and constructive relationship that enhances positive emotions and supports cardiovascular health. Consider this list of pointers a special bonus section to the Positive Emotions Prescription. After all, happy relationships make for happy hearts.

- **Keep communication channels open.** You can greatly reduce relationship negativity or, better yet, head it off before it develops by engaging in regular dialogue with your spouse or partner. Instead of the cold shoulder or harboring unspoken resentments, prevent emotional toxins from building up before they wreak havoc on your relationships and on your health. Address potential or brewing conflicts in a supportive, rather than combative, way.
- **Never say anything you might regret later.** As difficult as this may be at times, extricate yourself from those inevitable tense situations in relationships by leaving the area so you can take a deep breath and cool down. Not only will this prevent you from saying something hurtful, but you're also giving your revving cardiovascular system a much-needed time-out. Visualizing something that brings calm and peace to your mind also helps. Over the years, like anyone, I've been tempted to say something regrettable, but I now make it a practice to visualize the wise, kind, white-haired Kate McWilliams. It's a potent reminder for *me* to be wise, and I'm able to refrain from getting my relationship—and myself!—into trouble.
- **Help out around the house.** If your partner cooks, then assist in the preparation and/or cleanup. My wife, Lisa, likes to remind our children and me that she is not a short-order chef. In other words, if she cooks, we'd better help out—no excuses. There are endless ways to help with maintaining the house, so seek them out and follow through.
- **Give your partner a break.** Even if you travel for work, you are definitely not exempt from giving your spouse or partner a break upon your return. (Believe me, I learned this one the hard way!)
- **Don't brag about bringing home the bacon.** If you're the primary or sole breadwinner, don't underestimate your partner's contributions or overestimate your own. (I'll speak to traditional gender roles because that's been my experience, but naturally this applies to either sex.) Women care less about men "bringing home the bacon" if it comes at the expense of meaningful time spent with family. All too often, husbands believe that simply

having a job that provides for their spouse and family is sufficient to get a free pass to go and do as they please. Not so! If you want to hang out with your buddies once a week, a similar arrangement should be made for your wife to do the same. Ladies, the same applies to your husband if you're in the habit of having a regular girls' night out.

- **Show appreciation for everything you receive.** A simple "thank you" is fine, but whether it's simple or elaborate, show your appreciation by acknowledging and being grateful for the many things your spouse or partner routinely does for you and brings to your relationship.
- **Do not interrupt your spouse or partner when he or she is talking.** You may not realize it, but constantly interrupting your partner can damage an otherwise healthy relationship. It shows a lack of respect and precludes the possibility of a true dialogue. And *never, ever* criticize your partner in front of other people.
- **Find something that you both can laugh about.** Laughter is *great* for a healthy heart, but it's nonnegotiable for a healthy relationship. It creates true and meaningful connection. It is also one of the first things to go when a relationship sours, so pay attention when laughter starts to leave your relationship (see Chapter 3).
- **Listen, listen, and listen some more.** Listening to what your partner has to say without interrupting and with respect is essential for a healthy relationship.
- **Be kind.** Whether they have been together for 5, 15, or 50 years, my patients in successful relationships consistently remark that their spouse is kind to them in many ways that include being supportive, respectful, and appreciative on a daily basis.
- **Adore your partner, and don't take him or her for granted.** Compliment your spouse in front of other people. Try and break the common cycle of taking your spouse for granted by surprising her with something she'd truly appreciate. Small gestures go a long way. It can be a small token of appreciation, like bringing lunch to work or getting up a few minutes early to have a fresh pot of coffee waiting. Or surprise your spouse with a trip to the movies or a concert. Most importantly, it should be something that your *partner* likes and not what *you alone* would like.

The Role of Human Touch in Heart Health

The benefits of touch would've been next on the list of pointers, but human touch is such a powerful instrument of physical, mental, and emotional health that it's worth exploring in more detail. During childhood visits to the doctor, I remember feeling a sense that everything was going to be fine when my pediatrician would place his hand on my upper shoulder as he listened to my lungs. Early in my training, nearly 30 years ago, I made it a point to do the same thing to my patients during the lung examination, and it's a practice that I continue to this day. Over the years, I have consistently found that this simple gesture relaxes patients and makes them feel more comfortable during what can be an uncomfortable and intimidating experience. A gentle touch can help foster trust and build the doctor-patient relationship, especially when combined with talking to the patient in a soft and reassuring manner.

Several studies lend support to the concept that interpersonal touch has important heart health benefits. In one study, women who received frequent hugs from their partners evidenced reduced heart rate and blood pressure and higher levels of the powerful neurotransmitter oxytocin,[25] which has been referred to as "the love hormone," "the bonding hormone," and "the trust hormone." Oxytocin is released during physical contact such as hugging, touching, sexual intercourse, and orgasm. It results in feelings of contentment, decreased anxiety, increased empathy, bonding, and trust.

On a physiological level, the release of oxytocin leads to blood vessel dilation in a manner similar to endorphin release. And because oxytocin plays a role in reducing inflammation, it helps facilitate the healing of wounds. One study vividly demonstrated oxytocin's role in wound healing—and how positive social interactions cue the release of oxytocin—by giving couples small, superficial blister wounds and then having them interact with each other. The couples who had positive interactions not only enjoyed higher levels of oxytocin, but their blister wounds healed faster than the couples who engaged in conflict.[26]

Another study had 38 couples spend 10 minutes together sitting on a loveseat, during which they were asked to talk about mundane events that made them feel close as a couple, holding hands if desired. At the end of the 10-minute period, they gave each other a 20-second hug. Blood testing found higher levels of oxytocin and reduced systolic blood pressure compared to baseline measurements.[27] Unfortunately, the study didn't test shorter hug times, such as a 5- or 10-second hug or an "until you feel the love hug." Nor did it test the effect of hugging a non–emotionally attached partner for 20 seconds. (That study would likely require cortisol measurements as well—as that's sure to promote some stress!)

Can you still obtain the benefit of human touch if you're single or if your partner is out of town? While the positive *emotional* effect won't be the same, interestingly enough, hugging yourself can increase your oxytocin levels, your pain threshold, and your tolerance to pain.[28] You can also hug your pet, as affectionate contact with your pet releases oxytocin as well. And believe it or not, at least one study has found that hugging an inanimate object can reproduce the oxytocin effect by decreasing the stress hormone cortisol. Researchers recently found that hugging a human-shaped device (such as a Hugvie) after a conversation with a stranger resulted in lower levels of cortisol.[29]

The bottom line is that hugging, kissing, holding hands, and cuddling lead to the release of oxytocin and, like the release of endorphins we've discussed in the chapters on laughter and music, are good for your heart. Additionally, newly discovered properties of oxytocin have now been suggested to directly heal the heart, as we will explore further in Chapter 8.

Thus, for the Positive Emotions Prescription, the personal relationship goal is to maximize positive emotions by activating release of our natural protective neurochemicals, endorphins and oxytocin. To help accomplish this, here are three final tips to get you on the path to closer, more fulfilling relationships and robust cardiac health.

1. **Allot at least 10 minutes each day to touch, hold, and cuddle with your partner.** Don't ever miss out on the chance to give your partner and your kids a good 10- to 20-second hug. Both people enjoy the emotional and physical benefits, and a healthy marriage has been shown to provide better physical and mental health to children, even years down the road.[30]

2. **Be open and honest about your needs.** Solid relationships are built on compromise, respect, and trust. If your need for physical contact is not being fulfilled by your partner, gently ask him or her what you can do to make it happen. It's a two-way street, and you'll both enjoy the physical and emotional benefits of a closer, deeper relationship.

3. **Find a shared activity that you both enjoy.** I typically recommend that my patients incorporate an activity such as taking a long walk or a hike in nature where they can hold hands and enjoy the beautiful surroundings. Other activities might include watching a funny movie together, going to a coffee house, taking a

personal yoga class, giving each other a massage, or dancing. These simple activities will not only fortify your relationship, but also lower your blood pressure in much the same way as taking blood pressure medication, reduce your stress hormone level, and improve your overall heart and emotional health.[31]

The Positive Emotions Prescription: Relational Wellness

To boost positive emotions and heart health, engage your loved ones with respect, kindness, gratitude, and affection—and that includes giving a meaningful hug at least twice daily.

CHAPTER 7

My Job Is Killing Me

POSITIVE EMOTIONS AND YOUR PROFESSIONAL LIFE

WHEN I COWROTE my first book nearly 20 years ago, a manual for fellow physicians entitled *The Practice of Coronary Disease Prevention*, the chapter that garnered the most interest was on stress in the workplace. Many of my colleagues were astonished to learn that a relationship existed between one's occupation and cardiovascular health, because the prevailing wisdom was that only smoking, high blood pressure, diabetes, and high cholesterol were triggers for heart disease. How we managed stress wasn't even on most doctors' radars. And even though nearly 2 decades have elapsed since the publication of that book, I'm afraid that the field has still not advanced to the point where stress management has become intertwined with the other four primary triggers of heart disease.

Yet since I began my medical training more than 30 years ago, I can tell you that with few exceptions, *poor management of stress is by far the most important trigger of a heart attack.* As we discussed in Chapter 1, stress directly promotes inflammation "from the outside in" by converting completely innocent macrophages to angry macrophages, which leads to cholesterol plaque lining our blood vessels and to increased blood clot tendencies, both precursors for a heart attack. Stress also indirectly promotes heart disease by raising blood pressure and triglyceride levels; increasing the urge to smoke among cigarette smokers; and, often, increasing junk food consumption that can lead to weight gain, obesity, insulin resistance, and diabetes.[1] Needless to say, when other health professionals read our discussion about stress in the workplace, far more than a few eyebrows were raised.

It's really no wonder that chapter provoked so much discussion. The majority of most people's days (or nights, if they do shift work) from early adulthood until retirement is spent in the workforce. Our occupations and the stress levels they engender have a profound effect on our overall health, and certainly on our cardiovascular wellness. As we've seen, the risk of heart disease is dependent in great part on how we manage our daily stress levels. And as we spend so much time at our jobs—and that includes any time at home, working remotely—for many of us our place of work is our primary locus of health. If we're not healthy there, we're not healthy anywhere! Thus, one aspect of the Positive Emotions Prescription includes guidelines for managing job-related stress.

Stress in the Workplace

There are many causes of stress in the workplace, and you're no doubt familiar with at least some of them.

- Too much responsibility
- Lack of adequate information or training for your responsibilities
- Lack of support from coworkers or your boss
- An overbearing or "toxic" boss
- Conflict with coworkers
- Lack of job satisfaction—a job that feels meaningless, unchallenging, or as if you're a cog in a machine; a job that offers no possibility of advancement
- Poor working conditions—a job that exposes you to toxins or puts you in danger; a crowded or noisy environment; shift work that disrupts your body's normal circadian rhythm; a job that is physically strenuous, etc.

But by far the most often cited source of job-related stress, no matter your occupation, is having little or no control over your situation. It can be an incredibly frustrating experience if, for instance, you don't have enough input in when or how often you work, if fulfilling your job duties is largely dependent on a colleague who can't or won't get his or her job done, if you feel you're at the mercy of an unpredictable boss, or if you feel you have little or no impact on outcomes. Any scenario in which your decision-making power has been attenuated or removed is going to provoke stress.

A landmark study from the late 1980s examined the relationship between the incidence of myocardial infarction (heart attack) and job-related stress. The study found that job stress is based largely upon two characteristics: *decision making* and *job strain*.[2]

Jobs with the highest decision-making ability and lowest job strain were associated with the lowest risk of heart attack, and the reason is simple: In these cases, you are the decision maker or have power over the decisions that are cast, and thus you have control over your environment. A sense of control alleviates or precludes a great deal of stress and anxiety. And an occupation with low job strain is generally less demanding and/or offers a relatively low-stress environment.

The 10 jobs with the highest decision latitude (i.e., ability to make independent decisions) and the lowest job strain were architect, civil engineer, dentist, foreman, health technician, machinist, natural scientist, programmer, repair technician, and sales representative. On the other hand, the 10 jobs with the lowest decision latitude and highest job strain were cashier, electrician, factory worker, firefighter, freight handler, gas station attendant, mail carrier, nurse's aide, textile operator, and waiter.

The occupations that fall in between are those with high decision latitude but increased job strain—such as electrical engineer, farmer, high school teacher, physician, and public official—and those that are low in job strain but also low in decision latitude, such as billing clerk, carpenter, dispatcher, delivery person, and janitor.[3]

Other sources have compiled lists of the most stressful and least stressful jobs, as well. For a more current listing, see "The 2014 Top 10 Most Stressful and Least Stressful Jobs."

If you're like me, you may be surprised at some of the jobs on both lists, or you may want to take issue with some. (And you may want to add your own job, but I hope it's to the latter list.) Now clearly, lists like these mainly offer entertainment value, but for our purposes they bring up a couple of interesting points.

There's little doubt that jobs that put one's life in danger (such as firefighter, police officer, or a soldier on the front lines) are extremely stressful. But in terms of job-related stress *as it relates to cardiovascular health*, it's difficult to predict the extent to which a particular occupation may be the basis for accelerated cardiovascular disease. This is because there are so many different temperaments and different abilities to handle stress (which is why we don't see scores of police officers or newspaper reporters dropping dead of heart attacks).

One such example is my patient Tom, a retired City of Baltimore police officer

The 2014 Top 10 Most Stressful and Least Stressful Jobs

At the time of this writing, *Forbes* had just released its list of the 10 most stressful jobs for 2014. As you'll see, many of them are timeless:[4]

1. Enlisted military personnel
2. Military general
3. Firefighter
4. Airline pilot
5. Event coordinator
6. Public relations executive
7. Senior corporate executive
8. Newspaper reporter
9. Police officer
10. Taxi driver

Forbes also released the list of the 10 least stressful jobs for 2014: [5]

1. Audiologist
2. Hairstylist
3. Jeweler
4. University professor
5. Seamstress/tailor
6. Dietitian
7. Medical records technician
8. Librarian
9. Multimedia artist
10. Drill press operator

whom I've been treating for approximately 20 years. Prior to seeing me, Tom suffered a heart attack at the age of 42. Although he was routinely in high-stress situations on the job—including being shot at—Tom continued to serve dutifully for 27 years, until his retirement in 1999. In addition to reducing his sky-high cholesterol level with statin therapy, Tom became an active subscriber to the Positive Emotions Prescription Plan. He is an avid hunter and fisherman and engages in these activities for leisure and stress relief. He also watches funny movies with his wife and listens to music from the Grand Ole Opry on Friday and Saturday evenings. Since he added the Positive Emotion Prescription Plan to his lifestyle, he says that his overall outlook has improved. In fact, Tom continues to do well and has had no further heart problems since 1987. Now, some individuals may be attracted to a certain field because they have type A personalities and actually enjoy a stressful, demanding job that keeps their adrenaline revved—in other words, though their stress level may be high, so is their job satisfaction. For still others, a great sense of meaning or purpose—such as the soldier with a deep sense of patriotism or the firefighter dedicated to saving lives—can mitigate a high level of stress. The bottom line? *Our minds are inextricably and intimately related to our hearts.* We can affect the stress levels of our jobs, no matter what they are and no matter what our temperament is, with simple, mindfulness-based practices that are beneficial to our minds and our hearts.

WHEN YOUR JOB-RELATED STRESS BECOMES DANGEROUS

Now, the anecdotal evidence about job stress and temperament aside, what evidence-based research has established is that, generally speaking, *having a highly stressful occupation with little if any ability to make decisions increases your risk of cardiovascular disease.* A meta-analysis of 13 studies that looked at the relationship between job strain and coronary heart disease found that this deadly combination of high job stress and low decision-making latitude increased one's chances of having a heart attack by 23 percent.[6] The meta-analysis provided data from nearly 200,000 subjects.

Smaller, more focused studies have revealed the same link between job-related stress and heart disease. A study of female law enforcement officers found that the female officers experienced more stress than their male counterparts and, compared to the general female population, had a higher prevalence of high cholesterol and diabetes, both of which are cardiovascular disease risk factors. When asked their opinion on their biggest cardiovascular disease risk factor, 77 percent of the respondents replied "stress."[7]

Another study focusing on male professional drivers found that stress was highest in city bus drivers and next highest in intercity bus drivers. Truck drivers and taxi drivers reported lower stress than bus drivers, but all reported job-related stress. What's fascinating about this study is that the prevalence of cardiovascular risk factors showed up in direct proportion to the level of stress. In other words, those who experienced the highest levels of stress showed the highest levels of triglycerides, total cholesterol, LDL cholesterol, and blood pressure, and the lowest levels of desirable HDL cholesterol.[8]

Other studies have found that chronic stress can lead to a chronic inflammatory process. As we've seen, the endothelium is an amazing barometer of stress, and under stressful conditions, the walls of the arteries constrict due to sympathetic (or adrenaline) overdrive. When this happens, the production of nitric oxide, the crown jewel of protective heart chemicals, is impaired.[9] Impairment of nitric oxide limits its ability to carry out one of its most important jobs, which is to reduce inflammation. As a result, inflammation increases and the level of the inflammatory protein C-reactive protein (CRP) rises.[10] My colleague, Dr. Paul Ridker, director of the Center for Cardiovascular Disease Prevention at Brigham and Women's Hospital, and others have demonstrated that just a small rise in CRP (generally above 2 micrograms per liter) is associated with an increased risk of cardiovascular disease. This compares with higher levels of inflammation as occur with active arthritis or other inflammatory conditions, in which CRP levels can rise well above 10 micrograms per liter. Testing for high-sensitivity C-reactive protein, or hs-CRP, is done through a simple blood test to detect the lower levels of inflammation that may raise your risk of heart disease.

Is there a relationship between job strain and inflammation? You bet there is! In fact, studies conducted in Germany found not only a strong relationship between job strain and elevated CRP,[11] but also that the inflammatory burden caused by high job strain *doubled* heart attack risk.[12]

Yet another study found a significant relationship between job strain and the known cardiovascular risk factors hypertension, hyperlipidemia (an increased BMI), and cigarette smoking. In this study, job strain was defined as that familiar combination of high demand and low decision-making ability.[13] The results again demonstrate the synergistic interaction of stress and cardiovascular outcomes. Further, it's worth noting that these workers could very well be smoking in a misguided attempt to ameliorate their work-related stress—something that happens far too often. Physiologically speaking, smoking is simply *not* a stress reliever. Nicotine increases heart rate, constricts blood vessels, raises blood pressure, and causes a spike in adrenaline. These physical effects are the very antithesis of a calming effect and reduced stress.

Other Sources of Job-Related Stress

Before we move on to ways to manage stress while at work, I'd like to briefly touch on a few of the lesser-known sources of occupational stress. Those who work in a noisy environment can be exposed to stress that interferes with good heart rate variability (HRV). As we discussed in Chapter 1, HRV is an important measure of our ability to deal internally with stress. If your heart isn't sufficiently flexible to make appropriate adjustments in times of stress, your sympathetic nervous system, or fight-or-flight response, can go into overdrive and trigger an arrhythmia.[14, 15]

Noise has even been linked to potentially fatal cardiac events. Researchers in Denmark followed 55,000 middle-aged men and women (ages 50 to 64) for 10 years and found a strong relationship between residential traffic noise and an increased risk of a heart attack or stroke. For each 10-decibel increase in noise, the risk of a heart attack increased by 12 percent, while the risk of stroke increased by 14 percent.[16, 17] More generally, a Swedish study found that men and women living in locations with constant noise levels above 65 decibels (for reference, city traffic inside a car averages 85 decibels and whispering is 30 decibels) had a 45 percent higher likelihood of hypertension compared to those living in locations with lower noise levels.[18] If you work at a job that exposes you to high levels of noise, you'll want to take every precaution to protect your ears—and thus, believe it or not, protect your heart. (In the United States, OSHA guidelines require that exposure over 8 hours a day must not exceed 90 decibels. If the exposure lasts for only a quarter of an hour, OSHA allows workers to be exposed to 115 decibels.[19] The case could be made to lower these limits.)

In addition to noise pollution, some workers must deal with air pollution. At first glance, you may not think this applies to you unless you work in a mine or possibly in an office with "sick building syndrome," but air pollution is a real threat to those who work in congested cities, those who work in proximity to vehicles that emit carbon monoxide and other exhaust fumes, and certainly to those who work in factories or plants that deal with toxic chemicals and toxic fumes. Very recently, investigators in Germany found that both air pollution and noise pollution contribute to hardening of the arteries and blood clot formation. They evaluated more than 4,800 men and women and found that long-term exposure to fine particulate matter and traffic noise during the evening hours were associated with development of thoracic atherosclerosis. This suggests that exposure to toxic chemicals radiating from busy roads and the accompanying loud noises during evening hours (which disrupt sleep patterns) accelerate this process.[20, 21]

Just as with noise pollution, your place of employment should provide every means to minimize exposure to danger. Fortunately, tree leaves and vegetation are great at vacuuming up air pollutants,[22] and I recommend that during your lunch or other daytime breaks (when the weather is conducive) you sit away from the traffic and close to neighboring trees or plants, perhaps at a park that is within walking distance. This is one way you can enjoy the sunlight that not only provides natural vitamin D production, but also leads to endorphin release. It also allows you to experience urban nature, where exposure to foliage has been shown to improve mood.[23] Having indoor plants in your office or workplace has also been shown to reduce stress and improve concentration and mood.[24]

For some people, the daily commute will present the most noxious mix of noise pollution, air pollution, and stress. According to a study conducted in Sweden, simply driving to work increases heart attack risk by 70 percent compared to walking, biking, or taking public transportation. This alarming number reflects both the increased stress of driving as well as the loss of positive effects on weight, blood fats (triglycerides), and inflammatory markers that we'd gain through increased activity.[25]

Then, of course, if you drive through and/or work in a polluted metropolitan area, you're exposed to pollutants on an almost-daily basis. If this is the case for you, it's better to keep your windows rolled up and use your air conditioner rather than keeping the windows rolled down. A study conducted in Taipei examined 60 subjects who had 2-hour commutes and found that simply keeping their car windows shut improved heart rate variability. Why? Because they had reduced exposure to outside noise and pollutants.[26] Another study by the same investigators found that keeping the air conditioner on rather than opening the windows in the home or office was associated with reduced blood levels of inflammatory markers such as CRP, oxidative stress, blood clotting factors, and heart rate variability.[27] If you live or work in a congested city, it's far better for your heart if you keep out the noise and the toxic particulate matter.

Finally, no chapter on occupational stress would be complete without at least a glance at the one person we all want to avoid, the toxic boss. The toxic boss comes in all guises, from an overbearing supervisor to one who never shows any gratitude to one who berates employees to bosses who abuse power, are hypercritical, have little or no regard for needs outside of work, or have questionable ethics. And on occasion, bosses can be downright incompetent, which makes everyone's jobs more difficult. Well, as it turns out, science has now proven what we've all known intuitively: A toxic boss is hazardous to your health. A Swedish study of more than 3,100 male employees found that supervisors who were condescending, provided minimal direction and/or negative feedback, or were incompetent or egotistical (or "egotesticle," as my son memorably put it) raised their employees' risk of heart disease by up to 40 percent. The study followed the employees for 10 years and found that the longer the employee worked for the toxic boss, the greater the period of chronic stress and the greater the health risk.[28]

Whatever the source of your job-related stress, if the stress has reached unmanageable levels, it's well worth your time to consider finding a different job. It may be time for you to get out of a stressful job before too much plaque gets into your arteries.

Going to Work with the Positive Emotions Prescription

In this section, I'd like to tag along with you on a typical workday and show you some easy but impactful ways to ward off stress, deal with it when it occurs, and beat its harmful effects. Let's start with the beginning point for the vast majority of workers, the daily commute.

Commuting, for many people, is inherently stressful. There's traffic to deal with, maybe you're dropping kids off at school on the way to work (and maybe—no, check that, *probably*—they're bickering in the backseat), maybe you're running late, maybe you're preoccupied with problems at work or with deadlines to meet. In spite of everything coming at you, minimizing stress levels while in the driver's seat can be accomplished in several ways: Try listening to soothing music, relaxation tapes, recordings of white noise, or, if it won't distract you from your driving, comedy shows, as laughing is such a quick, effective stress-buster. Some of my patients subscribe to satellite radio, which provides endless choices. If you're so inclined, try singing, like my patient Doug; it quickly opens up blood vessels and gets your mind off of anything bothering you. Alternatively, your commute may be one of the few points in your day during which you can indulge in some silence. This can be a time to repeat a mantra, pray, do some deep breathing, or just enjoy a rare time of quiet.

Then, of course, there are alternatives to driving. They aren't available in all areas, but it may be worth your cardiovascular health and peace of mind to explore alternatives such as carpooling, public transportation, biking, or walking. And with increasing possibilities to work remotely, perhaps you can cut out or cut down on your commute by working from home or from your favorite local café.

Okay, so however you get there, you've now arrived at the workplace. What can you do to get your juices flowing and raise your positive emotion profile right off the bat? First, remember the emotional and physical benefits of exercise. If you work above ground level, try walking up at least one or two flights of stairs. But don't be afraid to add more if your level of fitness allows it! According to the Department of Health and Human Services, each flight of stairs burns 5 calories, so if you make a practice of walking up two flights of stairs two or three times daily, you'll burn 20 to 30 calories and get your blood flowing. This short burst of physical exertion also improves attention and concentration. In short, it's perfect for the start of the workday.

Upon entering the workplace, a simple smile to your coworkers can do wonders for your heart. The trick here is to deliberately manipulate your facial muscles to form a broad smile. It doesn't matter if the smile feels insincere—chances are it will become sincere as coworkers smile back at you, and in terms of physiological effect, your body doesn't know the difference. Believe it or not, researchers have found a direct link between a manipulated grin and a reduced heart rate. They also found that in stressful situations, smiling broadly precipitates a quicker recovery to normal heart rate.[29] This will serve you well, since your heart rate would have increased after walking up those stairs and burning some calories.

Smiling also activates brain centers such as the amygdala, which is essential for processing emotions and supporting emotional health. In addition, smiling while at the workplace will enhance overall morale and productivity.[30]

And while we're on the topic of smiling, let's not forget that good oral hygiene contributes to heart health. Poor oral health is not only linked to high levels of bacteria that cause gingival plaque, but it also spreads inflammation to cause plaque in the carotid arteries, which can raise the risk of stroke.[31] Periodontal disease also worsens glucose control in diabetics due to the release of inflammatory proteins that not only increase insulin resistance, but also raise the risk of heart attack and stroke.[32]

MANAGING STRESS AT WORK

Now that we've started the day on a positive note before work has even begun, let's look at some ways to deal with stress during those inevitable times when it does arise.

Aromatherapy. Lavender has long been touted for its calming properties. It's been used to help relax mothers in labor, counteract insomnia, and decrease anxiety. Enjoying a few drops of lavender oil in a warm bath is a wonderful way to give yourself some stress relief and promote a healthy night's sleep.

As for lavender in the workplace, a study concentrating on nurses had one group affix a small bottle of 3 percent lavender oil to their shirts, while a control group affixed a bottle containing no lavender. Not only did the lavender group experience a significant decrease in workplace stress that lasted 3 to 4 days, but the control group actually experienced a slight *increase* in stress symptoms.[33] Aromatherapy is an easy, inexpensive, and noninvasive means of bringing some stress relief to your workday. (And with any luck, its pleasant aroma will have a positive effect on your coworkers, too.)

Take note, however, that lavender should not be applied directly to skin unless it's well diluted, as it is an irritant. Ingesting the oil directly can be toxic and should also be avoided.[34]

Take a 15-minute time-out. A high school principal in a suburb of Baltimore came to see me because his blood pressure was out of control. He enjoys his job, but says that from the time he arrives at 7 a.m. until he leaves in the early evening, he has zero downtime. That's 11 to 12 hours of unrelenting stress! I explained to him that his heart could not take this constant level of stress and that his extremely high blood pressure was telling him so. After some discussion, we identified late morning, between 10:30 and 11:00 a.m., as a manageable time frame for him to have some peace and quiet. I instructed him to tell his assistant that he would not be available during this time unless there was an "absolute emergency." Otherwise, he was to lock his office door and relax on his couch in order to recharge and give his overworked cardiovascular system a break. When I saw him several months later, he was much more relaxed and his blood pressure had normalized. In fact, he no longer takes blood pressure medication at all!

Moral of the story? No matter how busy you are, take periodic breaks. Even taking just 5 minutes away from a frenetic workplace environment is beneficial. Your mind and body really need it.

Learn to single-task rather than multitask. In many workplace cultures, the ability to multitask earns us bragging rights, and in many cases demanding jobs make it unavoidable. (And by the way, I'm thinking not only of busy offices, labs, and some forms of manual labor, but also about stay-at-home parents, whose days are one long marathon of multitasking.) We live in a multitasking culture, and our devices help us with this and even implicitly encourage it. But there's something to be said for giving a single task our full and undivided attention. There's less chance for mistakes, and there can be greater pleasure and far less stress in immersing ourselves in one thing at a time, rather than juggling multiple balls at once.

For older workers, single-tasking becomes even more of a priority. Just as our reflexes slow down as we age, our brain's ability to multitask wanes. The problem here is that we have not been taught that we can no longer operate in multitask mode as we did when we were younger. Consequently, we become frustrated and angry when multiple balls are thrown in our direction and we can't juggle them as well as we used to. However, we can still do one thing at a time *very* well, and shifting into this mind-set will ease your stress in the workplace.

I recently saw a very successful executive whose stressful lifestyle was putting him at high risk for a heart attack or stroke. He had high blood pressure and had developed very poor sleep habits as a result of sometimes working into the night and, more often than not, being so stressed out he couldn't fall asleep. Over time, he'd become less proficient at multitasking and consequently was spending many more hours at work and less time at home, becoming less efficient and less fulfilled in both arenas. He found that despite the greater number of hours he was putting in, details were getting lost in the shuffle. After a thorough neurological evaluation confirmed that he was normal and not developing senile dementia, I suggested that he consider working on one task at a time rather than trying to do too many tasks simultaneously. He found that he far preferred doing one task at a time supremely well, rather than tackling many tasks with mediocrity—or simply leaving them unfinished!

In fact, a study using brain wave signaling found a slower brain wave pattern in adults over age 60 (compared to those under age 30), with impaired ability to recognize a previously shown nature scene after subjects were interrupted and asked to perform another task. In other words, older folks can do single tasks just as well as their grandkids, but they are less efficient in re-engaging functional connections to easily switch between tasks. This process probably starts sometime in our mid to late forties, so now that you are armed with this knowledge, take it easy on yourself.[35] And go for one thing at a time! Here are some helpful tips:

Do not sit for prolonged periods at work. And if you absolutely must, fidget. Sitting for prolonged periods during the day impairs our ability to efficiently process fat and increases the risk of a heart attack by more than 50 percent. Fidgeting will also rev up your metabolic engine and keep your fat-processing enzymes, like lipoprotein lipase, active.[36, 37] Look back to Chapter 5 for the benefits of fidgeting and other NEAT lifestyle advantages.

Stand up or walk around the office every 15 to 20 minutes. Keeping active even at a desk job will keep you in good metabolic shape. In fact, taking multiple breaks during the day is associated with $1\frac{1}{2}$-inch smaller waistlines, reduced triglycerides, reduced blood glucose, and reduced CRP.[38, 39] If you get bored walking around the corridor, consider walking up or down a flight of stairs to use the water fountain or restroom, or, if it's possible, take a short walk outside. Who knows, you may even make a new friend or two, and we know the benefit of social connection in promoting heart health!

Get juiced up. Eat a citrus fruit or three. Being stressed-out at work releases stress hormones and raises blood pressure and heart rate, especially if you are in a hostile, toxic environment. But you may be surprised to learn that vitamin C counteracts these effects. In one study, ascorbic acid (vitamin C) was given to volunteers who were subjected to stress-inducing situations. Each one experienced lower blood pressure and a lower subjective experience of stress than those in the control group, who did not receive ascorbic acid. Furthermore, their recovery from the stressful situation occurred more quickly than the control group's, as evidenced by salivary cortisol levels.[40] In this study, supplements were used at a very high dose of 3,000 milligrams per day, which is 30 percent more than our body can even store. I would recommend having several vitamin C–rich foods on hand for snacking or for lunch. They include red bell peppers, broccoli, kale, cauliflower, strawberries, and of course, oranges. Guava, papaya, and kiwifruit are even better sources of vitamin C, if available. Better yet, try some of the positive emotion elixirs that are part of the 28-Day Positive Emotions Prescription Plan discussed in Chapter 10.

Keep humor nearby. Whether it's funny photos, bookmarked humorous Web sites, a funny book you can read over lunch, or even a hilarious colleague you can chat with over break, find ways to laugh throughout the day. Giving yourself a good dose of laughter every now and again helps you to de-stress and dilates your blood vessels.

If at all possible, do not take your work home with you. Many people tell me that they can't avoid taking at least some work home. But I'd encourage you to find some way to prioritize spending time with your family and friends once you leave the office. You need to recharge and relax, and your heart needs to recharge and relax. Getting away from your work for a time will help you feel invigorated for the next day of work, and you'll approach your tasks with a clear mind and a fresh outlook.

Before you leave work, tidy up your desk. This simple habit makes a marked difference in stress level. If the first thing that greets you when you walk into the office is a mountain of disorder on your desk, you're beginning the day with unnecessary stress. Tidy everything up the afternoon before. Your desk *and* your mind won't feel cluttered and disorganized.

Learn to prioritize. Good time management skills are essential for managing stress levels. In fact, if you're on top of your tasks and meeting your deadlines, you're precluding a great deal of stress before it even begins. So after you tidy your work area, prepare a short list of the most important activities and tasks that require your attention when you arrive the next day. This will not only ease anxiety—you've got clearly delineated tasks right there in black and white—but will also help you shift readily into gear the next morning. Additionally, it will allow you to finish the workday feeling that you have a plan in place, and hopefully, it will give you a little latitude in spending time with friends and family after 5 o'clock.

The Positive Emotions Prescription: Work- and Job-Related Stress

To boost positive emotions and heart health, follow the suggestions beginning on page 136 for managing stress at work. They will make your workplace more tolerable and enjoyable, and who knows? They could just make your day.

CHAPTER 8

Recovering from a Broken Heart

REGAINING POSITIVE EMOTIONS AFTER A LIFE-ALTERING EVENT

IN CHAPTER 6, we learned about the value of close relationships for our heart health and overall wellness. But what happens when those relationships fracture, or one of our loved ones dies? How can we regain our positive emotions in times of distress and loss? And more importantly, how can we prevent further heart damage from occurring during these times?

Protecting Your Heart During Life's Most Stressful Events

The death of a spouse is commonly cited as the most stressful event a person can experience, with divorce coming in a close second. As stress inevitably undermines mental and physical wellness, I'd like to devote time in this chapter to these two stressful events. While prescription medications certainly have their place and are the subject of many books on grieving and depression, I'd like to offer a drug-free approach to regaining optimism after loss. The Positive Emotions Prescription will provide strategies for encouraging the return of positive emotions after serious loss and speeding your body's natural recovery process.

Dealing with Death

When you lose a spouse or other loved one, the term "broken heart" truly couldn't be any more apt. You've absorbed an emotional and physical blow—an excruciatingly painful blow, and at a time like this, you simply can't go it alone. You'll need your village, which includes your entire support network of family, dear friends, and loved ones.

So if you're the type of person who'd normally brush aside help or insist that you can manage on your own, resist this impulse. Not only will you need help with managing the regular details of life for a time, but also, on a physiological and neurochemical level, your heart and mind are actually calling out for the healing that social connection can provide.

What does this mean, exactly? It all goes back to that powerful hormone, oxytocin. Oxytocin facilitates bonding and trust between people, and it can evoke feelings of contentment, calm, and security. It's also been shown to improve mood, alleviate stress, and lower blood pressure. And when is oxytocin released? During times of positive social interaction. This can include anything from a conversation to a shared meal to hugging, to more intimate forms of contact, such as sex and orgasm. Massage therapy can also precipitate oxytocin release and can be very therapeutic following a loss.[1] The bottom line is that oxytocin isn't a solo neurochemical. Its release is dependent upon our being with and interacting with others.

But it also turns out that one of oxytocin's best-kept secrets is that it directly acts on the heart muscle to improve its pump function. Just as endorphins released by the brain interact with specialized blood vessels, leading to the release of cardioprotective nitric oxide, oxytocin binds to specialized receptors located directly on the heart muscle.[2] It's pretty amazing how the brain and heart are connected through receptor networks! Now throw in the autonomic nervous system, and you can visualize the various routes our emotions can take when driving down the highway that connects the nervous system and heart. Simply stated, what's on your mind is truly on your heart.

While we've known for many years of the importance of oxytocin during childbirth and breastfeeding, scientists now have proof that oxytocin also plays a cardioprotective role by exhibiting antioxidant, anti-inflammatory, and heart restorative properties.[3] This raises the tantalizing possibility that oxytocin can play an important role in helping to heal a broken heart. One of the most exciting recent discoveries is that the binding of oxytocin activates the regeneration of heart muscle cells that have sustained injury and damage from a heart attack.[4] Further study is already under way on this repair process, and a patent has been issued on a form of oxytocin that can be administered (via intranasal inhalation, pill form, injection, or infusion) to help regenerate heart muscle cells.[5]

Although the medical administration of oxytocin continues to undergo testing and is not currently available for prime-time use, the good news is that there's no need to wait for science to catch up to the miracle of the human body. Oxytocin and its healing effects are readily available the old-fashioned way, through hugging, kissing, cuddling, and intimate physical contact. Turns out the best things in life really are free! And once again, these new discoveries underscore the old truth that positive emotions directly benefit the health of your heart and your overall physical wellness.

It's worth remembering that you do not have to have intimate contact in order to produce the oxytocin effect. A sustained hug lasting about 20 seconds is more than sufficient to trigger the release of oxytocin and represents an important and meaningful therapy that you should "administer" throughout the grieving process.[6]

If you're not a "touchy-feely" person or if hugs just aren't feasible for whatever reason, you can still reap the benefits of oxytocin. Any kind of social interaction can get the oxytocin flowing—elevated blood levels of oxytocin have even been found in response to interacting with others on social media. It's best, however, to have in-person contact, and studies have found that another way to trigger the release of oxytocin is through volunteering. Believe it or not, *the high death rate (approximately 30 percent) following a major stress event is essentially eliminated by helping others*. This stress-buffering strategy of volunteering is most effective if you care about those whom you are helping, but either way, it dramatically demonstrates the powerful lifesaving role of oxytocin and social bonding.[7]

Helping Others through the Grieving Process

If you haven't yet experienced catastrophic loss but you've wondered how to provide meaningful help to someone who's grieving, reach out to him or her—quite literally!—and give a hug that lasts at least 10 seconds. Offer times of social interaction that your grieving loved one will appreciate—go out to lunch, go to a concert together, go for a walk or to the gym together, or just have your friend or family member over for some quiet conversation. And perhaps most importantly, try to respect your loved one's timetable for grieving. Even though we all recognize that emotional support following loss is critical to the healing process, it is all too commonly short-lived, and a week or two after a loved one passes away, family and friends not directly involved in the loss go on with their lives and may make less of an effort to check in and follow up with those who continue to grieve. Having a schedule among family members and friends that ensures daily contact and preferably a daily hug will greatly assist the grieving process.

This is precisely what one of my patients recently went through. Stu happens to be a world-class photographer of notables such as Willie Nelson, B. B. King, and John, Paul, and Ringo, just to name a few. Even though he has remained healthy (undoubtedly due to the great music he is exposed to, as I like to remind him during his yearly visits), he has a strong family history of premature heart disease. Tragically, both his brother and mother died within 6 months of each other, his brother at the age of 59. Stu told me that what helped him through that very difficult period was intentionally spending time with family. Just after his brother died, a cousin from Paris came to visit for 2 weeks. "She is the same age as my daughter," Stu said, "and planning what we would do with her allowed me to think of happier times." In that same time period, there was a family wedding and a 65th birthday party, and Stu attended both. These events "allowed me to be with my family on my mother's side to reminisce," Stu said. It's important that he took advantage of these social opportunities. His strong support network of family made a world of difference in getting him through this difficult time.

The Science behind Having a Support Network

The acute symptoms of grief generally resolve around 6 months following a loss, except in the approximately 15 percent of cases that require intensive therapy due to complicated grief.[8] Assisted by a strong support system and management of physical health, however, the resolution of the acute symptoms of grief will transition into hopefulness and a more optimistic outlook within that 6-month time period. A wealth of studies has indicated that having an optimistic outlook speeds healing and is a significant predictor of positive physical health. Experiencing positive emotions and having at least a moderately optimistic outlook offers the cardioprotective benefit of a 22 percent reduced risk of heart attack.[9, 10, 11]

A review of published studies also demonstrates that optimism and hopefulness not only protect our hearts, but also set into motion a healthier lifestyle that includes more nutritious eating, increased physical activity, and better sleep habits.[12] This would certainly seem to be the case with my patient Bernie. Bernie is

70 years old but is often mistaken for a person 20 years younger. After a quintuple bypass at age 48—that's *five* bypasses—and having to have his sternum wired together not once but twice, Bernie never looked back. "After something like that," he said, "I don't let anything bother me. I've got a second chance." Bernie began exercising and eating a healthy diet, but he attributes his continuing health to his positive attitude. "Everything is now 100 percent for me," he said. "I never once said, 'I can't do this or that because of my heart.'" His zest for life is apparent to anyone. Bernie has traveled all over the world, and he does adventurous trips like halibut fishing in Alaska, climbing fourteeners (mountains at or higher than 14,000 feet above sea level), and hunting big game in Alberta, Canada. His heart-healthy lifestyle is a synergy of good diet, exercise, lots of time with loved ones, and perhaps most of all, a positive attitude.

Following loss, it's easy to neglect one's health. Keeping to an exercise routine or eating healthy may feel pointless for a while, or perhaps you feel exhausted or simply uninterested in eating. These experiences are common and may even give your body and mind a chance to rest and absorb the shock of loss, but if they persist beyond a few weeks you should by all means reach out to your village for help. Though you may feel overwhelmed with grief, life goes on and *will* regain some sense of normalcy, and you need to tend to your own health. Studies have shown that grieving can raise the risk of a heart attack if there is preexisting heart disease or if risk factors are not under control. In other instances, some people forget to take or refill medications during a period of mourning, which obviously exacerbates a plethora of health conditions. Furthermore, there are plenty of medications that absolutely should not be stopped cold turkey. Some heart medications, for example, can produce a "rebound effect" when they're discontinued or withdrawn. A notable example is the beta-blockers used to treat angina, high blood pressure, and heart failure. Sudden discontinuation of these medications can not only raise your blood pressure and heart rate to levels higher than before treatment, but may also trigger a heart attack, exacerbate heart failure, or cause a stroke or even sudden death.[13]

Rely on your village! They're there to help you, and most people are happy to do anything to help following the loss of someone we love. This very stressful time in your life is exactly when you should accept all means of support, including help with activities of daily living (cooking, medication management, cleaning, transportation, etc.), help from bereavement support groups, help maintaining your health, activities that provide social interaction, and, as you're able, social engagements that will get the oxytocin flowing and keep you on the path to whole-body health and recovery from grief.

Dealing with Divorce

With approximately half of first marriages ending in divorce, there's an excellent chance that lots of you reading this book will have already "been there and done that."

I'm in this camp with you, and while everyone's situation is different, there were four important strategies I learned that helped me navigate this difficult period. I'll briefly summarize my story and comment on these strategies.

Strategy #1: Making plans for the future stimulates positive emotions and is an excellent way to defray the stress related to separation from a loved one. After my ex-wife and I separated, she relocated with our 5-year-old daughter to the West Coast, where her family resided. I made a promise to myself to maintain close contact with my daughter. Until the divorce settlement was reached the following year, I traveled to see her each month, with a primary goal of spending quality time with her. As each visit drew to a close, we were already planning our next visit.

At the time, what was occurring on a neurochemical level was the last thing on my, well, mind. But later I learned that the portion of the brain known as the prefrontal cortex, which is involved in planning for the future and helps to regulate dopamine activity, was activated every time my daughter and I were making plans for my next visit. Simply planning the next visit elevated my mood and helped to ease the pain of departure and temporary separation.[14]

Strategy #2: Surround yourself with understanding coworkers, and make sure to acknowledge your appreciation for their acts of kindness. Fortunately, I had a very understanding group of colleagues who switched their schedules to help accommodate my trips to the West Coast. If you're going through a tough time of any sort, I hope you have supportive colleagues and an understanding boss who are willing to help. It's worth having a conversation with your boss to ask for what you need to help you through this trying time (such as extended leave or to work part time for a while).

And, concerning gratitude, our old friend oxytocin turns up again. Studies have shown that expressing gratitude triggers the release of oxytocin, which automatically lifts our spirits.

Strategy #3: Reach out to family members and friends. Though it's a common tendency to isolate ourselves when we're in pain, just as we've seen with regard to dealing with death, this is the *least* advisable time to withdraw. Your heart and your mind need the support of loved ones and the neurochemical effects of social bonding, so don't be afraid of reaching out and asking for what you need. Friends and family are usually more than happy to help.

If you're in the midst of a divorce and there are children involved, visiting or taking trips with family and friends who have children of a similar age is a positive emotion win-win because it fosters a sense of normalcy and everyone gets the benefits of social bonding. A particularly memorable trip that my daughter Avery and I took was when we met up in Orlando with my brother Neil and his family. It was just our luck to hit a major storm en route to Disney World! While the rest of us passengers were holding on for dear life due to the severe air turbulence, Avery, a fearless kid, was having the time of her life riding the air bumps with laughter and finesse. Needless to say, the flight far surpassed Mr. Toad's Wild Ride. Despite persistent rain in Orlando, the trip was a great experience because it gave Avery bonding time with her cousins and allowed me to catch up with Neil and his wife, Karen. More importantly, it helped to foster our continued long-distance relationship despite our living on opposite sides of the country.

Strategy #4: Don't speak negatively to your child about a coparent. Never, ever speak negatively to your child about his or her other parent. Not only will it lead to the release of negative stress hormones, but it will also cause your child to feel confusion, anger, and resentment both in the short term and in later years.[15]

So how did it all turn out in my case? Well, it's been close to 20 years since Avery relocated to the West Coast. I'm proud to say that she is a very responsible young woman who is gainfully employed, having graduated from an Ivy League school before earning a master's degree. We've remained in close contact over the years and continue our visits. In fact, Avery and I recently enjoyed a father-daughter European holiday along with my younger daughter, Ilana, and my brother Neil and his family, who are currently living in Paris.

Other Strategies to Consider for Dealing with Loss

Loss of any type is inherently disruptive and stressful and can be literally heartbreaking. Here are three additional nonpharmacological strategies you can use to lift your spirits and jump-start the healing process for your broken heart.

1. Participate in spiritual and religious practices. Suffering a major loss can shake our sense of meaning and purpose. For many people, that sense of meaning and purpose comes from their religious beliefs, and taking refuge in spiritual practices and a spiritual community can provide inestimable comfort.

Science, however, has actually provided measurable means of demonstrating the healing power of spirituality. The support of a religious community will not only help to ease the pain after a major life crisis, but religious belief has also been shown to reduce the risk of dying from heart disease.[16] There have been numerous studies on the effect of religion and spirituality on cardiovascular health, and the majority found positive effects on cardiovascular functioning and outcomes, including improved heart rate variability, faster healing after cardiovascular surgery, and lower inflammatory markers such as C-reactive protein. Those who identify as religious or spiritual are also more apt to experience positive emotions such as a feeling of well-being, happiness, hope, optimism, a sense of meaning and purpose, and a sense of control.[17]

What about the role of religion in coping with and adjusting to a major stressful event such as death, cancer, or other life-changing event? A large review of this issue examined 49 studies that included more than 13,500 men and women. The primary conclusions of this meta-analysis can be boiled down to three points. First, there was a direct relationship between religious coping strategies and outcomes of the stressful event. Men and women who used positive strategies such as seeking spiritual support, religious forgiveness, or religious purification rituals generally experienced spiritual growth, positive mood, and higher self-esteem after a stressful, life-altering event. Second, the positive religious coping strategies were also associated with reduced depression and anxiety. Third, men and women who reported experiencing *negative* patterns of religious coping, such as spiritual discontent or interpreting their stressful event as the result of a punishing God, experienced more distress, anxiety, and depression in response to a major adverse life event. These data suggest that positive religious coping can play an important role in adjusting to and recovering from major life stressors.[18, 19]

In Chapter 9, we'll look at some specific forms of spiritual practice and how they have a salutary effect on the mind and the heart—and, as many would claim, on the spirit.

2. Know and respect your grief timetable. I'll begin with a caveat: There is no standard, one-size-fits-all timetable for recovering from a major loss. Personalities, temperaments, and levels of resiliency differ greatly from person to person, and well-intentioned efforts to put a loss behind you or to urge a grieving friend to "get back into the swing of things" before he or she is ready can do more harm than good.

That said, generally speaking, it takes about 6 months after a loss for life to resume some level of normalcy. During this initial 6 months, take measures to eliminate as much stress from your life as you can. This is a time of healing, and the needs of your body and mind should be respected.

If 6 months or so pass and you find that you're continuing to experience extreme or debilitating grief, you should seek professional help. You're putting your physical health at risk with this state of constant, high-level stress, and a good therapist, social worker, support group, healing practitioner, or religious leader can help with your emotional wellness. Finally, don't forget the value of friends and family. You need social interaction and the support of loved ones.

3. Alter your perception. Granted, this is easier said than done, but take a look at the evidence and maybe you'll be inspired to give it a try. A household survey conducted by the National Center for Health Statistics posed this question: "During the past 12 months, would you say that you experienced a lot of stress, a moderate amount of stress, relatively little stress, or almost no stress at all?" It also asked respondents about their own subjective perception of how stress affected their health: "During the past 12 months, how much effect has stress had on your health—a lot, some, hardly any, or none?"

While 35.3 percent reported experiencing a moderate amount of stress and 20.2 percent reported a lot of stress in the prior 12 months, the most surprising finding in this study was how *perception of stress* impacted health. That is, only those who experienced a lot of stress *and* who perceived that this stress adversely affected their health were at substantial risk. These participants experienced a *43 percent increased risk of premature death* compared to participants who experienced minimal if any stress at all. But the kicker was that participants who experienced a lot of stress but did not perceive that the stress affected their health were at the same low risk of death as the respondents who experienced little or no stress![20] It's a stunning and very vivid example of how the mind influences the body.

Similar results were seen in Britain, in a study in which men and women who reported that stress greatly affected their health also exhibited an approximately 50 percent higher risk of heart attack or death compared to those who did not believe that stress affected their health. These results were true even after researchers adjusted for biological, behavioral, and psychological risk factors.[21]

The Synergy of Mind and Heart

This brings us full circle back to our discussion in Chapter 1. The synergy between our minds and our hearts is apparent from every angle. Armed with this lifesaving knowledge, we can make lifestyle decisions right now to enhance our positive emotions and thus promote our cardiovascular wellness. Conversely, continuing to live in a constant state of anxiety leads to the continuous release of stress hormones that ultimately eats away at our hearts. Learning to manage stress in a positive way and to facilitate the occurrence of positive emotions will help us work through and recover from some of life's most trying experiences, including the catastrophic losses we experience through death and divorce. As grievously life-altering as serious loss is, our hearts and minds are equipped with the means to recover, and the hearts and minds of our village stand ready to help.

The Positive Emotions Prescription: Recovery from Loss

To boost positive emotions and heart health, you need to allow yourself time to heal. Rely on your village of loved ones, friends, and coworkers to nurture you through this difficult time and help you get back on your feet.

CHAPTER 9

What's on Your Mind Is on Your Heart

A SURVEY OF INTEGRATIVE THERAPIES

TODAY, DOCTORS ARE much more open to the idea of a holistic approach to health care that incorporates the tools used in integrative or complementary medicine. In a sense, they're following consumer interest: The use of alternative therapies in many countries is steadily on the rise.[1] When I was a medical student, the curriculum focused exclusively on traditional Western interventional medicine, and if any of us had an interest in therapies such as acupuncture or Reiki, we kept it to ourselves. But many of today's medical students are eager to learn about alternative approaches to healing. I know this well because I lecture to our 2nd-year medical students on the topic of preventing heart disease, and one of the most commonly asked questions is, "What is the role of alternative and complementary medicine in preventing a heart attack?"

Despite advancement in integrative medicine[2] and growing interest from doctors and patients, however, medical students largely continue to be trained using traditional approaches simply because this is where the bulk of the evidence exists. For many years, well-executed, peer-reviewed studies on alternative therapies simply weren't conducted. Much work still needs to occur in this area, but the good news is that in recent years, traditional Eastern medical approaches that have been used for millennia to heal and maintain good health are being put to the test.[3] While not all of these therapies may prove to reduce the risk of a heart attack, stroke, or other serious medical condition, the tools we'll cover in this chapter all have reasonable data supporting their efficacy. I'm also confident that integrative therapies will soon make their way to the forefront, alongside proven traditional medical therapies, to help us provide the best care possible.

Exploring the Heart Health Benefits of Alternative Approaches

A major step toward bringing alternative approaches to the forefront of traditional medicine occurred when the American Heart Association included complementary medicine in its scientific statement for evaluating high blood pressure. Written by a panel of experts who are well respected in the field of hypertension, including several of my own colleagues, the statement's bottom line is that it is reasonable for men and women who have blood pressure levels above 120/80 mm Hg to consider alternative approaches as an add-on method to help lower blood pressure. Currently, the best available information supports breathing exercises as the most effective therapy both for short- and long-term control of blood pressure. Simply breathing slowly and deeply at a pace of 5 seconds per breath for 30 seconds can reduce your systolic blood pressure by nearly 4 mm Hg.[4] Many of the practices that could fall under the rubric of alternative approaches—yoga, breathwork, tai chi, qigong, and various forms of meditation—promote healing through focused attention to slow, diaphragmatic breathing. But no special training or adherence to a particular school of thought is required to take advantage of the healthful effects of deep, regular breathing.

Let's look at the data collected on popular integrative therapies that are easy to find and that also promise emotional balance. They include Ayurveda, grounding, spirituality, touch therapy, Traditional Chinese Medicine (acupuncture, qigong, and tai chi), and yoga. Not only may these activities lead to spiritual or emotional healing, but they can also benefit your heart health without the use of medication.

Ayurveda

Ayurveda is a system of medicine that originated in India more than 3,000 years ago and is still practiced widely today. According to the Ayurvedic system, we are healthy when our three bodily constitutions, or *doshas*—kapha, pitta, and vata—are in balance, and we become ill when they go out of balance. Each of us has a unique combination of the three doshas, though one or two usually predominate. Once you know your dosha or body type, you can follow a diet and make other lifestyle choices to remain balanced and healthy. Our doshas become imbalanced due to external and internal factors such as stress, poor diet, lack of exercise, injury, and changes in climate. The goal of Ayurveda is to bring us back into balance. This balance brings us into harmony with ourselves physically, emotionally, intellectually, and spiritually. For example, if it's cold outside, the Ayurvedic system would have us grab a bowl of hot soup.

Though Ayurveda does treat disease when it occurs, its focus is on prevention, and its treatments, as we saw with the hot soup example, come from nonpharmacological means such as proper diet, herbs, massage, meditation, yoga, and various means of detoxification. Ayurvedic treatments are highly specific to the individual and based upon each person's unique constitution. While Ayurvedic medicine is a blessing because it provides comprehensive, individualized attention, it's also a curse from the standpoint of conducting clinical studies, as it's all but impossible to isolate single aspects of treatment to study and compare them to a control group. It should come as no surprise then that the number of studies conducted in the United States testing Ayurvedic therapies has been rather slim. After all, it's pretty straightforward to test a new drug to treat high blood cholesterol levels, for example. But it's a different story when it comes to measuring the effect of Ayurvedic medicine.

The general Western approach also commonly emphasizes a quick cure (i.e., prescription medication, surgery) for a specific complaint, whereas Ayurveda is an intentionally slow and holistic process. Most of us have not had the opportunity to be exposed to some of the wonderful Ayurvedic techniques that can calm our minds and soothe our hearts. Back in the mid-1990s, I had the opportunity to serve on a panel of educators in alternative medicine and found Ayurveda to be a very soothing treatment for stress and anxiety. My wife wanted to experience Ayurveda therapy during our visits to India, and she enjoyed these experiences so much that she continues to use warm oil and Ayurvedic massage after a long day at work.

The plant compound berberine, a mainstay in Ayurvedic medicine, has been shown to improve depression.[5] Berberine has also been shown to enhance glucose control in diabetics and lower LDL cholesterol by 21 percent and triglyceride levels by an impressive 36 percent.[6, 7] And Ayurvedic Abhyanga massage—a type of heated oil massage that lifts mood and enhances relaxation—has been shown to reduce heart rate and lower blood pressure.[8]

One of the most mood-uplifting Ayurvedic techniques that I have come across in my travels is Shirodhara. With this therapy, warm oil is gently poured over the "third eye" position of the forehead. Studies on people who receive Shirodhara have found significant improvement in mood scores that coincide with drops in blood pressure, pulse, and breathing rate.[9, 10] My wife uses both Abhyanga massage and Shirodhara treatments and finds both to be great de-stressors and mood elevators.

Though much more extensive testing on Ayurveda is needed, the anecdotal evidence—based on the thousands of years Ayurveda has been in use, as well as its current widespread use throughout the world—is strong. And we do know that many of the principles of Ayurveda, such as a healthy diet, the practice of yoga, and avoiding chronic stress, are proven ways to promote and maintain cardiovascular health. With proper guidance from your physician, Ayurveda can be an effective and noninvasive complementary therapy to your current health care regimen.

Grounding

Simply stated, grounding is walking barefoot on the earth. Taking a walk on the beach or a stroll through the grass on a summer's day is not only very relaxing, but also uplifts your mood and can promote a good night's sleep.[11] There is even scientific evidence that grounding may be good for your heart, as studies on grounding have shown significant reductions in the stress hormone cortisol.

Some have suggested that grounding may also have anti-inflammatory properties. When we are grounded, our bodies transfer the earth's negatively charged ions to help neutralize positively charged free radicals in the atmosphere. These free radicals, such as ozone, can cause oxidative stress and promote chronic inflammation.[12] Though this might seem like a far-fetched hypothesis, a dedicated fan base believes this theory to be worthy of further study.

And while we do not yet know whether grounding can reduce heart disease, one recent study found that it was associated with reduced blood thickness, or viscosity. We want to keep our blood "thin" because increased blood viscosity, more commonly found with high blood fat or triglyceride levels, is associated with increased risk of a heart attack.[13]

While more research is needed, we can all benefit from balance and equanimity, and to do so, we clearly need to start from the ground up. In the meantime, I recommend that—weather permitting—my patients spend some time each day in a "grounded state" by walking barefoot outside and listening to the sounds of nature. It will bring both momentous connection to the earth and calm into your day, and it will also help to balance your mood and reduce your heart's stress hormones.

Spirituality

Spirituality is a generalized term that reflects an intimate connection to an organized religion, the supernatural, or the mystical. Many research studies use the term interchangeably with *religion* (or *religiousness*), and some use both, in the form of *religion/spirituality*, or *R/S*. The terms encompass all faith traditions.

You may wonder why spirituality is included in a chapter on alternative therapies, since so many people identify themselves as religious or spiritual. The distinction here is the emphasis on turning to spiritual or religious means for healing. Among the means people have used over the centuries to seek healing for themselves or others are prayer, the laying on of hands, the application of holy water or holy oil, pilgrimages to holy sites, and the use of a healing mantra.

Fortunately for our purposes, spirituality is so prevalent in our culture that there have been numerous studies on its effect on health and well-being. Dr. Dean Ornish's Lifestyle Heart Trial was the first study to demonstrate that lifestyle intervention employing diet, exercise, meditation, and other healthy measures significantly reduced the progression of coronary plaques that cause fatal blockages, and in some cases, even induced modest regression of these plaques.[14]

Quite tellingly, the degree of spiritual well-being a person reported was correlated to the amount of new or reduced coronary blockages over a 4-year time period.[15]

Another study looked at the role of spirituality and religion in predicting complications after heart bypass surgery. Conducted at the University of Michigan, researchers examined 177 patients scheduled to have heart bypass surgery. Two weeks prior to surgery, patients completed questionnaires that included questions about the importance of religion and prayer. The study found that patients who prayed prior to surgery were 45 percent less likely to experience complications after surgery.[16] A similar study also found that men and women with strong religious beliefs who underwent heart bypass surgery had fewer complications after surgery, along with shorter hospital stays.[17]

How about the role of spirituality months after heart surgery? A study at Dartmouth Medical Center evaluated the impact of religiousness on death rates 6 months after heart bypass or heart valve replacement surgery on 232 men and women. Two factors were consistent predictors of death: not participating in social or community groups and the absence of comfort or strength from religion. Those who felt comfort or strength as a result of their religious beliefs experienced more than a threefold lower risk of death over the study period.[18]

Another study of heart failure patients found that a sense of "spiritual well-being"—that is, feeling a sense of harmony, meaning, peace, and purpose in life—was strongly associated with a lower risk of depression.[19] Depression in patients with heart failure is quite common and leads to repeat hospitalizations and increased risk of dying.[20] Being involved in a religious tradition and/or spiritual practice can reduce or prevent depression and improve emotional wellness and cardiovascular health.

But these benefits go beyond the realm of the clinical study. I've observed that patients who are spiritual are more likely to accept a potential bad health outcome and, therefore, feel more at peace rather than overwhelmed by fear and stress. If being overly fearful when facing stressful life events magnifies risk of death, as we previously discussed in Chapter 8, then spirituality is likely to benefit patients in overcoming life-threatening situations such as a heart attack or stroke. Over the years, I've treated many patients who, despite having suffered a heart attack, remained remarkably calm. When I would ask why they seemed so relaxed, the answer was commonly that their faith helped them get through the ordeal. A similar event occurred more than a dozen years ago when my father-in-law, Paul, called and told me that he was having chest pain. A deeply spiritual man, even as he was being admitted to the hospital with a heart attack, Paul told me that he "wasn't afraid to die." Throughout his course of treatment, the nurses were impressed by how "mellow and unfazed" he was. Paul made a complete recovery, continues to live independently into his late nineties, and is one of the most content individuals I've ever known.

Paul's story is reminiscent of a group of centenarians I had the opportunity to meet through Odessa Dorkins, PhD, Maryland Centenarians Committee founder. Centenarians now comprise the fastest-growing segment of the US population, with an estimated population approaching 75,000. For more than 20 years, Dr. Dorkins has studied hundreds of men and women who have reached and surpassed their 100th birthday, and she organizes a yearly lunch to celebrate this milestone with their families. At one of these luncheons, we asked about 50 centenarians what they attributed their longevity to, and almost universally their answer was their faith. (The second most popular response was, "I try to avoid doctors." Would that suggest that they've fared well without the use of traditional medical interventions? I'll let you be the judge!)

When it comes to the impact of spirituality and religion on health, the question always arises as to whether the positive results can be attributed to some supernatural or divine force, if people who identify as spiritual and/or religious are doing other things to promote health, if it's all a placebo effect, or if it's some combination of these factors. The truth is, we'll never know the exact answer. Researchers must rely on empirical evidence, and what we know is this: People who identify as spiritual or religious *tend* not to engage in unhealthy behaviors such as smoking, unprotected sex, excessive consumption of alcohol, or other risky lifestyle behaviors that can compromise health. We also know that people who are involved in a faith tradition are usually members of communities, so they're gaining the benefits of social involvement. Likewise, they tend to be involved in volunteering efforts and other altruistic activities, and we've seen the cardiac benefits of volunteering. Then, of course, there's the inevitable stress relief that comes from a practice of prayer or meditation. My patient Rick, who is 63 and started testing for borderline-high cholesterol in his thirties, maintains his health through exercise, diet, and a daily practice of meditation. Spirituality is an integral part of his life; he and his wife attend weekly meditation groups together and have gone through levels of Shambhala training. With a host of practices in place that benefit both his mind and his heart, it's no surprise that Rick is one of those patients I see only once a year—and that's mostly to tell him to keep up the good work. Bottom line? The myriad benefits associated with religion and spirituality certainly seem to suggest that for a variety of reasons, quantifiable or not, spirituality is good for your health.

Touch Therapy

Touch-based therapies like Healing Touch, Therapeutic Touch, and Reiki are used for stress reduction, relaxation, and the promotion of overall health and well-being. They each involve directing the universal life energy in each person to bring the energies back into balance and promote a person's natural healing ability.

The term *Healing Touch* is often used interchangeably with *Therapeutic Touch*, and indeed these two touch-based therapies are closely related. There are differences, however, in their origins and, in some cases, in the way they're practiced.

Healing Touch was developed by a nurse, Janet Mentgen, in the early 1980s. A Healing Touch practitioner lightly touches a person's body or places his or her hands inches from the body to intentionally direct energy in order to release pain, stress, and toxins from the body. Therapeutic Touch, developed by Dolores Krieger, PhD, RN, and Dora Kunz, an alternative healer, is another energy therapy that directs the flow of energy to advance the body's natural healing process. As with Healing Touch, a Therapeutic Touch practitioner will apply light touch or a sweeping motion to affected areas of the body over a 15- to 30-minute period. Both Healing Touch and Therapeutic Touch are performed with the recipient fully clothed and either sitting comfortably or lying down.

Reiki

Based on ancient Eastern philosophy, Reiki was rediscovered by a Japanese Buddhist monk in the 19th century. It flourished in Japan and began to be practiced regularly in the United States in the 1970s. The word *Reiki* means "life energy," and Reiki masters place their hands at various points on the recipient to allow the Reiki to flow wherever it needs to flow.[21] Reiki, in stark contrast to both Healing Touch and Therapeutic Touch, can be performed at a distance; a Reiki master can send Reiki to recipients wherever they're located. My colleague Joyce is the executive director of a major health care foundation and also a certified Reiki master. According to Joyce, the Reiki master helps the recipient to relax and rebalance the body's energies so the recipient can get rid of stress and activate his or her own natural healing abilities. The healing energy itself "goes where it's needed." Joyce has used Reiki to facilitate healing and stress reduction for people dealing with cancer and injury, and she has used Reiki on herself to help recover from injury and, as she described it, "bring me back to center."

There is little doubt that touch-based therapies reduce anxiety, improve relaxation, and facilitate positive emotions, resulting in an overall sense of improved well-being. Tension headaches and other stress-related ailments are reduced and in some cases cured. In an Iranian study, women with palpitations and other anxiety-based heart conditions experienced a cessation of their symptoms after receiving Therapeutic Touch.[22] Reiki has also been found to reduce blood pressure and heart rate, and to improve heart rate variability (HRV).[23, 24]

In the first published study of the effects of Reiki on patients hospitalized for an acute coronary syndrome, Reiki treatment was found to improve HRV and to produce a positive emotional state characterized by feelings of happiness and relaxation. Because poor HRV is a powerful predictor of worse outcomes after a cardiac event, Reiki therapy may be a promising nonpharmacological treatment after a heart attack.[25]

As energy-based healing therapies are used by up to 2 percent of men and women at risk for heart disease, it would be reasonable to conduct studies to determine whether such therapy can reduce the risk of a heart attack or stroke. Touch therapy came under fire more than a decade ago when an astute 9-year-old, Emily Rosa, conducted a study asking Therapeutic Touch practitioners to feel the energy from her hand. Using a screen to block the practitioners' view, Emily held her hand over one of their hands and asked them to pick the correct hand. The touch therapists were no better at selecting the correct hand (and energy source) than anyone, which suggests that the benefit of Therapeutic Touch on relieving stress is nothing more than a placebo effect.[26]

The Magic of the Placebo Effect

Instead of saying the benefit of touch therapy is nothing *more* than the placebo effect, perhaps I should say it's nothing *less* than the placebo effect. In my view, even if the benefits are derived from the placebo effect, that's still okay, because the same salutary benefits are still achieved. If stress is reduced through touch therapy for *whatever* reason, then ailments that may be induced by stress, such as headaches, fibromyalgia, gastrointestinal discomfort, and insomnia, not to mention the cardiovascular impairments caused by chronic stress, may be effectively treated.

Over the years I've conducted many clinical trials that test an active compound versus a placebo, and if you can't tell already, I've become a big fan of the placebo effect.[27] As it turns out, simply participating in medical research seems to be good for your heart! This isn't because people often receive an active compound that turns out to work well for them. In fact, these studies fail as often as they succeed, and only about 5 percent of drugs that make it to clinical trials ever get approved for use. So when I ask a patient whether he or she is interested in participating in one of our clinical trials, I simply say there is "a 50-50 chance of receiving the active compound." But it turns out that while the active compound is often disappointing, the placebo compound is virtually always a winner.

How can this be? It's because our desires, hopes, perceptions, and expectations—the power of our minds, in short—have profound effects on physical outcomes. Folks who participate in clinical trials have been shown to fare better than the natural history of their disease would otherwise dictate. We know, for example, that if you have a history of heart attack, your annual risk of having another cardiovascular-related problem is somewhere between 2 and 3 percent. However, in clinical trials, the annual risk of having another event in the placebo-treated patients is 30 to 50 percent lower![28, 29]

In part this reflects the fact that patients who participate in clinical trials are more closely monitored and tend to take better care of themselves, but these factors cannot entirely account for the large benefit observed. Another explanation is that the close bonds that commonly form between patient and study coordinator and members of the research team likely lead to the release of cardioprotective compounds such as oxytocin. In other words, the research team can serve as another "support group," and the more support, the lower the risk of a heart attack or stroke.

All that said, the placebo effect has been studied in many clinical trials and has been shown to be an effective means to reduce pain, mediate allergic responses, decrease stress, reduce heart rate, and even improve motor function in patients with Parkinson's disease.[30] In other words, the placebo effect is quite real and can certainly be used to mitigate negative symptoms and enhance the healing process.

So the next time you have an opportunity to participate in a medical research study, consider it a win-win situation. Having served as a volunteer in many studies over the years, I can attest that it is certainly a rewarding and enlightening experience!

Traditional Chinese Medicine: Acupuncture, Qigong, and Tai Chi

Acupuncture is generally a safe procedure, with side effects primarily limited to mild pain and bruising at the site of administration. Studies have suggested that acupuncture may be effective for patients with mild hypertension, or systolic blood pressure of 140 to 159 or diastolic blood pressure of 80 to 89 mm Hg.[31, 32] Acupuncture also improves HRV by stimulating a specific area (ST36) in the lower leg, leading to an increase of vagus nerve activity.[33]

Of the various forms of acupuncture available, the transmission of small electrical currents known as electroacupuncture (EA) may be the most effective for weight loss. In studies using EA in overweight women for 30 minutes daily over a 20-day period, there was a 4.8 percent reduction in weight compared to the 2.5 percent weight reduction in the diet-treated group. Other studies using EA also found significant weight loss compared to exercise alone. Pending larger confirmatory trials, EA may be a promising therapy for the treatment of obesity.[34, 35, 36] Acupuncture has also been shown to reduce cholesterol and triglycerides, insulin resistance, blood pressure, and inflammation.[37]

Acupuncture can be effective for treating depression, with significant improvement seen when acupuncture is received once or twice weekly. Because it stimulates the release of serotonin and opioids, including beta-endorphin, dynorphin, and enkephalin, overall mood is lifted and anxiety is reduced.[38]

Of all the nontraditional approaches, acupuncture has accumulated the most scientific data showing improvement in heart disease risk factors in conjunction with mood-elevating effects. Although very few studies have been conducted in the United States, the results appear promising and support future research efforts combining acupuncture with other lifestyle measures to support a healthy heart.[39]

Qigong is an ancient Chinese practice that integrates breathing, posture, and mental focus for inner healing and energy. Literally hundreds of types of Qigong exercises have been developed throughout China and serve different purposes for health maintenance and enhancement. One of the more popular branches of Qigong is tai chi, which has become very popular in the United States. Tai chi consists of graceful movements with a focused concentration on breathing timed to movement, all aimed at synchronizing the mind and body connection. I remember watching a perfectly choreographed group of men and women participating in low-impact tai chi exercises in front of our medical school when I was an undergraduate student back in the 1970s. Since that time, tai chi has continued to gain popularity in the United States, with more than 2 million Americans participating. When performed three times a week for 3 months, Qigong, and specifically tai chi, can reduce blood pressure by the same amount as taking one blood pressure medication.[40, 41]

Practicing tai chi for 1 year reduces inflammation, cholesterol, and triglyceride levels and improves exercise capacity. It also reduces insulin resistance and improves glucose control in diabetics.[42] Tai chi is very safe and effective for men and women who have suffered a heart attack.[43] Similarly, tai chi promotes weight loss and blood pressure reduction in patients with heart failure.[44]

A couple of Harvard University studies found improved quality of life and overall mood in heart failure patients practicing tai chi. This is extremely important because up to 40 percent of patients with heart failure suffer from major depression.[45, 46, 47] The practice of tai chi has been shown to reduce levels of the stress hormones cortisol and norepinephrine, and these effects likely account for some of the mood-altering benefits associated with this ancient Chinese practice.[48]

Yoga

Yoga is so prevalent in our culture that more than 20 million Americans practice it. Yoga is designed to improve our mood and our overall sense of well-being by achieving union and harmony in mind-body connections. And the amazing thing about yoga is that it has many different variations that can be tailored to your specific needs. For example, there are specific breathing exercises and postures that lower blood pressure, improve breathing capacity, and affect heart rate. There are also at least 13 different branches of yoga available throughout the United States. For more information, visit the University of Maryland Integrative Medicine Web site at http://umm.edu/health/medical/altmed/treatment/yoga.

When practiced for 6 months, yoga has been shown to decrease oxidative stress and improve both glucose and lipid control.[49] Triglycerides can be sky-high in poorly controlled diabetics, and several studies have demonstrated improvement in glucose control and insulin requirements in diabetics who practice yoga, suggesting that yoga is an excellent nonpharmacological way to manage high triglycerides. The magnitude of reduction in triglyceride levels that occurred (10 to 25 percent) is similar to that obtained with statin therapy.[50]

So can yoga also lead to weight loss? Even though yoga is not viewed as a traditional aerobic activity, weight reduction may occur. A recent review examining studies conducted in the United States, India, and Europe identified minimum requirements for a yoga program to translate into an effective strategy for weight loss. They include practicing yoga at least three times weekly, with each yoga session lasting between 75 and 90 minutes—including 5 to 15 minutes of breathing exercises (pranayama) and 10 minutes of deep relaxation (shavasana) at the end of the session—for a minimum of about 3 months (although one study showed significant changes in as little as 6 weeks). The types of yoga generally used in weight loss studies were traditional and updated, "Americanized" versions such as power yoga (known as ashtanga). Reductions of up to 3 percent of body weight and 6 percent of body fat have been observed in concert with significant mood improvement.[51]

Even if heart disease has been diagnosed, yoga can be good for the mind-heart relationship. Studies have found reduced coronary blockage with reduced heart attack risk and need for heart bypass surgery following 2 years in a yoga program.[52] Because coronary arteries fill when the heart relaxes (the period of diastole), techniques that increase this period, such as slowing the heart rate, help to maximize coronary flow; yoga is quite effective in this regard.

Practicing yoga also increases the brain's levels of thalamic gamma-aminobutyric acid (GABA), which is believed to contribute to the calm yet uplifted mood that yoga practitioners experience.[53] It also helps to open up the seven primary chakras, or energy centers, in our bodies. Try each of the seven chakra elixirs in Chapter 11 to boost your mood and energy level. Combining yoga with other enjoyable activities will help you get the most out of the five supermood chemicals (beta-endorphins, dopamine, GABA, oxytocin, and serotonin) and will keep your heart healthy and spirit energized.

The Positive Emotions Prescription: Alternative Therapies

Though much more research into complementary therapies is called for, we know that alternative therapies reduce anxiety and stress, improve energy levels, and enhance positive emotions and mood. Because they're noninvasive and nonpharmacological, complementary therapies represent fruitful routes to overall health and wellness when combined with traditional cardiology. To get the most from the Positive Emotions Prescription, choose an alternative therapy from this chapter and give it a try. You may be surprised by how much better you feel.

CHAPTER 10

The Positive Emotions Prescription

YOUR COMPREHENSIVE 4-WEEK PLAN FOR WHOLE-BODY WELLNESS

IN THIS CHAPTER, you'll find an easy-to-follow, comprehensive 4-week plan for following the Positive Emotions Prescription, complete with healthy menus and activities that incorporate positive emotions into everyday living. This plan encompasses three crucial elements that promote a sense of well-being: nutrition, physical activity, and mood-enhancing activities. But before you dive in, I've provided some tips and helpful advice to get you started on your way to healing your heart.

Nutrition Tips for Maximizing Positive Emotions

I recommend eschewing fruit juices in favor of natural fruits. Adding a slice of orange, lemon, lime, or apple to a glass of water each morning is delicious and invigorating—and it's a mainstay of the Positive Emotions Prescription elixirs provided in Chapter 11.

For milk products, stick with low-fat options such as skim or 1% milk, almond milk, hempseed milk, and brown rice milk. If you prefer soy milk, I recommend an organic soy milk free of both genetically modified organisms (GMOs) and carrageenan. Carrageenan is a food additive used to enhance the texture of dairy replacement products including soy, hempseed, and other plant-based milks, as well as yogurts and ice creams. There is scientific evidence linking carrageenan to inflammation and possible conversion of certain cells into cancer, as has recently been seen with the colon. Even though GMOs are widely used to protect crops like soybeans and corn from destructive pests, the evidence is still out on whether or not they are hazardous to our health. Until the health consequences of GMOs are established, I recommend sticking with non-GMO products.[1] It is not easy to find organic soy milk that is free of both GMOs and carrageenan, as popular brands such as Silk contain the latter. However, Organic Valley Soy is free of both.

Regarding coffee or tea, both beverages are rich sources of polyphenol antioxidants that help keep inflammation at bay. Caffeinated coffee can improve mental alertness, articulation, and memory recall. I recommend up to 2 cups of coffee (spaced 4 or 5 hours apart), making sure that the second cup is consumed at least 8 hours prior to bedtime. Caffeine contains the stimulant methylxanthine, which not only improves mood but also dilates bronchial vessels; this can literally be a breath of fresh air for asthmatics.[2]

Adding raw cacao powder and a dash of cinnamon to coffee or tea can also lift one's spirits and may even help to stave off diabetes. Simply adding cinnamon powder is less likely to be as effective, as freshly ground cinnamon bark is more likely to exert its salutary effects.

Exercise Tips for Maximizing Positive Emotions

In addition to eating well, we all need to move. Physical exercises activate the release of the major chemicals that promote positive emotions: beta-endorphin, dopamine, norepinephrine, oxytocin, gamma-aminobutyric acid (GABA), and serotonin. As we discussed in Chapter 5, aerobic activities provide the highest yield of positive emotions when it comes to physical activity. I recommend engaging in 30 minutes of physical activity daily. This can include aerobic activities, such as brisk walking (a pace of 3 to 4 miles per hour or a 15- to 20-minute mile), with a 5- to 10-minute warmup and cooldown period. See the list of activities in "Positive Emotions Through Exercise" (page 169) for some great recommendations—such as swimming, rebounding, or walking the equivalent of 10,000 steps daily—that will also fulfill your positive emotions requirement for that day.

Daily Living Tips for Maximizing Positive Emotions

While good nutrition and physical activity are two ingredients that are necessary to bolster your heart health, the third ingredient (or the icing on the cake) is learning to experience positivity in your personal and professional life. You may know a loved one or coworker who eats well, exercises daily, and is still excessively stressed out and miserable. Despite seemingly doing all the right things (as we discussed in earlier chapters), these folks are still at increased risk of heart disease. You can enhance your positive emotions and, ultimately, your heart health through intentional activities of daily living.

Start by finding activities that stimulate each of your senses, as well as those that draw upon holistic and social-based interactions. Aim to enhance positive emotions while working toward ferreting out some of the negative emotions that may stifle you. This might include developing or strengthening friendships with positive, upbeat people rather than pessimistic people. Also, choose activities that bring you joy and contentment, rather than going through the motions of activities you really do not enjoy doing.

Charting Positive and Negative Emotions in Your Daily Life

Below is a chart of positive emotions you are likely to encounter through nutrition, traditional exercise (such as walking or bicycling), and daily living activities (such as listening to joyful music or engaging in social activities or spiritual or holistic practices). The chart is simply intended to provide a road map to boost your overall Positive Emotions Quotient (PEQ) score. Activities with the most positive points (3 to 5) are going to produce the strongest positive emotional responses, while activities with the lowest values (–3 to –5) will produce the strongest negative emotional responses. Getting at least 15 points each day (5 points through nutrition, 5 points through exercise, and at least 5 points through activities of daily living) will lift your spirits and give you a strong dose of cardiovascular health. For example, here is a day's worth of activities enhancing positive emotions.

	ACTIVITY	POINTS
EXERCISE	Walked 30 minutes at a pace of 3 miles per hour	5
NUTRITION	Followed Day 1 of the 28-Day Nutrition Plan	5
DAILY LIVING	Hugged my husband and kids before work	1
	Had an uplifting lunch with my coworkers	2
	Played with my dog upon returning home	1
	Played joyful music while cooking	4
	Had an enjoyable family dinner	1
	Total PEQ	**19**

After you read through both the positive and negative emotions activities, use this chart to calculate your current PEQ before you begin the Positive Emotions Prescription Plan. You can also utilize this chart to check in and see how you're progressing each day.

Positive Emotions through Nutrition (aim for 5 points each day)

TASK	ALLOTTED POINTS	MY POINTS
Eat 5 positive emotion–inducing foods for the day (see Chapter 11 for recipes that contain a minimum of 5 positive emotion–inducing foods each day).	5	

Total Nutrition Points ________

Positive Emotions through Exercise (aim for 5 points each day)

TASK	ALLOTTED POINTS	MY POINTS
AEROBIC ACTIVITY LASTING 30 OR MORE MINUTES AND RESULTING IN FATIGUED MUSCLES		
Brisk walking or jogging	5	
Swimming	5	
Water aerobics	5	
Bicycling	5	
Hiking	5	
Jumping rope or rebounding	5	
Horseback riding	5	
Rowing	5	
Skating	5	
Skiing	5	
Singles tennis	5	
Basketball	5	
OTHER ACTIVITIES		
Dancing (includes ballroom dancing, Zumba, and freestyle)	5	
Walking 10,000 steps daily	5	
Fishing	3	

(continued)

Positive Emotions through Exercise (*cont.*)

TASK	ALLOTTED POINTS	MY POINTS
OTHER ACTIVITIES (*cont.*)		
Gardening	4	
Weight lifting or toning	4	
Golfing (without frustration)	3	
Doubles tennis	3	
Bowling	2	
Tai chi	2	
Yoga	2	
Pilates	2	
Walking up two or more flights of stairs daily	1	
Table tennis	1	
Golfing (with frustration)	–1	

Total Exercise Points _________

Positive Emotions through Daily Living (aim for a minimum of 5 points each day)

TASK	ALLOTTED POINTS	MY POINTS
AUDITORY-BASED POSITIVE EMOTIONS		
Listening to music that induces chills down the spine	4	
Playing a musical instrument and singing aloud	4	
Singing in a group (as in a choir)	4	
Slow dancing with a partner	3	
Singing to yourself (in a shower, car, etc.)	2	
Being sung to or serenaded	2	
Playing a musical instrument	2	

TASK	ALLOTTED POINTS	MY POINTS
AUDITORY-BASED POSITIVE EMOTIONS ***(cont.)***		
Dancing alone	1	
Listening to the sounds of nature	1	
Listening to relaxing music	1	
OLFACTORY-BASED POSITIVE EMOTIONS		
Experiencing aromatherapy	1	
Smelling fresh flowers or other pleasing fragrances, such as citrus fruits	1	
Smelling herbs and pleasant spices	1	
TOUCH-BASED POSITIVE EMOTIONS		
Receiving or giving a massage	2	
Participating in touch therapy (as either the instructor or patient)	2	
VISUAL-BASED POSITIVE EMOTIONS		
Experiencing visually appealing colors or scenery	1	
Visualizing an upcoming trip or remembering pleasurable past experiences	1	
Looking at pictures of family or loved ones	1	
Looking at photo albums/videos of memorable and pleasurable trips and experiences	1	
Watching a comedy	1	
Drawing or painting	1	
HOLISTIC AND SPIRITUAL POSITIVE EMOTIONS		
Spiritual prayer in a house of worship	3	
Participating in Ayurvedic oil massage	2	
Participating in Traditional Chinese Medicine, such as acupuncture, tai chi, or qigong	2	
Spiritual prayer alone	2	
Walking barefoot (grounded) on the beach	1	
RELATIONSHIP BUILDING AND SUSTAINING POSITIVE EMOTIONS		
Falling in love	5	
Sexual intimacy	5	

(continued)

Positive Emotions through Daily Living (*cont.*)

TASK	ALLOTTED POINTS	MY POINTS
RELATIONSHIP BUILDING AND SUSTAINING POSITIVE EMOTIONS (*cont.*)		
Laughing with your spouse or partner enough to cause eye tearing	4	
Dressing up to go out *or* date night with spouse or partner and/or friends	3	
Showing gratitude to your partner (for helping out)	3	
Receiving gratitude from your partner (for helping out)	3	
Writing a poem, letter of gratitude, letter of love, or love song	2	
Apologizing to a loved one or friend	2	
Forgiving a loved one or friend	2	
Reading a love letter from a loved one	1	
Hugging a loved one or friend	1	
Holding hands or putting an arm around another	1	
RELAXATION-BASED POSITIVE EMOTIONS		
Taking a warm bath with soft music, aromatherapy, and lit candles	3	
Taking a warm bath	2	
Feeling well rested after a good night's sleep	2	
Individual or group meditation	2	
Taking a power nap (15 to 30 minutes)	1	
SOCIAL-BASED POSITIVE EMOTIONS		
Intense laughter that causes eye tearing	4	
Volunteering for the less fortunate (such as at a soup kitchen, Ronald McDonald House, etc.)	3	
Doing a good deed for no reason	2	
Volunteering at a community function	2	

TASK	ALLOTTED POINTS	MY POINTS
SOCIAL-BASED POSITIVE EMOTIONS (***cont.***)		
Socializing with upbeat people	2	
Showing kindness to a stranger (such as smiling or holding open a door)	1	
Enjoying a family meal	1	
Enjoying a sitcom with family or friends	1	
Playing a card or board game with friends or family	1	
Playing with a pet	1	
Showing good sportsmanship	1	
Feeling appreciated	1	
MISCELLANEOUS-BASED POSITIVE EMOTIONS		
Taking a 2-minute cold shower	4	
Completing a major project or goal	3	
Mastering a skill	3	
Enjoying a hobby	2	
Feeling passionate about your job	2	
Completing a minor project or goal	2	
Maintaining a sense of control (organized daily structure)	2	
Keeping a personal journal that includes a highlight of each day	2	
Playing fun and challenging computer games (such as QuizUp)	1	
Learning a new skill	1	
Experiencing something new (trying a new food, taking a different route to work)	1	
Teaching others	1	
Reading an enjoyable book	1	
Practicing good posture	1	
Being out in the sun (15 minutes)	1	
Sitting or having lunch or a snack under a tree or in a garden	1	

(continued)

Positive Emotions through Daily Living (*cont.*)

TASK	ALLOTTED POINTS	MY POINTS
MISCELLANEOUS-BASED POSITIVE EMOTIONS (*cont.*)		
Taking 5 slow, deep breaths (inhale for 4 seconds and exhale for 2 seconds)	1	
Doing absolutely nothing; recharging (15 or more minutes)	1	

Total Daily Living Points ________

Negative Emotions (subtract these points from positive emotion points earned above)

TASK	ALLOTTED POINTS	MY POINTS
MILD-TO-MODERATE NEGATIVE STRESSORS		
Sitting for more than 15 minutes at a time (unless in meditation)	–1	
Feeling bloated	–1	
Viewing repulsive images	–1	
Watching TV shows or movies that are stressful	–1	
Smelling displeasing or repulsive aromas	–1	
Listening to music that is stressful to you	–1	
Losing a game that matters to you	–1	
Acting like a bad sport	–1	
Practicing poor posture	–1	
Socializing with negative people	–2	
Acting defensively	–2	
Feeling sensory overload	–2	
Feeling ignored	–2	
Feeling loss of control (such as being stuck in traffic)	–2	
Feeling rushed for time (such as being late for an appointment)	–2	

TASK	ALLOTTED POINTS	MY POINTS
MODERATE-TO-SEVERE NEGATIVE STRESSORS (*cont.*)		
Getting less than 6 hours of uninterrupted sleep	–2	
Watching 4 or more hours of TV	–3	
Feeling angry and/or hostile	–3	
Feeling overwhelmed	–3	
Feeling like a loser (displaying poor posture, poor hygiene, being unkempt)	–3	
Feeling resentful	–3	
Feeling stressed-out by family member(s), friend(s), or acquaintances	–3	
Yelling at or being yelled at by your partner or loved ones	–3	
Having your "buttons pushed"	–3	
Needing but not getting sufficient downtime	–3	
Feeling emotionally drained	–4	
Feeling rejected or unloved	–4	
Feeling disrespected or unduly criticized	–4	
Feeling ill due to stress (headache/stomachache/acne)	–4	
MOST SEVERE STRESSORS		
Experiencing verbal or physical abuse	–5	
Experiencing a relationship breakup	–5	
Experiencing job loss or financial distress	–5	
Experiencing a major health issue (personal or immediate family)	–5	
Experiencing a tragic loss	–5	

Total Negative Emotions Points ________

TOTAL SCORE________

(continued)

OVERALL SCORE	POSITIVE EMOTION QUOTIENT (PEQ)
15 or more	High; no adjustments needed (Heart Healthy)
10–14	Good; minimal adjustments needed (Heart Stable)
5–9	Low; moderate adjustments needed (Heart at Risk)
<5	Very low; major adjustments needed (Heart Stressed)

Your 28-Day Positive Emotions Quotient Tracker

What is your Positive Emotions Quotient? Use the chart below to keep track of your current PEQ and then monitor how it changes as you participate in the Positive Emotions Prescription Plan over the next 4 weeks. This is a great accountability tool, helping you to make any necessary adjustments each day to maintain a heart-healthy score.

	MON.	TUES.	WED.	THURS.	FRI.	SAT.	SUN.
WEEK 1 PEQ SCORES							
WEEK 2 PEQ SCORES							
WEEK 3 PEQ SCORES							
WEEK 4 PEQ SCORES							

Applying the Positive Emotions Prescription to Daily Life

Now let's go through some examples of how the Positive Emotions Prescription Plan can help change your mood and improve your PEQ score. The three cases that follow are fictitious examples to illustrate how small adjustments in our responses to events that occur during a typical day can have a dramatic effect on mood that, over the long term, can decrease the risk of heart disease. The four success stories that begin on page 180, however, feature real patients who have improved their heart health and PEQ scores by following the Positive Emotions Prescription Plan.

CASE 1: Mary

Mary is a single professional who had a falling-out with a coworker yesterday. She is irritable upon awakening but is thinking about making up with her coworker. After having a cup of coffee *(+1 point)*, she heads off to work. En route to work, she runs into traffic due to a highway accident, gets stressed out *(–2 points; feeling loss of control)*, feels rushed because she knows that she will be late to her morning meeting *(–2 points; rushed for time)*, and has a sense of being overwhelmed *(–3 points)*, believing that she will never be able to get all of her daily tasks done.

At work, she arrives at the tail end of the meeting with slumped shoulders *(–1 point; poor posture)*, looking at the floor and feeling like a loser. She blows off a coworker who approaches her and spends her day feeling sorry for herself. She goes home and instead of exercising, as she had planned, she eats junk food, watches 4 hours of TV *(–2 points)*, and tosses and turns all night *(–2 points)*.

Mary's PEQ score for the day is a depressing –11 points. If her emotional outlook does not change, then over time, she is putting herself at increased risk of heart disease.

With an intention toward enhancing positive emotions, let's see how Mary might now respond to the same events.

She prepares a green elixir *(+1 point)* because she is in a mood to forgive her coworker. For breakfast, she has old-fashioned oatmeal *(+1 point)* with a cup of coffee *(+1 point)* containing a teaspoon of cacao powder *(+1 point)*. En route to work, she runs into traffic due to a highway accident. Realizing that there is nothing she can do about it, she takes five slow, deep breaths *(+1 point)*, collects her thoughts, and calls the office to alert them that she will be late for the meeting. She plays a

CD of joyful music that she has not heard in several months and she experiences euphoria, with chills down her spine *(+4 points).*

At work, she arrives at the tail end of the meeting but stands up straight *(+1 point; excellent posture)*, looks directly at the group, and smiles as she sits down *(+1 point).* She apologizes to her coworker for dismissing her *(+2 points)* and they go out for coffee later in the afternoon *(+1 point).* She enjoys a 30-minute light jog after work *(+5 points),* has a relaxing dinner *(+1 point),* and gets a restful night's sleep *(+2 points).*

Her revised PEQ score for the day is an impressive 22 points. Just a few small adjustments in her emotional outlook can drastically affect her PEQ score. If maintained over time, they should translate into a reduced risk of heart disease.

CASE 2: JAKE

Jake is a middle-aged male who works in a business that requires overnight travel. His wife is a stay-at-home mom of twin elementary school–age girls. He has been working hard to advance his career and has been on a business trip all week, but he's returning this evening in time for dinner. He calls his wife in the morning to check in, but feels rushed for time *(–2 points)* due to a 9 a.m. meeting that he needs to finish preparing for. He tells her that he will call later, but ends up having lunch and drinks with coworkers *(+1 point; feeling appreciated)* before catching his flight back home. Upon returning home that evening, his children run up to give him a hug *(+1 point),* but his wife is exhausted and has a headache, and no dinner has been prepared. Not understanding his wife's plight, Jake becomes angry *(–3 points)* and resentful *(–3 points)* that dinner has not been made. He feels disrespected *(–4 points)* and ignores his wife for the rest of the evening.

Jake's PEQ score for the day is a depressing –10 points. In the long run, it doesn't really matter how ambitious or successful he is because, if no adjustments are made, Jake will put himself at increased risk of heart disease. With an intention to enhance positive emotions, let's see how Jake might now respond.

Jake's wife is a stay-at-home mom of twin elementary school–age girls. Jake understands that his wife works really hard at home, so he calls her first thing in the morning not only to check in, but also to voice his gratitude for her taking great care of the kids and the house while he is away *(+3 points).* He is prepared for his 9 a.m. meeting *(+1 point; completing a minor goal),* so he doesn't rush the phone call. Upon returning home that evening with a bouquet of flowers to show his gratitude *(+3 points)* to his wife, his children run up to give him a hug *(+1 point)*, but his wife is exhausted and has a headache, and no dinner has been prepared. Understanding his wife's plight, Jake gives his wife a hug *(+1 point)* and recruits his daughters to assist as they prepare the Sesame Chicken Stir-Fry (page 244; *+1 point*). The family enjoys a meal together *(+1 point)*.

His revised PEQ score for the day is a solid 11 points. These small, simple adjustments can make a big difference for Jake's overall heart health if he maintains these habits over time.

CASE 3: JEN

Jen is a middle-aged stay-at-home mom of twin elementary school–age girls. You guessed it . . . Jen is Jake's wife (from Case 2). While she understands that his job requires overnight travel, she feels somewhat resentful *(−3 points)* that he gets to come and go as he pleases and that she doesn't get sufficient downtime *(−3 points)*. Today, Jake will be coming home after a week on the road. He calls to check in, but before Jen can go into detail about the stress-related headaches that she's been experiencing *(−4 points)*, Jake tells her he's running late for his 9 a.m. meeting and that he needs to finish preparing and will call her later. When Jake doesn't call, Jen feels angry *(−3 points)*. When he returns home that evening, Jen has a bad headache and is emotionally drained *(−4 points)*.

Jen's PEQ score for the day is a very concerning −17. Jen is very stressed out and feels that she is not appreciated. Over time, if things don't change, she runs the risk of experiencing poor heart health. With an intention to enhance positive emotions, let's see how Jen might now respond.

While Jen understands that Jake's job requires overnight travel, she knows that when he returns he will give her a break. She is reassured when Jake calls to check in and voice his gratitude *(+3; feeling appreciated)* for taking great care of the kids and home while he is away.

After Jen gets the kids off to school, she has some time for a brisk walk *(+5 points)* in bright sunlight *(+1 point)* and later, a lunch date with two of her upbeat friends *(+2 points)*. She has just enough time to pick up the kids from school, but by late afternoon, she's exhausted from taking care of them all week and takes a 15-minute power nap *(+1 point)* while the girls color.

When Jake returns home, Jen has a bad headache and has not gotten around to dinner. Jen suggests a kid-friendly restaurant where Jake can take the kids out for dinner while she stays at home. Instead, Jake recruits his daughters to assist in preparing Sesame Chicken Stir-Fry for dinner *(+1 point)*. The family enjoys a meal together *(+1 point)* and Jen feels appreciated *(+1 point)*. Her headache recedes.

Her revised PEQ score for the day is a sound +15. With just a few minor tweaks, Jen is well on her way to excellent positive emotional and physical health.

PATIENT SUCCESS STORY #1: DONALD

My patient Donald is a 61-year-old who worked for a governor but then lost his prestigious position following the election, when the governorship changed hands. Shortly after the election, he became stressed-out *(–3 points)* with a feeling of loss of control *(–2 points)*, started eating late at night, gained weight, and became hypertensive and ill with headaches and back pain *(–4 points)*. When he returned for a follow-up visit, he had just been hired as a consultant and was ready to make the lifestyle changes that would restore his health and wellness. These changes included restricting carbs in the evening and following other dietary suggestions in the 28-Day Positive Emotions Prescription Plan, starting slowly on an exercise program, listening to soothing music, and experiencing laughter with his wife.

Within 6 months, Donald's results were dramatic. He lost 18 pounds by cutting out carbs and some of his late-night snacking, got off his blood pressure medicine, and lowered his triglyceride level from over 250 to under 90 mg/dL. In addition, he ate at least five Positive Emotions Foods daily *(+5 points)*, alternated rowing *(+5 points)* with lifting light weights every other day *(+4 points)*, stood up straight *(+1 point)*, listened to joyful music *(+4 points)*, and enjoyed a good daily laugh *(+4 points)*. But just as important were his renewed vigor and energy for life, with a PEQ score that went from –9 during the darkest hours to +23. At one of his recent office visits, Donald exclaimed, "I haven't felt this great in years!"

PATIENT SUCCESS STORY #2: CLARA

Clara has been a patient of mine for the past 18 years. She had a history of high cholesterol and high blood pressure, both of which are now under control. After her husband passed away following 55 years of marriage, thanks to a villageful of family and friends she has been able to experience positive emotions in her life again. "I have many good memories of my life with Dick," she said. "We had respect for each other and definitely never took ourselves too seriously. Humility and humor were always a part of our lives. We seemed to know instinctively that what was on our minds was also on our hearts."

Clara consumes at least five Positive Emotions Foods each day *(+5 points)*, and when the weather is conducive, she spends a lot of time outdoors gardening *(+4 points)* and devotes 15 minutes each day to sitting and enjoying the sunshine *(+1 point)*. Among the most important sources of her positive emotions is the time she spends each weekend with her granddaughter, when they work on fun projects together *(+2 points)* and laugh frequently *(+4 points)*. "The Positive Emotions program has helped me to enjoy the simple things in life again," she says. Clara's daily PEQ score is virtually always positive and in the 10 to 18 range. She looks 20 years younger than her chronological age of 81 years and today remains healthy and very active.

PATIENT SUCCESS STORY #3: MARK

Mark's wife passed away from a heartrending lung condition known as primary pulmonary hypertension. When he began seeing me, he was slightly overweight, with high triglycerides, high blood pressure, and a high coronary calcium score, plus he was emotionally drained *(−4 points)*. Following lifestyle changes provided in the Positive Emotions Prescription Plan, Mark improved his diet by eating a predominately vegetarian and fish-based diet *(+5 points)*, started exercising on a regular basis *(+5 points)*, and improved his emotional outlook by watching and laughing through repeats of the situational comedy *Seinfeld (+4 points)*. He owns racehorses and is at peace "when feeding the horses carrots and peppermint and seeing how well everyone gets along at the racetrack" *(+1 point)*.

Since starting the Positive Emotions Prescription Plan, Mark shares, "I have lost more than 15 pounds and am close to my weight as a young adult." In addition, he now has normal blood pressure, triglycerides well below 100, and has been able to eliminate most of his medications. His PEQ score usually exceeds 15 on a daily basis, as compared to a PEQ score commonly in the negative range prior to starting the Positive Emotions Prescription Plan. But the most impressive fact is that Mark has sustained these changes for the past 12 years!

PATIENT SUCCESS STORY #4: MARGIE

Margie says that she never thought that she would survive into late adulthood, as she vividly recalls the day her pediatrician diagnosed her with rheumatic heart disease. The two things she remembers most from that day are her mother's devastation at the news of Margie's illness and the beautiful new parrot at her pediatrician's office. That was 75 years ago. Ultimately, Margie defied her doctor's orders to remain sedentary, which was recommended for her illness at the time. By the time I began treating her nearly 15 years ago, Margie was still in good health despite progressive deterioration of her aortic valve.

Margie's lifestyle already mimicked the Positive Emotions Prescription Plan in large part, but she now intentionally follows the plan, and her health and outlook have improved over the past decade and a half. Her lifestyle includes eating lots of fish and fruits—mostly strawberries and blueberries *(+5 points)*, exercising daily by walking briskly and biking *(+5 points)*, and participating in mindful activities like yoga *(+2 points)*, all of which have contributed to her good health for many years. But equally important to her positive outlook is being in control of her daily activities. "I only do things I enjoy doing since retiring," she said. After she underwent inevitable heart valve surgery several years ago (which was likely delayed for many years due to her exceptional lifestyle habits), Margie's outlook on life changed. "I don't complain," she told me recently during her semiannual visit. "And if you don't complain, there's nothing to worry about."

When I told her I was writing a book, this 80-year-old who's beaten the odds asked if she could share her secrets to good health. "Don't be a hypochondriac," she advised, recalling a brother who fell into that category and died at age 64. In addition to receiving the maximum 5 points daily for positive emotions through nutrition, Margie does not eat after 7 p.m. She also walks briskly at least 30 minutes daily *(+5 points)*, continues to do yoga *(+2 points)*, has good friendships *(+2 points)*, laughs readily when watching comedies *(+4 points)*, and volunteers *(+2 points)*. Margie maintains her emotional equilibrium by "never keeping things bottled up." Her PEQ score is a solid 20 on a daily basis. And although her pediatrician is long gone, she recently learned that the parrot is still alive and well!

The 28-Day Positive Emotions Prescription Nutrition Plan

To maximize the heart health benefits of positive emotions, this nutrition plan incorporates all of the Top 50 Foods and food groups that we discussed in Chapter 2 (each worth 1 point in your PEQ score). In addition, each day's meals contain a minimum of five positive emotion foods and provide the optimal balance of proteins, carbohydrates, fats, and other nutrients. Oh, and you also get to have both snacks and desserts! When it comes to your nutritional needs, the goal is to consume foods that are delicious, heart healthy, and mood uplifting. Each week, you'll find three *'til your heart's content* meals—these are your "cheat meals." While some nutritionists voice skepticism about recommending cheat meals, principally due to the concern that a person will inevitably fall off the wagon, research in fact indicates that dietary cheating on weekends does not negatively impact weight gain. In other words, good weight control is not offset by mild calorie increases that may occur during weekend diet cheating—provided, of course, that normal dietary behavior resumes during the week.[3]

I've taken that a little further to include a cheat meal during the week as well. Including the *'til your heart's content* meals is my way of throwing my patients a bone (rather than a carrot stick). But as discussed in Chapter 2, please don't go hog wild. I also enjoy a good steak, but keep the portion size in check. The same goes for ice cream—after all, you only tend to remember the first and last spoonfuls anyway. Permitting three meals a week of your choice gives you something to look forward to, thereby making it easier to follow a heart-healthy diet for the remaining 17 meals each week. I've recommended eating *'til your heart's content* for lunch on Wednesday, dinner on Friday, and brunch on Sunday. Of course, you are free to use any of these three weekly cheat meals on days that work best for you, though I recommend that they occur on separate days. This way you will still get a minimum of five of the Positive Emotions foods each day.

Also feel free to mix and match meals. For example, some of my patients prefer old-fashioned oatmeal as their breakfast staple because it is an excellent source of soluble fiber, is filling for several hours, and goes extremely well with a variety of mood-elevating fruits and nuts. And some of these patients prefer hot oatmeal during winter months and then switch to cold oat-based cereals such as Cheerios during the warmer months. The Positive Emotions Prescription Nutrition Plan offers a variety of heart-healthy and emotionally empowering selections to choose from, so you should be able to adapt the plan to your own tastes and needs.

The menus are devised to be carb enriched during the day, when you are most physically and mentally active, and lower in carbs in the evening, to avoid impairing a good night's sleep and loading up on extra calories your body doesn't need.

During the workweek, I recognize that food preparation is all about time management, and therefore Positive Emotions Prescription Nutrition Plan meals are designed to be easy and reasonably quick to prepare (10 minutes or less for breakfast and 30 minutes or less for lunch and dinner). Easy preparation for a busy family cuts down on the stress level for the primary cook in the house. The more time-consuming meals are reserved for the weekends (for example, see Week 1, Days 6 and 7 on pages 190 and 191). Also, keep in mind that listening to joyful music while preparing your dishes can make cooking even more pleasurable. If you have an Internet connection at home, there is a world of possibilities for streaming free music. For example, the app Songza enables you to create playlists based on your mood to enhance positive emotions.

I've also provided recipes for 15 different Positive Emotion elixirs in Chapter 11. Seven of the elixirs are named for chakras, or energy centers, and you may wish to select one of these depending upon your daily aspiration, as shown below.

CHAKRA	GOAL
Violet (Crown) Elixir	Spirituality
Indigo (Third-Eye) Elixir	Imagination
Blue (Throat) Elixir	Speech and communication
Green (Heart) Elixir	Compassion and forgiveness
Yellow (Solar Plexus) Elixir	Willpower and self-control
Orange (Abdomen) Elixir	Intimacy and desire
Red (Root) Elixir	Grounding and stability

I hope that you find the Positive Emotions Prescription Nutrition Plan to be energizing, uplifting, delicious, and most importantly, sustainable. Enjoy . . . *'til your heart's content!*

WEEK 1

DAY 1

BREAKFAST:

Overnight oats (Bircher muesli) or old-fashioned oatmeal (½ cup) with low-fat milk of your choice, topped with a handful of blueberries

Tea or coffee (caffeinated or decaf) with low-fat milk of your choice, 1 to 2 teaspoons cacao powder (mix well), and dash of cinnamon (optional)

MIDMORNING SNACK:

Your choice of Positive Emotions Elixir (pages 283–288)

LUNCH:

Tuna with Veggies (page 223)

Side salad with balsamic vinaigrette

Tea or coffee (caffeinated or decaf) with low-fat milk of your choice and 1 to 2 teaspoons cacao powder (mix well)

AFTERNOON SNACK:

Your choice of Positive Emotions Elixir (pages 283–288)

¼ cup pistachios (approximately 25 nuts)

DINNER:

Sesame Chicken Stir-Fry (page 244)

Orange-Spinach Salad (page 227)

DESSERT:

1-inch square dark chocolate (70% cacao or higher)

Mint tea

DAY 2

BREAKFAST:

Banana-Mango-Ginger Smoothie (page 215)

1 teaspoon almond butter on 1 slice Ezekiel bread (optional)

Tea or coffee (caffeinated or decaf) with low-fat milk of your choice, 1 to 2 teaspoons cacao powder (mix well), and dash of cinnamon (optional)

MIDMORNING SNACK:

Your choice of Positive Emotions Elixir (pages 283–288)

LUNCH:

Arugula-Avocado-Almond Salad (page 223)

2 or 3 slices turkey with mustard on 1 slice Ezekiel bread

Tea or coffee (caffeinated or decaf) with low-fat milk of your choice, and 1 to 2 teaspoons cacao powder (mix well)

AFTERNOON SNACK:

Your choice of Positive Emotions Elixir (pages 283–288)

Handful of grapes

DINNER:

Moroccan-Seasoned Wild Salmon (page 245)

Roasted Broccoli (page 272)

DESSERT:

4 to 6 strawberries with mint

Lemon ginger tea

DAY 3

BREAKFAST:

1 to 2 tablespoons sunflower seed butter on 2 slices toasted Ezekiel bread, topped with 1 thinly sliced apple or banana. Sprinkle with 1 teaspoon hempseeds (optional).

Tea or coffee (caffeinated or decaf) with low-fat milk of your choice, 1 to 2 teaspoons cacao powder (mix well), and dash of cinnamon (optional)

MIDMORNING SNACK:

Your choice of Positive Emotions Elixir (pages 283–288)

LUNCH:

'Til your heart's content

AFTERNOON SNACK:

Your choice of Positive Emotions Elixir (pages 283–288)

1 sliced apple and 2 to 4 dates

DINNER:

Flounder in Garlic White Wine Sauce (page 245)

Green Beans with Walnuts and Thyme (page 264)

Sautéed cabbage

DESSERT:

Amaretto Amore (page 274)

Peppermint tea

DAY 4

BREAKFAST:

Spinach omelet with mushrooms, onions, and tomatoes

Tea or coffee (caffeinated or decaf) with low-fat milk of your choice, 1 to 2 teaspoons cacao powder (mix well), and dash of cinnamon (optional)

MIDMORNING SNACK:

Your choice of Positive Emotions Elixir (pages 283–288)

LUNCH:

Grilled chicken breast

Heavenly Hearts of Palm Salad (page 224)

Tea or coffee (caffeinated or decaf) with low-fat milk of your choice, and 1 to 2 teaspoons cacao powder (mix well)

AFTERNOON SNACK:

Your choice of Positive Emotions Elixir (pages 283–288)

Sweet Potato–Miso Spread with crackers (page 267)

DINNER:

Rockfish Cakes (page 246)

Sautéed string beans

Side salad with tomatoes

DESSERT:

Ana's Blueberry-Cashew Treat (page 275)

Linden flower tea

DAY 5

BREAKFAST:

Deeply Satisfying Kasha Porridge (page 214), topped with handful of blueberries (optional)

Tea or coffee (caffeinated or decaf) with low-fat milk of your choice, 1 to 2 teaspoons cacao powder (mix well), and dash of cinnamon (optional)

MIDMORNING SNACK:

Your choice of Positive Emotions Elixir (pages 283–288)

LUNCH:

Stuffed Sweet Potatoes with Beans (page 225)

Turkey sandwich (3 slices turkey, ½ teaspoon Dijon mustard, ¼ avocado, spread, and sliced tomato on pita)

Tea or coffee (caffeinated or decaf) with low-fat milk of your choice and 1 to 2 teaspoons cacao powder (mix well)

AFTERNOON SNACK:

Your choice of Positive Emotions Elixir (pages 283–288)

1 sliced apple with almond butter or handful of walnuts

DINNER:

'Til your heart's content

DAY 6

BREAKFAST:

Ginger-Date Smoothie (page 215)

1 teaspoon almond butter on 1 slice Ezekiel bread (optional)

Tea or coffee (caffeinated or decaf) with low-fat milk of your choice, 1 to 2 teaspoons cacao powder (mix well), and dash of cinnamon (optional)

MIDMORNING SNACK:

Your choice of Positive Emotions Elixir (pages 283–288)

LUNCH:

Avocado spread (½ avocado, mashed, sprinkled with black pepper, and mixed with a squeeze of lime) on toasted Ezekiel bread with shredded romaine lettuce and slice of tomato

Tea or coffee (caffeinated or decaf) with low-fat milk of your choice and 1 to 2 teaspoons cacao powder (mix well)

AFTERNOON SNACK:

Your choice of Positive Emotions Elixir (pages 283–288) or Maca Date Shake (page 274)

DINNER:

Cedar-Planked Wild Salmon (page 247)

Spinach-Mango Salad with Hempseeds (page 226)

Steamed asparagus

DESSERT:

1 square dark chocolate (70% cacao or higher)

Hibiscus tea

DAY 7

BEFORE BRUNCH:

Your choice of Positive Emotions Elixir (pages 283–288)

BRUNCH:

'Til your heart's content

BEFORE-DINNER SNACK:

Your choice of Positive Emotions Elixir (pages 283–288)

DINNER:

Baked Rainbow Trout with Dates and Almonds (page 248)

Side salad with balsamic vinaigrette

Steamed green beans

DESSERT:

Baked Apples with Cinnamon (page 279)

Wild berry tea

WEEK 2

DAY 8

BREAKFAST:

Overnight oats (Bircher muesli) or old-fashioned oatmeal (½ cup) with low-fat milk of your choice, topped with 3 to 5 dried plums

Tea or coffee (caffeinated or decaf) with low-fat milk of your choice, 1 to 2 teaspoons cacao powder (mix well), and dash of cinnamon (optional)

MIDMORNING SNACK:

Your choice of Positive Emotions Elixir (pages 283–288)

LUNCH:

Spinach Salad with Berries and Honey Pecans (page 236)

1 can sardines (4 to 5 ounces in water or olive oil) on 1 or 2 slices rye toast or crackers

Tea or coffee (caffeinated or decaf) with low-fat milk of your choice and 1 to 2 teaspoons cacao powder (mix well)

BEFORE-DINNER SNACK:

Your choice of Positive Emotions Elixir (pages 283–288)

Almond-Chocolate Bark (page 279)

DINNER:

Pesto-Portobello Pizza (page 249)

Roasted Jerusalem Artichokes with Herbs (page 269)

Side salad with balsamic vinaigrette

DESSERT:

4 to 6 strawberries with vanilla sauce (¼ cup Greek fat-free vanilla yogurt and 1 teaspoon honey)

Chamomile tea

DAY 9

BREAKFAST:

2 scrambled eggs with sliced red bell pepper in tortilla wrap

Tea or coffee (caffeinated or decaf) with low-fat milk of your choice, 1 to 2 teaspoons cacao powder (mix well), and dash of cinnamon (optional)

MIDMORNING SNACK:

Your choice of Positive Emotions Elixir (pages 283–288)

LUNCH:

Green Bean, Artichoke, and Tuna Salad (page 228)

Tea or coffee (caffeinated or decaf) with low-fat milk of your choice and 1 to 2 teaspoons cacao powder (mix well)

AFTERNOON SNACK:

Your choice of Positive Emotions Elixir (pages 283–288)

1 ounce walnuts (about 14 halves)

DINNER:

Asian Baked Halibut (page 259)

Saffron Split Pea Soup (page 238)

DESSERT:

Pineapple Carpaccio (page 282)

Sage tea

DAY 10

BREAKFAST:

1 to 2 tablespoons almond butter and 1 small, thinly sliced banana on 2 slices Ezekiel bread

Tea or coffee (caffeinated or decaf) with low-fat milk of your choice and 1 to 2 teaspoons cacao powder (mix well)

MIDMORNING SNACK:

Your choice of Positive Emotions Elixir (pages 283–288)

LUNCH:

'Til your heart's content

AFTERNOON SNACK:

Your choice of Positive Emotions Elixir (pages 283–288)

DINNER:

Grilled Portobello Burgers (page 250)

Spicy Sweet Potato Fries (page 271)

DESSERT:

Almond-Chocolate Bark (page 279)

Pomegranate tea

DAY 11

BREAKFAST:

Overnight oats (Bircher muesli) or old-fashioned oatmeal (½ cup) with low-fat milk of your choice and handful of blueberries

Tea or coffee (caffeinated or decaf) with low-fat milk of your choice, 1 to 2 teaspoons cacao powder (mix well), and dash of cinnamon (optional)

MIDMORNING SNACK:

Your choice of Positive Emotions Elixir (pages 283–288)

LUNCH:

Avocado Turkey Burger Sprout Wrap (page 229)

1 small baked sweet potato

Tea or coffee (caffeinated or decaf) with low-fat milk of your choice and 1 to 2 teaspoons cacao powder (mix well)

AFTERNOON SNACK:

Your choice of Positive Emotions Elixir (pages 283–288)

Handful of nuts

DINNER:

Rejuvenating Red Lentil Soup (page 239)

Artichoke Frittata (page 222)

Roasted Lotus Root (page 266)

DESSERT:

1 sliced apple dipped in honey

Cinnamon tea

DAY 12

BREAKFAST:

Pumpkin Pie Smoothie (page 216)

Tea or coffee (caffeinated or decaf) with low-fat milk of your choice, 1 to 2 teaspoons cacao powder (mix well), and dash of cinnamon (optional)

MIDMORNING SNACK:

Your choice of Positive Emotions Elixir (pages 283–288)

LUNCH:

Leftovers from Rejuvenating Red Lentil Soup (see Dinner, Day 11)

Leftovers from Artichoke Frittata (see Dinner, Day 11)

Tea or coffee (caffeinated or decaf) with low-fat milk of your choice and 1 to 2 teaspoons cacao powder (mix well)

AFTERNOON SNACK:

Your choice of Positive Emotions Elixir (pages 283–288)

2 Almond Cookies (page 275)

DINNER:

'Til your heart's content

DAY 13

BREAKFAST:

Almond Flour Banana Waffles (page 220)

Tea or coffee (caffeinated or decaf) with low-fat milk of your choice, 1 to 2 teaspoons cacao powder (mix well), and dash of cinnamon (optional)

MIDMORNING SNACK:

Your choice of Positive Emotions Elixir (pages 283–288)

LUNCH:

Heartwarming White Bean Soup (page 240)

Glazed Beet and Red Grapefruit Salad (page 229)

Tea or coffee (caffeinated or decaf) with low-fat milk of your choice and 1 to 2 teaspoons cacao powder (mix well)

AFTERNOON SNACK:

1 fresh apple

Your choice of Positive Emotions Elixir (pages 283–288)

DINNER:

Miso Soup (page 243)

Seared Mahi Mahi with Mango Black Bean Sauce (page 251)

Steamed green beans

DESSERT:

Orange slices

Mint tea

DAY 14

BEFORE BRUNCH:

Your choice of Positive Emotions Elixir (pages 283–288)

BRUNCH:

'Til your heart's content

BEFORE-DINNER SNACK:

Your choice of Positive Emotions Elixir (pages 283–288)

10 to 12 baby carrots with ¼ cup hummus

DINNER:

Mediterranean Salmon with Sun-Dried Tomatoes, Capers, and Olives (page 252)

Orange, Lime, and Grapefruit Salad with Honey Mint Dressing (page 235)

DESSERT:

Egyptian licorice tea

WEEK 3

DAY 15

BREAKFAST:

Deeply Satisfying Kasha Porridge (page 214) and handful of walnuts (optional)

Tea or coffee (caffeinated or decaf) with low-fat milk of your choice, 1 to 2 teaspoons cacao powder (mix well), and dash of cinnamon (optional)

MIDMORNING SNACK:

Your choice of Positive Emotions Elixir (pages 283–288)

LUNCH:

Egg and avocado salad (2 hard-cooked eggs mashed with ½ avocado, seasoned with pepper and a pinch of salt, and served on crackers)

Tea or coffee (caffeinated or decaf) with low-fat milk of your choice and 1 to 2 teaspoons cacao powder (mix well)

AFTERNOON SNACK:

Your choice of Positive Emotions Elixir (pages 283–288)

½ cup edamame

DINNER:

Grilled chicken breasts

Steamed broccoli

Grilled polenta

DESSERT:

2 Almond Cookies (page 275)

Lemon tea

DAY 16

BREAKFAST:

Strawberry-Pineapple-Kale Smoothie (page 219)

Tea or coffee (caffeinated or decaf) with low-fat milk of your choice, 1 to 2 teaspoons cacao powder (mix well), and dash of cinnamon (optional)

MIDMORNING SNACK:

Your choice of Positive Emotions Elixir (pages 283–288)

LUNCH:

Tuna and Chickpea Salad (page 230)

Tea or coffee (caffeinated or decaf) with low-fat milk of your choice and 1 to 2 teaspoons cacao powder (mix well)

AFTERNOON SNACK:

Your choice of Positive Emotions Elixir (pages 283–288)

1 ounce raw almonds

DINNER:

Sesame Miso Cod (page 253)

Steamed sugar snap peas

DESSERT:

Frozen Coconut-Chia-Blueberry Parfait (page 276)

Lemon and ginger tea

DAY 17

BREAKFAST:

Peach and Blueberry Cobbler (page 221)

Tea or coffee (caffeinated or decaf) with low-fat milk of your choice, 1 to 2 teaspoons cacao powder (mix well), and dash of cinnamon (optional)

MIDMORNING SNACK:

Your choice of Positive Emotions Elixir (pages 283–288)

LUNCH:

'Til your heart's content

AFTERNOON SNACK:

Your choice of Positive Emotions Elixir (pages 283–288)

1 medium apple

DINNER:

Stir-fried chicken with broccoli, carrots, mushrooms, and summer squash

---

DESSERT:

Sesame Bars (page 276)

Vanilla almond tea

DAY 18

BREAKFAST:

Overnight oats (Bircher muesli) or old-fashioned oatmeal (½ cup) with low-fat milk of your choice and handful of walnuts

Tea or coffee (caffeinated or decaf) with low-fat milk of your choice, 1 to 2 teaspoons cacao powder (mix well), and dash of cinnamon (optional)

MIDMORNING SNACK:

Your choice of Positive Emotions Elixir (pages 283–288)

LUNCH:

1 can sardines (4 to 5 ounces in water or olive oil) on 2 slices Ezekiel toast

Gingered Carrot Soup (page 241)

Tea or coffee (caffeinated or decaf) with low-fat milk of your choice and 1 to 2 teaspoons cacao powder (mix well)

AFTERNOON SNACK:

Your choice of Positive Emotions Elixir (pages 283–288)

1 medium orange

DINNER:

Super-Easy Steelhead Trout Teriyaki (page 253)

Roasted Asparagus with Shallots (page 265)

DESSERT:

1 peeled and thinly sliced mango dipped in vanilla sauce (¼ cup Greek fat-free vanilla yogurt and 1 teaspoon honey)

Vanilla tea

DAY 19

BREAKFAST:

Ravens Purple Pride Smoothie (page 217)

Tea or coffee (caffeinated or decaf) with low-fat milk of your choice, 1 to 2 teaspoons cacao powder (mix well), and dash of cinnamon (optional)

MIDMORNING SNACK:

Your choice of Positive Emotions Elixir (pages 283–288)

LUNCH:

Persimmon-Mozzarella Panini (page 231)

Tea or coffee (caffeinated or decaf) with low-fat milk of your choice and 1 to 2 teaspoons cacao powder (mix well)

AFTERNOON SNACK:

Your choice of Positive Emotions Elixir (pages 283–288)

Handful of almonds

DINNER:

'Til your heart's content

DAY 20

BREAKFAST:

Pumpkin-Almond Smoothie (page 218)

1 teaspoon of almond butter on 1 slice Ezekiel toast (optional)

Tea or coffee (caffeinated or decaf) with low-fat milk of your choice, 1 to 2 teaspoons cacao powder (mix well), and dash of cinnamon (optional)

MIDMORNING SNACK:

Your choice of Positive Emotions Elixir (pages 283–288)

LUNCH:

Quinoa Salad (page 232)

Tea or coffee (caffeinated or decaf) with low-fat milk of your choice and 1 to 2 teaspoons cacao powder (mix well)

AFTERNOON SNACK:

Your choice of Positive Emotions Elixir (pages 283–288)

Sun-Dried Tomato Dip (page 267) with celery, bell pepper (red or yellow), or crackers

DINNER:

Salmon with Asparagus and Artichoke-Mustard Sauce (page 254)

Honey- and Maple-Glazed Brussels Sprouts (page 269)

Lightly Sautéed Purslane (page 266)

DESSERT:

Apple-Blueberry Crisp (page 277)

Apple cider tea

DAY 21

BEFORE BRUNCH:

Your choice of Positive Emotions Elixir (pages 283–288)

BRUNCH:

'Til your heart's content

MIDMORNING SNACK:

Your choice of Positive Emotions Elixir (pages 283–288)

DINNER:

Moroccan Chicken (page 256)

Sautéed Kale (page 265)

DESSERT:

Ultimate Date Cake (page 278)

Egyptian licorice tea

WEEK 4

DAY 22

BREAKFAST:

Overnight oats (Bircher muesli) or old-fashioned oatmeal (½ cup) with low-fat milk of your choice and handful of slivered almonds or walnuts

Tea or coffee (caffeinated or decaf) with low-fat milk of your choice, 1 to 2 teaspoons cacao powder (mix well), and dash of cinnamon (optional)

MIDMORNING SNACK:

Your choice of Positive Emotions Elixir (pages 283–288)

LUNCH:

Leftovers from Moroccan Chicken (see Dinner, Day 21)

Side salad with balsamic vinaigrette

Tea or coffee (caffeinated or decaf) with low-fat milk of your choice and 1 to 2 teaspoons cacao powder (mix well)

AFTERNOON SNACK:

Your choice of Positive Emotions Elixir (pages 283–288)

Handful of Brazil nuts

DINNER:

Gazpacho Soup (page 242)

Black Bean Burrito (page 257)

DESSERT:

¾ to 1 cup watermelon or ½ cup fresh peach slices

Mint tea

DAY 23

BREAKFAST:

Chamomile Smoothie (page 218)

1 teaspoon sunflower seed butter on 1 slice Ezekiel toast (optional)

Tea or coffee (caffeinated or decaf) with low-fat milk of your choice, 1 to 2 teaspoons cacao powder (mix well), and dash of cinnamon (optional)

MIDMORNING SNACK:

Your choice of Positive Emotions Elixir (pages 283–288)

LUNCH:

Grilled Chicken and Celery Salad à la Marcella (page 233)

Side salad with balsamic vinaigrette

Tea or coffee (caffeinated or decaf) with low-fat milk of your choice and 1 to 2 teaspoons cacao powder (mix well)

AFTERNOON SNACK:

Your choice of Positive Emotions Elixir (pages 283–288)

2 tablespoons each blueberries and walnuts

DINNER:

Roasted Salmon with Orange-Herb Sauce (page 258)

Curried Cauliflower (page 270)

DESSERT:

Raspberries and vanilla sauce (¼ cup Greek fat-free vanilla yogurt and 1 teaspoon honey)

Lemon tea

DAY 24

BREAKFAST:

Artichoke Frittata (page 222)

Tea or coffee (caffeinated or decaf) with low-fat milk of your choice, 1 to 2 teaspoons cacao powder (mix well), and dash of cinnamon (optional)

MIDMORNING SNACK:

Your choice of Positive Emotions Elixir (pages 283–288)

LUNCH:

'Til your heart's content

AFTERNOON SNACK:

Your choice of Positive Emotions Elixir (pages 283–288)

Cashew Butter Granola Bar (page 282)

DINNER:

Fish Taco (page 260)

Spicy Sweet Potato Fries (page 271)

Sautéed Spinach with Lemon and Pine Nuts (page 268)

DESSERT:

Sage tea

DAY 25

BREAKFAST:

Orioles Orange Smash Smoothie (page 219)

Tea or coffee (caffeinated or decaf) with low-fat milk of your choice, 1 to 2 teaspoons cacao powder (mix well), and dash of cinnamon (optional)

MIDMORNING SNACK:

Your choice of Positive Emotions Elixir (pages 283–288)

LUNCH:

Apple-Spinach Salad (page 233)

Tea or coffee (caffeinated or decaf) with low-fat milk of your choice and 1 to 2 teaspoons cacao powder (mix well)

AFTERNOON SNACK:

Your choice of Positive Emotions Elixir (pages 283–288)

1 square Almond-Chocolate Bark (page 279)

DINNER:

Roasted Butternut Squash and Black Bean Tacos (page 261)

Prepared guacamole

Lightly Sautéed Purslane (page 266)

DESSERT:

1 sliced apple

Chamomile tea

DAY 26

BREAKFAST:

Overnight oats (Bircher muesli) or old-fashioned oatmeal (½ cup) with low-fat milk of your choice, topped with walnuts and cinnamon as desired

Tea or coffee (caffeinated or decaf) with low-fat milk of your choice, 1 to 2 teaspoons cacao powder (mix well), and dash of cinnamon (optional)

MIDMORNING SNACK:

Your choice of Positive Emotions Elixir (pages 283–288)

LUNCH:

Mouthwatering Watermelon Salad (page 234)

Turkey sandwich with mustard, sliced tomato, and avocado on pita

Tea or coffee (caffeinated or decaf) with low-fat milk of your choice, 1 to 2 teaspoons cacao powder (mix well), and dash of cinnamon (optional)

AFTERNOON SNACK:

Your choice of Positive Emotions Elixir (pages 283–288)

2 or 3 figs

DINNER:

'Til your heart's content

DAY 27

BREAKFAST:

Egg white omelet with tomato, onion, and herbs (oregano, basil, or thyme)

1 slice toasted Ezekiel bread with 1 tablespoon hummus

Tea or coffee (caffeinated or decaf) with low-fat milk of your choice, 1 to 2 teaspoons cacao powder (mix well), and dash of cinnamon (optional)

MIDMORNING SNACK:

Your choice of Positive Emotions Elixir (pages 283–288)

LUNCH:

Strawberries and Watercress Salad (page 234)

Tea or coffee (caffeinated or decaf) with low-fat milk of your choice, 1 to 2 teaspoons cacao powder (mix well), and dash of cinnamon (optional)

AFTERNOON SNACK:

Your choice of Positive Emotions Elixir (pages 283–288) or Chai Hot Chocolate (page 280)

¼ cup roasted chickpeas

DINNER:

Pistachio-Crusted Tilapia with Strawberry Salsa (page 262)

Butternut Squash with Baby Spinach (page 272)

DESSERT:

Chocolate Chip–Beet Cake (page 281)

Orange tea

DAY 28

BEFORE BRUNCH:

Your choice of Positive Emotions Elixir (pages 283–288)

BRUNCH:

'Til your heart's content

AFTERNOON SNACK:

Your choice of Positive Emotions Elixir (pages 283–288)

DINNER:

Mediterranean Kale Tart (page 255)

Celestial Celery Root and Apple Soup (page 237)

Roasted Green Beans with Garlic and Thyme (page 273)

DESSERT:

½ ruby red grapefruit

Honey tea

CHAPTER 11

Recipes for Your Mind and Your Heart

THESE RECIPES FOR BOTH your mind and your heart come directly from my own kitchen. Each uses the whole foods and spices that have been scientifically proven to uplift your mood and keep your blood vessels dilated and healthy. To receive the greatest benefit for your mind, heart, and taste buds, try to use only the freshest ingredients, and choose organic foods whenever possible.

You've probably noticed that the 28-Day Positive Emotions Prescription Nutrition Plan tends to shy away from bread products. When bread is called for, I suggest using Ezekiel 4:9 bread because it tastes good (especially when toasted), has no added sugar, is GMO free, and contains sprouted grains, which provide good nutritional value. Ezekiel bread does contain gluten, however, so if you have gluten sensitivity, it's best to stay away from breads in general. In order to make the desserts friendly for those who suffer from gluten sensitivity, the baking recipes you'll find here call for gluten-free flours such as almond, soy (which needs to be certified gluten-free due to cross-contamination with farmed wheat products), teff, and arrowroot flour.

The recipes are based on the principles of the Mediterranean diet because of its proven ability to reduce heart disease and risk factors such as high blood pressure, high glucose, and high triglycerides. And just as important, traditional Mediterranean foods and products containing olive oil, fish, vegetables, and nuts are delicious, filling, and mood enhancing. In other words, they represent the quintessential ingredients of the Positive Emotions Prescription Plan, and I can personally attest that the results are delectable! Happy and healthy eating, from my home to yours. *Mangia!*

BREAKFAST

Deeply Satisfying Kasha Porridge

TOTAL TIME: 15 minutes *Makes 2 servings*

- 2 teaspoons olive oil
- ½ cup kasha (fine granulation)
- 1½ cups almond, coconut, hemp, or soy milk
- 3 dried dates or cherries, pitted and chopped
- ½ teaspoon ground cinnamon
- ½ teaspoon ground ginger
- 1 teaspoon maple syrup
- ¼ teaspoon Himalayan pink salt

In a medium saucepan, warm the oil over medium heat. Add the kasha and cook, stirring, for 2 minutes, or until toasted. Add the milk, dates or cherries, cinnamon, ginger, and maple syrup, and bring to a boil. Cook uncovered, stirring frequently, while maintaining a gentle boil for 10 minutes. If desired, add extra milk and maple syrup. Season with the salt and fluff with a fork. Serve warm.

Per serving: 326 calories, 6 g protein, 62 g carbohydrates, 8 g total fat, 1 g saturated fat, 8 g fiber, 141 mg sodium

Banana-Mango-Ginger Smoothie

TOTAL TIME: 10 minutes

Makes 2 servings

- 2 frozen bananas
- 1½ teaspoons finely chopped fresh ginger
- ¾ cup frozen mango slices
- ¼ cup almond, coconut, hemp, or soy milk
- Juice of ½ lemon
- ¼ teaspoon ground cardamom (optional)
- 4–5 blueberries (optional)
- Sprinkling of hempseeds (optional)

In a blender, combine the bananas, ginger, mango, milk, lemon juice, and cardamom (if using). Blend on high speed until smooth. Serve immediately. For an added heart healthy option, top with the blueberries and hempseeds.

Per serving: 151 calories, 2 g protein, 38 g carbohydrates, 1 g total fat, 0 g saturated fat, 4 g fiber, 25 mg sodium

Ginger-Date Smoothie

TOTAL TIME: 10 minutes

Makes 1 serving

- 1 cup almond, coconut, hemp, or soy milk
- 2–4 ice cubes
- 1–2 Medjool dates
- 1 frozen banana
- ½–1 teaspoon agave nectar
- ½ teaspoon ground ginger
- ½ teaspoon vanilla extract
- 1 scoop vanilla protein powder (optional)

In a blender, combine the milk, ice cubes, dates, banana, agave nectar, ginger, vanilla extract, and protein powder (if using). Blend on high speed until smooth, and enjoy!

Per serving: 249 calories, 3 g protein, 55 g carbohydrates, 3 g total fat, 0 g saturated fat, 6 g fiber, 183 mg sodium

Pumpkin Pie Smoothie

TOTAL TIME: 10 minutes

Makes 2 servings

- 1½ cups almond milk
- 1 scoop vanilla protein powder (I recommend Sunwarrior)
- ½ cup cooked fresh or canned pumpkin*
- ½ teaspoon maca powder
- 1 teaspoon ground cinnamon
- 2 dates, pitted
- 1 teaspoon ground vanilla bean
- ¼ cup water
- ¼ teaspoon ground cloves
- ¼ teaspoon pumpkin pie spice

In a blender, combine the almond milk, protein powder, pumpkin, maca powder, cinnamon, dates, and vanilla. Adding the water as needed to achieve the desired consistency, blend on high speed until smooth. Sprinkle with the cloves and pumpkin pie spice, and serve.

Per serving: 162 calories, 10 g protein, 30 g carbohydrates, 3 g total fat, 0 g saturated fat, 6 g fiber, 165 mg sodium

**Note: Do not use pumpkin pie filling.*

Ravens Purple Pride Smoothie

TOTAL TIME: 10 minutes

Makes 1 serving

- 1 cup fresh blueberries
- ½ cup water or almond, coconut, hemp, or soy milk
- 2–4 ice cubes
- 1 frozen banana
- 1½ teaspoons finely chopped fresh ginger
- Juice of 1 lime
- Handful of raw walnuts or cashews
- Sprinkling of hempseeds or chia seeds

In a blender, combine the blueberries, water or milk, ice cubes, banana, ginger, lemon juice, and nuts. Blend on high speed until smooth. Pour into a glass and top with the seeds. Serve immediately.

Per serving: 422 calories, 9 g protein, 57 g carbohydrates, 8 g total fat, 2 g saturated fat, 9 g fiber, 9 mg sodium

Pumpkin-Almond Smoothie

TOTAL TIME: 10 minutes

Makes 2 servings

- 1 cup almond milk
- 2 frozen bananas
- 1 cup canned pumpkin*
- 1 teaspoon ground allspice
- 1 teaspoon vanilla extract
- Pinch of sea salt

In a blender, combine the milk, bananas, pumpkin, allspice, vanilla, and salt. Blend on high speed until smooth, and enjoy!

Per serving: 175 calories, 3 g protein, 39 g carbohydrates, 2 g total fat, 0 g saturated fat, 7 g fiber, 172 mg sodium

**Note: Do not use pumpkin pie filling.*

Chamomile Smoothie

TOTAL TIME: 10 minutes

Makes 2 servings

- 1 cup chilled chamomile tea or 4 large chamomile-tea ice cubes
- 1 cup almond, coconut, hemp, or soy milk
- 1 frozen banana
- 1 teaspoon honey
- Juice of ½ lemon
- ¼ teaspoon ground turmeric
- ¼ teaspoon ground cinnamon

In a blender, combine the chamomile tea or ice cubes, milk, banana, honey, lemon juice, turmeric, and cinnamon. Blend on high speed until smooth, and serve immediately.

Per serving: 88 calories, 1 g protein, 19 g carbohydrates, 2 g total fat, 0 g saturated fat, 2 g fiber, 91 mg sodium

Strawberry-Pineapple-Kale Smoothie

TOTAL TIME: 10 minutes

Makes 2 servings

- 2 cups water or almond, coconut, hemp, or soy milk
- ½–¾ cup kale
- 1 cup fresh or frozen strawberries
- ½ cup fresh or frozen pineapple
- ½ cup cucumber chunks
- Juice of ½ lemon

In a blender, combine the water or milk, kale, strawberries, pineapple, cucumber, and lemon juice. Blend on high speed until smooth, and serve immediately.

Per serving: 58 calories, 2 g protein, 14 g carbohydrates, 1/2 g total fat, 0 g saturated fat, 3 g fiber, 18 mg sodium

Orioles Orange Smash Smoothie

TOTAL TIME: 10 minutes

Makes 1 serving

- 1 scoop vanilla protein powder (I recommend Sunwarrior)
- 1 cup almond, coconut, hemp, or soy milk
- 2–4 ice cubes
- 2 oranges, peeled
- 2 dates, pitted, or 1 teaspoon honey
- 1 frozen banana
- 1 teaspoon vanilla powder
- ¼ teaspoon ground turmeric
- Dash of ground cinnamon
- Dash of ground nutmeg

In a blender, combine the protein powder, milk, ice cubes, oranges, dates or honey, banana, vanilla powder, turmeric, cinnamon, and nutmeg. Blend on high speed until smooth. Serve immediately.

Per serving: 474 calories, 22 g protein, 102 g carbohydrates, 5 g total fat, 0 g saturated fat, 15 g fiber, 233 mg sodium

Almond Flour Banana Waffles

TOTAL TIME: 15 minutes

Makes 2 servings (or 1 large waffle)

- 1 ripe banana
- 1 egg
- 1½ cups almond flour
- ½ teaspoon baking soda
- ½ teaspoon ground cinnamon
- ¼ teaspoon ground nutmeg
- 1½ teaspoons maple syrup
- 2 tablespoons milk (optional)
- Handful of blueberries

In a medium bowl, mash the banana with a fork. Add the egg, flour, baking soda, cinnamon, nutmeg, and maple syrup, and stir well. Add the milk, if using, to moisten.

Fill a lightly greased waffle iron with the batter and cook for 5 minutes, or until golden brown. Top with the blueberries and enjoy!

Per serving: 584 calories, 22 g protein, 36 g carbohydrates, 45 g total fat, 4 g saturated fat, 11 g fiber, 381 mg sodium

Peach and Blueberry Cobbler

TOTAL TIME: 40 minutes

Makes 8 servings

- 6 fresh or frozen peaches, peeled and pitted
- Juice of ½ lemon
- 1 cup blueberries
- 1 vanilla bean, scraped
- 1½ teaspoons ground cinnamon, divided
- 2 cups almonds
- ½ cup chopped dates
- 2 tablespoons honey

Preheat the oven to 350°F. Cut the peaches into bite-size chunks and place them in a large bowl. Sprinkle with the lemon juice, gently mix in the blueberries, vanilla, and ½ teaspoon of the cinnamon, and set aside.

In a smaller bowl, combine the almonds, dates, honey, and the remaining 1 teaspoon of the cinnamon.

Pour the peaches and blueberries into a 9" deep-dish pie pan and top with the almonds and dates. Bake for 20 minutes, or until heated through. Serve warm.

Per serving: 303 calories, 9 g protein, 33 g carbohydrates, 18 g total fat, 1 g saturated fat, 7 g fiber, 2 mg sodium

Artichoke Frittata

TOTAL TIME: 55 minutes

Makes 6 servings

- 2 tablespoons olive oil
- 4 scallions, chopped
- 2 cloves garlic, chopped
- 1 red bell pepper, finely chopped
- 4 ounces sliced mushrooms
- 1 can (14 ounces) artichoke hearts, drained and coarsely chopped
- 6 eggs, beaten
- 2 slices organic soy mozzarella, finely chopped
- Salt
- Ground black pepper

Preheat the oven to 350°F. Coat a 9" deep-dish pie pan with cooking spray. In a medium skillet, heat the olive oil over medium heat. Add the scallions, garlic, red pepper, mushrooms, and artichokes, and cook, stirring frequently, for 4 minutes, or until soft.

Transfer the vegetables to a large mixing bowl and add the eggs, soy mozzarella, and salt and pepper to taste. Mix thoroughly, then pour into the pan. Bake for 35 minutes, or until golden brown.

Per serving: 155 calories, 10 g protein, 8 g carbohydrates, 10 g total fat, 2 g saturated fat, 2 g fiber, 409 mg sodium

LUNCH

Tuna with Veggies

TOTAL TIME: 10 minutes

Makes 4 servings

- 2 cans (10 ounces each) water-packed solid white albacore tuna, drained
- ¼ cup shredded carrots
- ¼ cup frozen green peas, thawed
- 3 tablespoons mayonnaise
- ½ teaspoon garlic powder

In a medium serving bowl, mix the tuna, carrots, peas, mayonnaise, and garlic powder. Serve on lettuce or crisp, whole grain crackers.

Per serving: 208 calories, 27 g protein, 2 g carbohydrates, 10 g total fat, 1 g saturated fat, 1 g fiber, 153 mg sodium

Arugula-Avocado-Almond Salad

TOTAL TIME: 15 minutes

Makes 1 serving

DRESSING

- 2 tablespoons extra-virgin olive oil
- Juice of 1 lemon
- ¼ teaspoon minced garlic
- ½ teaspoon honey (optional)

SALAD

- ½ head romaine lettuce, chopped into bite-size pieces
- ½ cup arugula
- ½ avocado, chopped into ½" cubes
- 1 radish, thinly sliced
- 2 tablespoons sliced raw almonds, soaked overnight

To make the dressing: In a large bowl, whisk together the oil, lemon juice, garlic, and honey (if using).

To make the salad: Add the romaine, arugula, avocado, radish, and almonds to the bowl with the dressing. Toss and enjoy.

Per serving: 524 calories, 9 g protein, 23 g carbohydrates, 47 g total fat, 6 g saturated fat, 14 g fiber, 36 mg sodium

Heavenly Hearts of Palm Salad

TOTAL TIME: 25 minutes

Makes 4 servings

SALAD

1 can (14 ounces) hearts of palm, drained and cut into ½" matchsticks
1 cucumber, peeled and sliced
2 Roma (plum) tomatoes, sliced
1 small red onion, finely chopped
2 cups baby spinach leaves

VINAIGRETTE

1 large clove garlic, minced
1 teaspoon grated lemon peel
2 tablespoons lemon juice
2 tablespoons balsamic vinegar
⅓ cup extra-virgin olive oil
Sea salt
Ground black pepper

To make the salad: In a large bowl, combine the hearts of palm, cucumber, tomatoes, and onion.

To make the vinaigrette: In a small bowl, whisk together the garlic, lemon peel, lemon juice, vinegar, and oil. Add salt and black pepper to taste.

Pour the vinaigrette over the vegetables and mix well. Let marinate for at least 1 hour in the refrigerator, and toss well. Serve over the spinach leaves.

Per serving: 218 calories, 3 g protein, 10 g carbohydrates, 19 g total fat, 3 g saturated fat, 3 g fiber, 303 mg sodium

Stuffed Sweet Potatoes with Beans

TOTAL TIME: 1 hour 30 minutes

Makes 4 servings

- 4 sweet potatoes
- 2 tablespoons olive oil
- ¼ cup chopped sweet onion
- 2 cloves garlic, minced
- 1 teaspoon dried oregano
- ¼ teaspoon red-pepper flakes
- 1½ cups canned or fresh black beans, cooked and drained
- 6 cups baby spinach
- 1 tablespoon white wine vinegar
- Salt
- Freshly ground black pepper

Preheat the oven to 400°F.

Scrub the sweet potatoes and pierce them in a few places with a fork. Place them on a baking sheet and bake for 1 hour, or until soft all the way through.

About 15 to 20 minutes before the sweet potatoes are done, in a wide, deep saucepan, heat the olive oil over medium heat. Add the onion and cook for 5 minutes, or until softened. Add the garlic, oregano, and red-pepper flakes and cook, stirring, for 1 minute. Add the beans and cook for 5 minutes, stirring occasionally. Add the spinach, cover the pan, and cook, stirring occasionally, for 5 minutes, or until the spinach is wilted. Stir in the vinegar and season to taste with the salt and pepper.

Slice open the sweet potatoes and stuff them with the spinach and bean mixture.

Per serving: 256 calories, 8 g protein, 43 g carbohydrates, 7 g total fat, 1 g saturated fat, 11 g fiber, 510 mg sodium

Spinach-Mango Salad with Hempseeds

TOTAL TIME: 10 minutes

Makes 4 servings

- 1 tablespoon avocado oil or olive oil
- 2 tablespoons balsamic vinegar
- 1 bag (6 ounces) baby spinach leaves
- 2 mangoes, cut into chunks
- ½ cup very thinly sliced red onion
- ½ cup blueberries
- 1 tablespoon hempseeds

In a small bowl, whisk the oil and vinegar until blended. In a large bowl, toss the spinach, mangoes, onion, and blueberries. Pour the oil and vinegar mixture over the spinach mixture, toss gently to coat, and top with the hempseeds.

Per serving: 187 calories, 4 g protein, 35 g carbohydrates, 5 g total fat, 1 g saturated fat, 5 g fiber, 72 mg sodium

Orange-Spinach Salad

TOTAL TIME: 10 minutes

Makes 6 servings

SALAD

- 1 package (12 ounces) spinach, washed
- 2 cans (11 ounces each) mandarin oranges, drained
- ½ cup slivered almonds or candied pecans
- Pomegranate seeds (optional)

VINAIGRETTE

- 1 teaspoon mustard powder
- 1 tablespoon honey
- 2 tablespoons cider vinegar
- 3½ tablespoons olive oil or avocado oil
- ½ tablespoon orange juice or lemon juice

To make the salad: In a large bowl, combine the spinach, oranges, nuts, and seeds, if using.

To make the vinaigrette: In a small bowl, whisk together the mustard powder, honey, vinegar, oil, and orange or lemon juice.

Pour the vinaigrette over the salad and mix well. Top with additional pomegranate seeds, if desired.

Per serving: 177 calories, 4 g protein, 13 g carbohydrates, 13 g total fat, 2 g saturated fat, 3 g fiber, 49 mg sodium

Green Bean, Artichoke, and Tuna Salad

TOTAL TIME: 15 minutes

Makes 2 servings

- 1 can (5 ounces) water-packed solid white albacore tuna, drained
- ½ cup coarsely chopped canned artichoke hearts
- ½ cup green beans, lightly steamed
- ¼ cup coarsely chopped pitted kalamata olives
- ½ cup quartered cherry tomatoes
- 2 tablespoons extra-virgin olive oil
- 2 tablespoons lemon juice
- Pinch of Himalayan salt
- Pinch of freshly ground black pepper
- 4 leaves fresh basil, thinly sliced

In a medium serving bowl, combine the tuna and the artichoke hearts. Add the green beans, olives, and tomatoes.

In a small bowl, whisk together the oil, lemon juice, salt, and pepper. Place the tuna mixture on a serving platter. Drizzle with the dressing and top with the basil leaves.

Per serving: 339 calories, 16 g protein, 12 g carbohydrates, 26 g total fat, 3 g saturated fat, 2 g fiber, 864 mg sodium

Avocado Turkey Burger Sprout Wrap

TOTAL TIME: 10 minutes

Makes 1 serving

- 1/4 avocado, sliced
- 1 brown rice tortilla wrap
- 1 grilled turkey burger (preferably organic)
- 1/4 cup sprouts
- 2 slices tomato
- 1 baby carrot, sliced
- 1 tablespoon sauerkraut

Place the avocado in the middle of the wrap. Put the turkey burger, sprouts, tomato, carrot, and sauerkraut on top. Fold and enjoy.

Per serving: 299 calories, 13 g protein, 38 g carbohydrates, 13 g total fat, 1 g saturated fat, 11 g fiber, 669 mg sodium

Glazed Beet and Red Grapefruit Salad

TOTAL TIME: 15 minutes

Makes 8 servings

- 3 packets (8.8 ounces each) prepared organic Love Beets*
- 2 ruby red grapefruits, peeled and separated into segments
- 1/4 cup olive oil
- 2 tablespoons white wine vinegar
- 2 teaspoons light brown sugar
- 2 tablespoons finely chopped pistachios

Drain the beet juice from the beets. Cut the beets into quarters.

Arrange the grapefruit sections on a platter and add the quartered beets to the platter. In a small bowl, whisk together the olive oil, vinegar, and brown sugar. Drizzle the sauce over the beets and grapefruit. Garnish with the pistachios.

Per serving: 138 calories, 2 g protein, 17 g carbohydrates, 8 g total fat, 1 g saturated fat, 3 g fiber, 73 mg sodium

**Note: The Love Beets brand can be found at Costco, Whole Foods Market, and other health food markets.*

Tuna and Chickpea Salad

TOTAL TIME: 10 minutes

Makes 4 servings

- 1 can (15 ounces) chickpeas, rinsed and drained
- 1 cup halved cherry or grape tomatoes
- ¼ cup chopped red onion
- ¼ cup olive oil
- 2 tablespoons red wine vinegar
- 2 teaspoons spicy brown mustard
- 2 tablespoons chopped flat leaf parsley
- ¼ teaspoon salt
- ¼ teaspoon ground black pepper
- 2 cans (5 ounces each) water-packed solid white albacore tuna, drained

In a large bowl, combine the chickpeas, tomatoes, and onion.

In a small bowl, whisk together the oil, vinegar, mustard, parsley, salt, and pepper. Pour the dressing over the chickpea mixture and toss to coat. Gently stir in the tuna. This can be eaten as a salad or in a sandwich, topped with lettuce and tomato.

Per serving: 262 calories, 17 g protein, 12 g carbohydrates, 16 g total fat, 2 g saturated fat, 4 g fiber, 401 mg sodium

Persimmon-Mozzarella Panini

TOTAL TIME: 20 minutes

Makes 2 servings

- 2 small handfuls of fresh arugula
- 4 slices Ezekiel bread
- 2–4 ounces mozzarella cheese, sliced
- 1 persimmon, cut into 8 thin slices
- 1 teaspoon olive oil

Place the arugula over 2 slices of the bread. Top each with half of the mozzarella cheese, 4 persimmon slices, and another slice of bread.

In a small skillet, heat the oil over medium heat. Place the panini in the pan and place a heavier pan on top to press them down. Cook for 3 minutes, or until the bottoms are golden brown. Flip the panini over and cook for another 3 minutes, or to desired doneness.

Remove the panini from the skillet. Slice them in half and serve immediately.

Per serving: 287 calories, 15 g protein, 36 g carbohydrates, 10 g total fat, 4 g saturated fat, 6 g fiber, 333 mg sodium

Quinoa Salad

TOTAL TIME: 35 minutes

Makes 2 servings

- ½ cup quinoa
- 1¼ cups water
- 2 cups broccoli florets, steamed
- 2 carrots, finely chopped and steamed
- 2 golden or red beets, finely chopped, steamed, and cooled
- 1 small red onion, finely chopped
- 2 tablespoons chopped parsley
- 3 tablespoons extra-virgin olive oil
- ¼ cup orange juice
- 2 tablespoons chopped fresh basil
- 1 clove garlic, minced
- Sea salt
- Ground black pepper

In a medium pot, combine the quinoa and water. Bring to a soft boil over high heat. Reduce to a simmer and cover. Stir every few minutes for 15 minutes, or until you see the outer ring of the quinoa separate.

In a large bowl, combine the broccoli, carrots, beets, onion, and parsley. Once the quinoa is cooked, add it to the bowl and toss to combine.

In a small bowl, whisk together the olive oil, orange juice, basil, and garlic. Drizzle the dressing over the salad. Season to taste with the salt and pepper.

Per serving: 458 calories, 11 g protein, 52 g carbohydrates, 24 g total fat, 3 g saturated fat, 10 g fiber, 211 mg sodium

Grilled Chicken and Celery Salad à la Marcella

TOTAL TIME: 10 minutes

Makes 1 serving

- 3 ounces grilled chicken breast, cut into ½" cubes
- 3 ribs celery, chopped
- ¾ cup red seedless grapes
- 1 teaspoon canola mayonnaise
- ½ teaspoon dried oregano
- ½ teaspoon salt
- ½ teaspoon ground black pepper
- ½ teaspoon garlic powder
- Salad greens (optional)

In a large bowl, combine the chicken, celery, grapes, mayonnaise, oregano, salt, pepper, and garlic powder. Stir together until just combined.

Serve on a bed of salad greens, if desired.

Per serving: 287 calories, 29 g protein, 27 g carbohydrates, 7 g total fat, 1 g saturated fat, 3 g fiber, 775 mg sodium

Apple-Spinach Salad

TOTAL TIME: 10 minutes

Makes 6 servings

- 1 package (10 ounces) fresh spinach, washed
- 2 Fuji apples, chopped
- ½ cup cashews
- ¼ cup golden raisins
- ¼ cup coconut sugar
- ¼ cup cider vinegar
- ¼ cup canola oil
- ¼ teaspoon celery salt
- ¼ teaspoon garlic salt

In a large bowl, mix together the spinach, apples, cashews, and raisins.

In a medium jar, combine the sugar, vinegar, oil, celery salt, and garlic salt. Cover and shake thoroughly. Pour the dressing over the spinach mixture and toss gently.

Per serving: 248 calories, 3 g protein, 29 g carbohydrates, 15 g total fat, 2 g saturated fat, 3 g fiber, 130 mg sodium

Strawberries and Watercress Salad

TOTAL TIME: 5 minutes

Makes 4 servings

- 1 tablespoon balsamic vinegar
- ¼ cup extra-virgin olive oil
- Ground black pepper
- 3 bunches watercress, stems removed
- 1 pint fresh strawberries, hulled and sliced

In a small bowl, whisk together the vinegar, oil, and pepper to taste. Place the watercress in a large bowl and add the strawberries and any residual strawberry juice. Pour the dressing over the salad, toss well, and serve.

Per serving: 157 calories, 1 g protein, 7 g carbohydrates, 14 g total fat, 2 g saturated fat, 2 g fiber, 18 mg sodium

Mouthwatering Watermelon Salad

TOTAL TIME: 10 minutes

Makes 2 servings

- 2 cups seeded, bite-size watermelon cubes
- 2 cups finely sliced arugula
- ¼ cup finely chopped jicama
- 1 tablespoon raw pumpkin seeds, soaked overnight
- Juice of 1 lime

In a large bowl, combine the watermelon, arugula, jicama, and pumpkin seeds. Add the lime juice and mix well.

Per serving: 88 calories, 3 g protein, 18 g carbohydrates, 3 g total fat, 0.5 g saturated fat, 2 g fiber, 12 mg sodium

Orange, Lime, and Grapefruit Salad with Honey Mint Dressing

TOTAL TIME: 20 minutes

Makes 6 servings

SALAD

- 6–8 mixed seasonal citrus fruits (any combination of oranges, blood oranges, tangerines, or clementines with limes and ruby red grapefruit)
- 2 cups melon cubes

DRESSING

- ¼ cup orange juice
- 2 tablespoons olive oil
- 1 tablespoon rice wine vinegar
- 1 tablespoon honey
- 4 mint leaves, chopped

To make the salad: Peel all of the citrus fruits and cut them into thin slices. Arrange the slices in layers on a plate and top with the melon cubes.

To make the dressing: In a small bowl, combine the orange juice, oil, vinegar, honey, and mint leaves. Serve alongside the citrus salad, so everyone can use as much dressing as desired.

Per serving: 130 calories, 2 g protein, 23 g carbohydrates, 5 g total fat, 1 g saturated fat, 3 g fiber, 51 mg sodium

Spinach Salad with Berries and Honey Pecans

TOTAL TIME: 20 minutes

Makes 4 servings

- 6 tablespoons olive oil, divided
- 3 tablespoons orange juice, divided
- 3 tablespoons honey
- 1 cup pecan halves
- 1 bag (6 ounces) baby spinach leaves
- 2 cups hulled and sliced strawberries or fresh blueberries
- Ground black pepper

Coat a sheet of foil with cooking spray. In a medium skillet over medium heat, heat 1 tablespoon of the oil, 1 tablespoon of the orange juice, and the honey. Stir for 2 minutes, or until syrupy. Add the pecans and cook, stirring, for 5 minutes, or until the nuts are toasted and coated with the syrup.

Transfer the pecans to the foil. Separate them and allow them to cool.

In a large bowl, combine the spinach, berries, and cooled pecans. In a small bowl, whisk together the remaining 5 tablespoons of oil and 2 tablespoons of orange juice. Season the oil and juice mixture with the pepper to taste. Drizzle the dressing over the salad and serve.

Per serving: 447 calories, 4 g protein, 29 g carbohydrates, 38 g total fat, 4 g saturated fat, 6 g fiber, 70 mg sodium

SOUPS

Celestial Celery Root and Apple Soup

TOTAL TIME: 1 hour

Makes 8 servings

- 2 tablespoons olive oil
- 1 clove garlic, chopped
- 3 ribs celery with leaves, sliced
- 2 large onions, chopped
- 2 Fuji apples, peeled, cored, and cut into 1"–2" cubes
- Sea salt
- Ground black pepper
- 1 pound celeriac, trimmed, peeled, and cubed
- 1 bay leaf
- 4 cups vegetable broth
- 1 cup white wine
- ½ cup plain soy yogurt
- Scallions, sliced

In a large soup pot, heat the oil over low heat. Add the garlic, celery, onions, and apples, and season to taste with the salt and pepper. Cook, stirring frequently, for 5 minutes, or until the vegetables are soft.

Add the celeriac, bay leaf, broth, and wine, and bring to a boil. Reduce the heat and cook at a gentle simmer for 25 minutes, or until the celeriac is soft. Remove the bay leaf.

In a blender or food processor, blend or process the soup until smooth. Taste and add additional salt and pepper, if desired.

Divide among 8 bowls. Stir 1 tablespoon of the yogurt into each serving and garnish with the scallions.

Per serving: 130 calories, 2 g protein, 18 g carbohydrates, 4 g total fat, 0.5 g saturated fat, 4 g fiber, 354 mg sodium

Saffron Split Pea Soup

TOTAL TIME: 3 hours

Makes 8 servings

- 2 pinches of saffron
- 1 tablespoon extra-virgin olive oil
- 1 teaspoon ground cumin
- 1 large onion, chopped
- 3 medium carrots, chopped
- 2 ribs celery, finely chopped
- ½ tablespoon minced garlic
- 1 cup yellow split peas
- 1 cup green split peas
- 5 cups fat-free chicken or vegetable broth
- 1 teaspoon salt
- Ground black pepper

In a small bowl, cover the saffron with a couple of tablespoons of hot water. Let sit for about 10 minutes, then strain the saffron, reserving the water.

In a large pot, heat the olive oil over medium heat. Add the cumin, onion, carrots, celery, and garlic, and cook for 5 minutes, or until the onion becomes translucent. Stir in the yellow and green split peas, broth, saffron water, salt, and pepper to taste. Cover and bring to a boil, then reduce the heat and simmer for 2½ hours, stirring frequently.

(Alternative pressure-cooking method: Follow the cooking instructions above, through the addition of black pepper. Lock the lid in place and, over high heat, bring the pressure cooker to high pressure. Lower the heat enough to maintain high pressure, and cook for 15 minutes. Allow the pressure to come down naturally. Remove the lid, tilting it away from you to allow any excess steam to escape. Add the black pepper and follow the remaining directions.)

Use an immersion blender or a food processor or blender to blend or process until smooth, working in batches if necessary. Add a pinch of the saffron, taste, adjust the seasoning if desired, and serve.

Per serving: 204 calories, 11 g protein, 34 g carbohydrates, 3 g total fat, 0 g saturated fat, 16 g fiber, 598 mg sodium

Rejuvenating Red Lentil Soup

TOTAL TIME: 50 minutes

Makes 8 servings

- 1 tablespoon extra-virgin olive oil
- 3 carrots, chopped
- 1 onion, finely chopped
- 1 sweet potato, peeled and chopped
- 1 tablespoon ground cumin
- 1 teaspoon ground ginger
- 1 teaspoon dried oregano
- ¼ teaspoon ground turmeric
- Juice of 1 orange or ⅓ cup orange juice
- 4 cups water or vegetable broth
- 1 cup red lentils, well rinsed
- Salt
- Ground black pepper
- 2–3 tablespoons finely chopped parsley or fresh cilantro

In a large pot over medium heat, heat the oil. Stir in the carrots, onion, and sweet potato. Cook, stirring frequently, for 10 minutes. Add the cumin, ginger, oregano, and turmeric, and stir well. Add the orange juice, water or broth, and lentils, and cook for 20 minutes, or until the lentils and carrots are tender. Add water as needed as the lentils soften and expand.

Remove from the heat and use an immersion blender, blender, or food processor to blend or process until smooth, working in batches if necessary. If the soup is too thick, add more water. Season with salt and pepper to taste. Garnish with the parsley or cilantro and serve hot.

Per serving: 137 calories, 7 g protein, 22 g carbohydrates, 3 g total fat, 0 g saturated fat, 5 g fiber, 52 mg sodium

Note: The soup will thicken considerably after overnight refrigeration. Use it as a sauce for steamed or roasted vegetables, or thin it with stock or water and reheat to serve as a soup.

Heartwarming White Bean Soup

TOTAL TIME: 25 minutes

Makes 2 servings

- 2 teaspoons extra-virgin olive oil
- 1 clove garlic, minced
- 2 scallions, thinly sliced
- ½ teaspoon finely chopped fresh oregano or rosemary
- 1 can (19 ounces) white beans, rinsed and drained
- 1 can (14.5 ounces) vegetable broth
- 1½ teaspoons fresh lemon juice
- Ground black pepper
- Sea salt

In a medium saucepan, heat the oil over medium heat. Cook the garlic, scallions, and oregano or rosemary, stirring frequently, for 3 minutes, or until the scallions start to soften. Add the beans and broth and cook for 4 minutes. Lightly mash some of the beans to thicken the soup. Stir in the lemon juice and season to taste with the pepper and salt. Serve hot or store in an airtight container in the refrigerator for 2 to 3 days.

Per serving: 265 calories, 13 g protein, 42 g carbohydrates, 5 g total fat, 1 g saturated fat, 10 g fiber, 511 mg sodium

Gingered Carrot Soup

TOTAL TIME: 55 minutes

Makes 8 servings

- 2 tablespoons olive oil
- 2 medium onions, sliced
- 2 cloves garlic, coarsely chopped
- 2 tablespoons dark brown sugar
- 1½ pounds carrots, scrubbed and sliced
- 1 teaspoon ground ginger
- ¼ teaspoon ground turmeric
- 5 cups vegetable stock
- ½ teaspoon Himalayan pink salt
- 2 tablespoons chopped fresh cilantro (optional)

In a large pot, heat the oil over medium heat. Add the onions, garlic, and brown sugar. Stir to combine.

Reduce the heat to medium-low and cook for 12 minutes, or until lightly browned. Add the carrots, ginger, turmeric, vegetable stock, and salt. Cover the pot and cook for 10 minutes, or until the vegetables are tender.

Use an immersion blender, blender, or food processor to blend or process until smooth, working in batches if necessary. Garnish with the cilantro, if desired.

Per serving: 100 calories, 1 g protein, 16 g carbohydrates, 4 g total fat, 0.5 g saturated fat, 4 g fiber, 441 mg sodium

Gazpacho Soup

TOTAL TIME: 40 minutes

Makes 6 servings

- 6–8 medium yellow and red tomatoes, halved
- 1 large cucumber, coarsely chopped
- 1 yellow bell pepper, coarsely chopped
- 1 scallion, finely chopped
- ½ cup orange juice or 2 tablespoons frozen orange juice concentrate
- 3 tablespoons extra-virgin olive oil
- 2 tablespoons Champagne vinegar or white wine vinegar
- 2 cloves garlic, chopped
- 1 medium jalapeño chile pepper with seeds, chopped (wear plastic gloves when handling)
- Pinch of salt
- Ground black pepper
- 1 avocado, pitted and chopped
- 1 bunch fresh cilantro, chopped

Set a strainer over a small bowl. Squeeze the tomatoes over the strainer so that the bowl catches the juice and the strainer catches the seeds. Chop the juiced tomatoes.

In a small bowl, reserve ½ cup of the chopped tomatoes, ¼ cup of the cucumber, and ¼ cup of the bell pepper. In a food processor, combine the remaining tomatoes, cucumber, and bell pepper. Add the tomato juice, scallion, orange juice, oil, vinegar, garlic, and jalapeño. Process until smooth. Season with the salt and pepper to taste, and transfer to a large pitcher or bowl. Add the reserved vegetables and chill overnight. Serve chilled, topped with the avocado and cilantro.

Per serving: 154 calories, 3 g protein, 13 g carbohydrates, 11 g total fat, 2 g saturated fat, 4 g fiber, 58 mg sodium

Miso Soup

TOTAL TIME: 45 minutes

Makes 4 servings

- 1 tablespoon hijiki (dried seaweed)
- 1 tablespoon sesame oil
- 1 carrot, sliced into thin rounds
- 1 piece (¼") fresh ginger, peeled and grated
- 1 clove garlic
- 3 tablespoons miso paste (I recommend South River Garlic Red Pepper Miso)
- ½ package (7 ounces) firm tofu, drained, pressed, and cut into cubes
- Handful of spinach leaves

In a small bowl, place the hijiki and enough water to rehydrate it. Let it sit while you prepare the soup.

In a large pot, heat the sesame oil over medium heat. Add the carrot, ginger, and garlic, stirring frequently. Reduce the heat to a simmer and partially cover. Let cook for 8 minutes, or until the carrot rounds are cooked through and soft.

Spoon some hot water and the miso paste into a small bowl and gently whisk until the miso dissolves.

Pour the miso mixture into the pot, then add the tofu and spinach. Stir once or twice, then let sit for 1 minute, or until the tofu is heated through. Top with the rehydrated hijiki and serve.

Per serving: 190 calories, 11 g protein, 10 g carbohydrates, 12 g total fat, 2 g saturated fat, 3 g fiber, 782 mg sodium

DINNERS

Sesame Chicken Stir-Fry

TOTAL TIME: 40 minutes

Makes 4 servings

- 3 tablespoons reduced-sodium soy sauce
- 1 teaspoon toasted sesame oil
- 3 tablespoons honey
- 1 pound boneless, skinless chicken breasts, cubed
- 2 tablespoons cornstarch
- 2 tablespoons extra-virgin olive oil, divided
- 1 sweet onion, thinly sliced
- 1 clove garlic, minced
- 4 cups thinly sliced bok choy
- Pinch of sea salt
- 2 tablespoons sesame seeds (black or regular)
- 2 tablespoons sliced scallions

In a small bowl, whisk together the soy sauce, sesame oil, and honey. Set aside.

In a shallow dish, toss the chicken with the cornstarch to coat. In a large skillet or wok, heat 1 tablespoon of the olive oil over medium-high heat. Add the chicken and cook for 6 minutes, or until browned. Transfer to a clean dish and set aside.

Add the remaining 1 tablespoon of oil and the onion and garlic, and cook for 2 minutes. Add the bok choy and cook for 1 minute. Add the chicken back to the pan, along with the soy sauce mixture. Simmer for 2 minutes, or until the sauce has thickened. Sprinkle with the salt, sesame seeds, and scallions, and serve.

Per serving: 305 calories, 28 g protein, 18 g carbohydrates, 13 g total fat, 2 g saturated fat, 2 g fiber, 650 mg sodium

Moroccan-Seasoned Wild Salmon

TOTAL TIME: 35 minutes

Makes 4 servings

- 2 cloves garlic, minced
- ¾ teaspoon ground cinnamon
- ¾ teaspoon ground cumin
- ½ teaspoon ground ginger
- ¼ teaspoon ground nutmeg
- Dash of ground red pepper
- 1 teaspoon extra-virgin olive oil
- 4 wild salmon fillets
- ¼ cup chopped pistachios
- 1 tablespoon lime juice

Preheat the oven to 425°F. In a small bowl, combine the garlic, cinnamon, cumin, ginger, nutmeg, pepper, and oil. Place the salmon fillets on a nonstick baking sheet and sprinkle them with the spice mixture and the pistachios. Allow them to sit at room temperature for 10 minutes. Drizzle with the lime juice and bake for 12 minutes, or until the salmon is opaque.

Per serving: 262 calories, 30 g protein, 4 g carbohydrates, 14 g total fat, 2 g saturated fat, 1 g fiber, 66 mg sodium

Flounder in Garlic White Wine Sauce

TOTAL TIME: 20 minutes

Makes 4 servings

- 1 tablespoon olive oil
- 2 cloves garlic, chopped
- ¼ cup white wine
- 2 tablespoons lemon juice
- 1 teaspoon Italian seasoning
- ¼ teaspoon ground black pepper
- 1–1½ pounds flounder fillets
- Sea salt

Preheat the oven to 425°F. Heat the olive oil in an ovenproof skillet over medium heat. Add the garlic and cook for 1 minute. Add the wine, lemon juice, Italian seasoning, and pepper, and whisk until combined. Gently place the fillets in a single layer in the skillet and transfer to the oven. Bake for 10 minutes, or until the fish turns opaque and flakes easily. Season to taste with the salt.

Per serving: 126 calories, 14 g protein, 2 g carbohydrates, 6 g total fat, 1 g saturated fat, 0 g fiber, 374 mg sodium

Rockfish Cakes

TOTAL TIME: 1 hour

Makes 4 servings

- 1 pound rockfish fillets
- Salt
- Ground black pepper
- Juice of 1 lemon
- 3 tablespoons white wine
- Peel of 1 lemon, grated
- 1 egg
- 2 tablespoons mayonnaise
- 1 tablespoon yellow mustard
- 1 teaspoon mustard powder
- 1 teaspoon Old Bay seasoning
- 3 tablespoons Worcestershire sauce
- 2 tablespoons chopped parsley
- ¼ cup chopped red bell pepper
- 3½ tablespoons bread crumbs or cracker crumbs
- Dash of paprika

Preheat the oven to 350°F. Place the fish in a baking dish and season with the salt, black pepper to taste, lemon juice, and wine. Bake for 10 minutes. Remove the fish from the oven and increase the oven temperature to 400°F.

Flake the fish off the skin and into a bowl. (Discard the skin.) Add the lemon peel, egg, mayonnaise, mustard, mustard powder, Old Bay seasoning, Worcestershire sauce, parsley, bell pepper, and bread or cracker crumbs. Mix well and form into 4 patties. Sprinkle each lightly with paprika. Place the patties in a broiler pan and bake for 10 minutes, then increase the oven temperature to broil. Broil the patties for 2 minutes to finish. Serve with a condiment such as stone-ground mustard or cocktail sauce.

Per serving: 228 calories, 24 g protein, 10 g carbohydrates, 9 g total fat, 2 g saturated fat, 1 g fiber, 528 mg sodium

Cedar-Planked Wild Salmon

TOTAL TIME: 30 minutes

Makes 6 servings

- 1 cedar plank, soaked in water per directions
- 1 teaspoon extra-virgin olive oil
- 1 teaspoon honey
- 1 teaspoon garlic powder
- 1 teaspoon dried oregano
- 1 teaspoon smoked paprika
- ¼ teaspoon sea salt
- ¼ teaspoon freshly ground black pepper
- 1 teaspoon coconut sugar
- 6 wild salmon fillets with skin

Preheat the grill. When it is hot, place the wet plank on the grill for 10 minutes, or until fragrant.

In a small bowl, combine the oil, honey, garlic powder, oregano, paprika, salt, pepper, and sugar. Pat the spice rub over the tops of the fillets. Place the salmon on the plank and cover the grill. Cook for 8 to 10 minutes. Serve the salmon directly from the cedar plank or wait until the plank is cool enough to transfer the salmon to a platter.

Alternatively, bake the planked salmon in a 425°F oven for 8 to 10 minutes, or until the fish is opaque.

Per serving: 218 calories, 29 g protein, 2 g carbohydrates, 10 g total fat, 2 g saturated fat, 0 g fiber, 128 mg sodium

Note: Mix a large batch of the spice blend and keep it in a covered glass jar so dinner is ready quickly when you're on the go.

Baked Rainbow Trout with Dates and Almonds

TOTAL TIME: 40 minutes

Makes 4 servings

- 1 cup blanched almonds
- 1½ cups pitted dates
- 1 teaspoon ground cinnamon
- 1 teaspoon maple syrup
- 1 teaspoon extra-virgin olive oil
- Pinch of salt
- Pinch of ground black pepper
- 4 rainbow trout fillets, butterflied

Preheat the oven to 350°F. In a food processor, combine the almonds, dates, cinnamon, maple syrup, oil, salt, and pepper. Process the mixture until it forms a smooth paste, scraping down the sides of the processor as needed. Place the fillets in a baking dish and spread the paste over them. Bake for 25 minutes, or until the fish flakes easily and is light golden brown on top.

Per serving: 505 calories, 26 g protein, 50 g carbohydrates, 26 g total fat, 3 g saturated fat, 8 g fiber, 88 mg sodium

Pesto Portobello Pizza

TOTAL TIME: 35 minutes

Makes 2 servings

- 2 large portobello mushroom caps, cleaned, stems removed
- 1 teaspoon olive oil
- 1 cup broccoli florets, steamed
- ¼ cup prepared or homemade pesto
- ¼ cup shredded organic soy mozzarella
- 1 teaspoon parsley

Preheat the oven to 375°F. Brush the bottom of each mushroom cap with the oil. Place the mushrooms oil side down on an ungreased baking sheet. Bake for 10 minutes.

Divide the broccoli between the mushrooms and top each with 2 tablespoons of the pesto. Sprinkle the cheese over each mushroom and return them to the oven for 10 minutes, or until the broccoli is heated through and the cheese is melted. Sprinkle with the parsley.

Per serving: 231 calories, 10 g protein, 10 g carbohydrates, 18 g total fat, 3 g saturated fat, 3 g fiber, 477 mg sodium

Grilled Portobello Burgers

TOTAL TIME: 20 minutes

Makes 6 servings

- 6 portobello mushrooms, cleaned, stems removed
- ¼ cup olive oil
- 1 tablespoon chopped fresh basil
- 1 tablespoon chopped fresh oregano
- 2 cloves garlic, mashed
- 2 tablespoons balsamic vinegar
- Salt
- Ground black pepper
- Prepared guacamole
- 1 tomato, diced
- 1 onion, diced

Preheat the grill or grill pan to high heat.

Pour the olive oil into a small bowl. Add the basil, oregano, garlic, vinegar, salt, and pepper to taste. Stir to combine.

Grill the mushrooms for 4 minutes on each side, brushing with the marinade while grilling. Serve the portobello burgers on romaine lettuce, topped with prepared guacamole, tomatoes, and onion.

Per serving: 114 calories, 2 g protein, 6 g carbohydrates, 9 g total fat, 1 g saturated fat, 1 g fiber, 31 mg sodium

Seared Mahi Mahi with Mango Black Bean Salsa

TOTAL TIME: 40 minutes

Makes 6 servings

SALSA

- 2 large ripe mangoes, peeled and cut into small cubes
- 1 can (15 ounces) black beans, drained and rinsed
- 1 small red onion, finely chopped
- 1 tablespoon finely chopped fresh ginger
- ¼ cup olive oil
- 2 tablespoons sugar
- Grated peel and juice of 2 limes

MAHI MAHI

- 2 pounds mahi mahi fillets
- 2 tablespoons extra-virgin olive oil
- Ground black pepper
- 2 tablespoons finely chopped pistachios

To make the salsa: In a large bowl, combine the mangoes, beans, onion, ginger, ¼ cup oil, sugar, and lime peel and juice. Chill until ready to serve.

To make the mahi mahi: Preheat the oven to 400°F. Coat a baking sheet with cooking spray. Place the fillets on the baking sheet, brush them with the 2 tablespoons of oil, and season with the pepper to taste. Bake for 25 to 30 minutes, or until the fish flakes easily and is cooked through. Remove from the oven, place on a serving platter, and sprinkle with the chopped pistachios. Serve with the salsa.

Per serving: 396 calories, 32 g protein, 32 g carbohydrates, 17 g total fat, 2 g saturated fat, 5 g fiber, 299 mg sodium

Mediterranean Salmon with Sun-Dried Tomatoes, Capers, and Olives

TOTAL TIME: 35 minutes

Makes 4 servings

- 4 salmon fillets
- Himalayan salt
- Freshly ground black pepper
- Juice of ½ lemon
- ¼ cup white wine
- 3 tablespoons chopped sun-dried tomatoes
- 1 tablespoon capers, rinsed
- 3 black olives, pitted and sliced

Preheat the oven to 375°F. Place the salmon, skin side down, in a shallow baking dish. In a small bowl, combine the salt and pepper to taste, lemon juice, wine, tomatoes, capers, and black olives. Pour the mixture over the salmon and marinate it for at least 10 minutes. Drain the marinade and bake the salmon for 15 minutes, or until the fish is opaque.

Per serving: 242 calories, 29 g protein, 6 g carbohydrates, 10 g total fat, 1 g saturated fat, 1 g fiber, 334 mg sodium

Sesame Miso Cod

TOTAL TIME: 2 hours 30 minutes

Makes 4 servings

- 2 tablespoons white miso (I recommend South River brand)
- 2 tablespoons extra-virgin olive oil
- 2 tablespoons grated fresh ginger
- 1 tablespoon honey
- 1 teaspoon toasted sesame oil
- 1 teaspoon chopped garlic
- 1–1½ pounds cod fillets (1"–1½" thick)

In a medium bowl, whisk together the miso, olive oil, ginger, honey, sesame oil, and garlic. Place the cod in a baking dish, pour the miso mixture over it, and marinate the cod for 2 hours. The miso will caramelize during this time to create a delicious flavor.

Preheat the oven to 375°F. Bake the cod for 15 minutes, or until the fish is opaque.

Per serving: 226 calories, 27 g protein, 8 g carbohydrates, 9 g total fat, 1 g saturated fat, 0 g fiber, 751 mg sodium

Super-Easy Steelhead Trout Teriyaki

TOTAL TIME: 25 minutes

Makes 4 servings

- 1½ pounds steelhead trout or salmon fillets
- 2 tablespoons Soy Vay Veri Veri Teriyaki or Trader Joe's Island Soyaki

Preheat the oven to 375°F. Coat a baking dish with cooking spray, or line it with parchment paper or nonstick foil. Place the fish in the baking dish and pour the teriyaki sauce over it. Bake for 10 to 15 minutes, or until the fish flakes easily. You can also grill the fish, if you prefer.

Per serving: 267 calories, 35 g protein, 3 g carbohydrates, 12 g total fat, 2 g saturated fat, 0 g fiber, 248 mg sodium

Salmon with Asparagus and Artichoke-Mustard Sauce

TOTAL TIME: 30 minutes

Makes 6 servings

SALMON

- 1½ pounds wild salmon fillets (1" thick)
- 1 tablespoon olive oil
- Freshly ground black pepper
- Pinch of sea salt

ARTICHOKE-MUSTARD SAUCE

- 2 tablespoons Dijon mustard
- ¼ cup warm water
- ½ cup extra-virgin olive oil
- 2 teaspoons lemon juice
- Freshly ground black pepper
- 2 cups asparagus tips, steamed
- 1 can (14 ounces) artichoke hearts, drained and chopped

Coat a grill rack with cooking spray. Preheat the grill to medium heat.

To make the salmon: Brush the salmon lightly with the 1 tablespoon olive oil, and season to taste with pepper and salt. Grill for 20 minutes, or until the fish is opaque. Set aside.

To make the artichoke-mustard sauce: Place the mustard in a small saucepan over medium-low heat and gradually add the water, whisking constantly. In a slow but steady stream, add the oil, continuing to whisk constantly. Stir in the lemon juice and pepper to taste, mixing well. Add the asparagus tips and artichoke hearts and stir to coat. Serve warm over the grilled salmon.

Per serving: 385 calories, 25 g protein, 7 g carbohydrates, 28 g total fat, 4 g saturated fat, 2 g fiber, 440 mg sodium

Mediterranean Kale Tart

TOTAL TIME: 1 hour 30 minutes

Makes 6 servings

CRUST

- 2 cups almond flour
- ½ teaspoon Himalayan pink salt
- 1 tablespoon finely chopped fresh oregano
- ¼ cup extra-virgin olive oil
- 1 tablespoon honey

FILLING

- 1 tablespoon olive oil
- 2 tablespoons thinly sliced garlic
- 3 cups coarsely chopped kale
- ½ teaspoon Himalayan pink salt
- 3 large eggs, beaten
- ¼ cup chopped oil-packed sun-dried tomatoes
- ¼ cup chopped kalamata olives
- ½ teaspoon lemon peel

To make the crust: Preheat the oven to 350°F. In a large bowl, combine the almond flour, ½ teaspoon salt, and oregano. In a medium bowl, whisk together the ¼ cup oil and honey. Stir the oil mixture into the almond flour mixture until thoroughly combined. Press the dough into a 9" tart pan and bake for 15 to 20 minutes, or until golden brown. Remove from the oven and let cool completely before filling.

To make the filling: Preheat the oven to 350°F. In a large skillet, heat the 1 tablespoon oil over medium heat. Cook the garlic and kale for 3 minutes, or until the kale begins to wilt. Remove from the heat. In a large bowl, beat the ½ teaspoon salt with the eggs. Add the tomatoes, olives, and kale mixture. Stir in the lemon peel. Pour the mixture into the crust and bake for 20 minutes, or until a knife inserted in the center comes out clean. Let the tart cool in the pan for 15 minutes before serving.

Per serving: 459 calories, 15 g protein, 16 g carbohydrates, 38 g total fat, 4 g saturated fat, 5 g fiber, 409 mg sodium

Moroccan Chicken

TOTAL TIME: 1 hour

Makes 4 servings

- 1 lemon, thinly sliced
- 1 onion, thinly sliced
- ½ cup dried apricots
- 6 pitted green Spanish olives
- 1 tablespoon extra-virgin olive oil
- 1 teaspoon ground cumin
- ½ teaspoon ground turmeric
- ½ teaspoon ground ginger
- ¼ teaspoon ground red pepper
- 4 boneless, skinless chicken breasts
- ½ teaspoon dried thyme

Preheat the oven to 350°F. Fill the bottom of a 13" x 9" baking dish with a single layer of the combined lemon slices, onion slices, and apricots. Top with the olives. In a small bowl, combine the oil, cumin, turmeric, ginger, and red pepper. Stir to make a paste, then rub the paste over each piece of chicken. Place the chicken on top of the olives and sprinkle it with the thyme. Bake for 30 to 40 minutes, depending on the thickness of the chicken, or until a thermometer inserted in the thickest portion registers 160°F and the juices run clear.

Per serving: 321 calories, 37 g protein, 20 g carbohydrates, 9 g total fat, 2 g saturated fat, 4 g fiber, 263 mg sodium

Black Bean Burritos

TOTAL TIME: 40 minutes

Makes 4 servings

- 2 teaspoons extra-virgin olive oil
- ½ white onion, finely chopped
- 1 clove garlic, smashed
- ½ teaspoon ground cumin
- 1 tablespoon ground red pepper or ¼ teaspoon crushed red pepper
- 1 can (15 ounces) black beans, drained
- 1 tablespoon apple cider vinegar
- 1 teaspoon coconut sugar
- Salt
- Ground black pepper
- 2 tablespoons chopped fresh cilantro
- 4 brown rice tortillas
- 1 avocado, sliced (optional)
- Dash of hot sauce (optional)

In a medium Dutch oven or pot, heat the oil over medium to high heat. Add the onion and cook, stirring frequently, for 6 minutes, or until soft. Add the garlic, cumin, and red pepper, and continue cooking for another 2 minutes. Add the beans, reduce the heat to medium, and cook for 10 minutes, stirring occasionally. After the bean mixture is heated, reduce the heat to a simmer and add the vinegar, sugar, and salt and pepper to taste. Stir in the cilantro.

In a skillet over medium heat, warm the tortillas very gently for 5 seconds on each side before filling with the black bean mixture. Serve with the sliced avocado and hot sauce, if using.

Per serving: 218 calories, 6 g protein, 37 g carbohydrates, 5 g total fat, 0.5 g saturated fat, 6 g fiber, 552 mg sodium

Roasted Salmon with Orange-Herb Sauce

TOTAL TIME: 45 minutes

Makes 6 servings

- 1 large orange, unpeeled and thinly sliced
- ½ fennel bulb, sliced
- 1½ tablespoons extra-virgin olive oil
- Salt
- Ground black pepper
- 6 skinless salmon fillets
- 3 tablespoons chopped fresh fennel fronds, divided
- ½ cup orange juice
- ¼ cup thinly sliced scallions
- Additional orange slices (optional)

Preheat the oven to 400°F. In a 13" x 9" glass baking dish, arrange the orange and fennel slices in a single layer. Drizzle with the oil. Season to taste with the salt and pepper. Roast for 25 minutes, or until the fennel is browned and tender.

Increase the oven temperature to 450°F. Push the orange and fennel slices to the sides of the baking dish and place the salmon in the center of the dish. Sprinkle with 1½ tablespoons of the fennel fronds and a pinch of salt and pepper. Spoon the orange and fennel slices on top of the salmon. Bake for 8 minutes, or until the salmon is opaque in the center.

In a small bowl, combine the orange juice, scallions, and the remaining 1½ tablespoons fennel fronds. Transfer the salmon to a platter and spoon the cooked fennel slices alongside it. Discard the cooked orange slices. Pour the orange sauce over the fish and garnish with additional orange slices, if desired. Serve immediately, or refrigerate and serve cold the next day.

Per serving: 251 calories, 29 g protein, 4 g carbohydrates, 13 g total fat, 2 g saturated fat, 1 g fiber, 99 mg sodium

Asian Baked Halibut

TOTAL TIME: 30 minutes

Makes 2 servings

- 1 pound halibut fillets
- Freshly ground black pepper
- Pinch of sea salt
- 3 cloves garlic, smashed
- 1 tablespoon grated fresh ginger
- ¼ teaspoon crushed red-pepper flakes
- ¼ cup coarsely chopped cilantro + additional for garnish
- ¼ cup white wine
- 2 tablespoons reduced-sodium soy sauce
- 1 teaspoon toasted sesame oil
- Chopped scallions

Heat the oven to 450°F. Pat the fish dry and place it in a ceramic or glass baking dish. Season it lightly with the black pepper and salt.

In a food processor, combine the garlic, ginger, red-pepper flakes, and ¼ cup of cilantro. Add the wine, soy sauce, and sesame oil and pulse until blended. Pour the sauce over the fish and bake for 10 to 15 minutes, or until the fish flakes easily and is cooked through. Garnish with the scallions and additional cilantro before serving.

Per serving: 277 calories, 44 g protein, 5 g carbohydrates, 5 g total fat, 1 g saturated fat, 1 g fiber, 786 mg sodium

Fish Tacos

TOTAL TIME: 25 minutes

Makes 8 servings

- 2/3 cup mashed avocado
- 2 cups tomato salsa, divided
- 1 sole fillet (1 pound)
- 8 corn tortillas
- 2 cups shredded red or green cabbage
- 3/4 cup chopped fresh cilantro
- 4 limes, quartered

In a small bowl, combine the avocado and 1 cup of the salsa. Mix well and set aside.

Coat a grill pan or electric grill with cooking spray. Grill the fillet for 3 minutes per side, or until the fish flakes easily. In a skillet over medium heat, warm the tortillas for 5 seconds on each side. Cut the fillet into 8 pieces and place a piece in the center of each warm tortilla. Top each piece with 1/4 cup of cabbage and a sprinkle of cilantro. Fold each taco in half and squeeze the juice from 2 lime quarters over it. Serve the tacos with the remaining 1 cup of salsa on the side.

Per serving: 141 calories, 10 g protein, 17 g carbohydrates, 5 g total fat, 1 g saturated fat, 4 g fiber, 632 mg sodium

Roasted Butternut Squash and Black Bean Tacos

TOTAL TIME: 1 hour 15 minutes

Makes 5 servings

- 2 pounds butternut squash, peeled and sliced into 1" cubes
- 3 tablespoons olive oil, divided
- Freshly ground black pepper
- ¼ teaspoon sea salt + additional to taste
- 1 red onion, chopped
- 2 teaspoons ground cumin
- 1 small jalapeño chile pepper, chopped (wear plastic gloves when handling)
- 2 cans (15 ounces each) black beans, rinsed and drained (or 4 cups cooked black beans)
- ½ cup water
- 1 teaspoon sherry vinegar
- 10 small (6") corn tortillas
- Toasted pepitas

Preheat the oven to 425°F. On a baking sheet, toss the squash with 2 tablespoons of the oil, the black pepper to taste, and ¼ teaspoon salt. Arrange the squash in a single layer and bake for 30 minutes, turning halfway through the baking time, until the squash cubes are tender and caramelizing at the edges.

In a large saucepan over medium heat, warm the remaining 1 tablespoon oil. Cook the onion, stirring occasionally, for 5 minutes, or until it turns translucent. Add the cumin and jalapeño chile pepper and cook for 30 seconds while stirring. Pour in the beans and water. Stir, cover, and reduce the heat to a simmer. Cook for 5 minutes, then remove the lid and use the back of a fork to mash about half of the beans. Remove from the heat, stir in the vinegar, season with additional salt and pepper to taste, and cover until you're ready to serve.

Heat a cast-iron skillet over medium heat and warm each tortilla individually, flipping occasionally. Fill the tortillas with the squash and bean mixture. Top with the pepitas and serve.

Per serving: 329 calories, 11 g protein, 53 g carbohydrates, 11 g total fat, 1 g saturated fat, 12 g fiber, 515 mg sodium

Pistachio-Crusted Tilapia with Strawberry Salsa

TOTAL TIME: 30 minutes

Makes 6 servings

- 6 tilapia fillets (4 ounces each)
- Freshly ground black pepper
- Sea salt
- 5 tablespoons extra-virgin olive oil, divided
- 1 cup crushed pistachios
- 1 pound strawberries, cut into ¼" cubes
- ¼ cup chopped red onion
- 2 tablespoons lime juice
- 2 tablespoons chopped fresh cilantro

Preheat the oven to 350°F. Brush a baking sheet with olive oil or coat it with cooking spray. Season the tilapia fillets with the pepper and a pinch each of sea salt. Pour 4 tablespoons of the olive oil into a shallow dish. Dip each fillet in the olive oil and then in the pistachios. Place the fillets on the baking sheet and bake for 10 minutes, or until the fish is opaque.

In a medium bowl, toss the strawberries, onion, lime juice, the remaining 1 tablespoon oil, and salt to taste. Serve the fish with the salsa and garnish with the cilantro.

Per serving: 354 calories, 28 g protein, 13 g carbohydrates, 23 g total fat, 3 g saturated fat, 4 g fiber, 95 mg sodium

SIDES

Baked Sweet Potato Fries

TOTAL TIME: 30 minutes

Makes 4 servings

- 2 medium sweet potatoes, peeled
- 2 tablespoons extra-virgin olive oil
- 1 tablespoon maple syrup
- ½ teaspoon freshly ground black pepper
- Pinch of sea salt

Preheat the oven to 450°F. Cut the sweet potatoes in half lengthwise and then slice each half into 3 long spears. Spread the potatoes in a single layer on a baking sheet and lightly coat them with the oil, turning them with a spatula to evenly distribute the oil.

Drizzle the maple syrup over the potatoes and sprinkle them with the pepper. Bake for 15 minutes. Turn with the spatula and bake for another 5 minutes, or until lightly browned. Season with the salt. Serve hot.

Per serving: 127 calories, 1 g protein, 15 g carbohydrates, 7 g total fat, 1 g saturated fat, 2 g fiber, 60 mg sodium

Green Beans with Walnuts and Thyme

TOTAL TIME: 45 minutes

Makes 12 servings

- 3½ pounds green beans, trimmed and halved diagonally, lengthwise
- 3 tablespoons extra-virgin olive oil
- 2 shallots, finely chopped
- 1 cup toasted walnuts
- 3 tablespoons fresh thyme leaves
- Ground black pepper
- Sea salt

Bring a large pot of salted water to a boil. Add the green beans and cook until crisp-tender, about 5 minutes. Drain, then place the beans in a large bowl of ice water to cool them quickly and maintain their vibrant green color.

In a large skillet, heat the oil over medium-high heat. Add the shallots and cook, stirring frequently, for 30 seconds. Add the beans and continue to cook, stirring frequently, for another 7 minutes. Add the walnuts and thyme and cook, stirring, for 2 minutes. Season to taste with black pepper and sea salt and serve.

Per serving: 125 calories, 4 g protein, 10 g carbohydrates, 9 g total fat, 1 g saturated fat, 4 g fiber, 16 mg sodium

Roasted Asparagus with Shallots

TOTAL TIME: 25 minutes

Makes 4 servings

- 1 pound asparagus, woody ends trimmed
- 1 shallot, thinly sliced
- ½ yellow bell pepper, finely chopped
- 1½ tablespoons extra-virgin olive oil
- Salt
- Ground black pepper
- Splash of balsamic vinegar

Preheat the oven to 450°F. On a baking sheet, place the asparagus, shallot, and yellow pepper. Toss with the oil and season to taste with salt and pepper. Bake for 10 minutes. Remove from the oven, add a splash of balsamic vinegar, toss to coat, and place back in the oven for 3 minutes. Serve hot or warm.

Per serving: 76 calories, 2 g protein, 7 g carbohydrates, 5 g total fat, 1 g saturated fat, 1 g fiber, 38 mg sodium

Sautéed Kale

TOTAL TIME: 35 minutes

Makes 4 servings

- 2 tablespoons extra-virgin olive oil
- 1 sweet onion, finely chopped
- 1 bunch kale, trimmed and chopped
- ¼ teaspoon Himalayan pink salt

In a large pan, heat the oil over medium heat. Reduce the heat to medium-low and add the onion. Cook, stirring frequently, for 15 minutes, or until caramelized.

Add the kale and cook, stirring frequently, for 5 minutes. Cover the pot with a lid and cook for 2 minutes longer, or until wilted. Add the salt and serve.

Per serving: 108 calories, 3 g protein, 9 g carbohydrates, 8 g total fat, 1 g saturated fat, 2 g fiber, 75 mg sodium

Lightly Sautéed Purslane

TOTAL TIME: 25 minutes *Makes 4 servings*

- 2 tablespoons extra-virgin olive oil
- 1 shallot, chopped
- 1 pound purslane, chopped
- ¼ teaspoon Himalayan pink salt
- ¼ teaspoon freshly ground black pepper

In a large pan, heat the oil over medium heat. Reduce the heat to medium-low and add the shallot. Cook, stirring frequently, for 7 minutes, or until caramelized.

Add the purslane and cook, stirring frequently, for 3 minutes. Season with the salt and pepper and serve.

Per serving: 82 calories, 2 g protein, 3 g carbohydrates, 7 g total fat, 1 g saturated fat, 0 g fiber, 88 mg sodium

Roasted Lotus Root

TOTAL TIME: 30 minutes *Makes 4 servings*

- 1 lotus root, thinly sliced
- 1 tablespoon extra-virgin olive oil
- 1 teaspoon salt
- ½ teaspoon ground black pepper

Preheat the oven to 425°F.

In a roasting pan, toss the lotus root slices with the oil, salt, and pepper before arranging in a single layer. Roast for 20 minutes, or until light brown and crispy.

Per serving: 53 calories, 1 g protein, 5 g carbohydrates, 4 g total fat, 0.5 g saturated fat, 1 g fiber, 593 mg sodium

Sweet Potato–Miso Spread

TOTAL TIME: 10 minutes

Makes 4 servings

- 1 roasted sweet potato
- 1 tablespoon miso (I recommend South River Garlic Red Pepper Miso)
- ½ teaspoon dried oregano

Remove the flesh from the sweet potato and mash it. In a bowl, mash together the sweet potato, miso, and oregano. Spread on toast or use as a dip for veggies.

Per serving: 32 calories, 1 g protein, 7 g carbohydrates, 0 g total fat, 0 g saturated fat, 1 g fiber, 203 mg sodium

Sun-Dried Tomato Dip

TOTAL TIME: 10 minutes

Makes 8 servings

- ¼ cup chopped oil-packed sun-dried tomatoes
- ½ cup soy yogurt
- ½ cup toasted pine nuts
- 1 teaspoon dried basil
- Sea salt
- Ground black pepper

In a food processor, combine the tomatoes, yogurt, nuts, basil, salt, and pepper to taste. Process until smooth. Add a little water if needed to form a thick paste. Serve with crackers or veggies. This dip can also be used as a delicious sandwich spread and will keep in the refrigerator for 1 week.

Per serving: 74 calories, 2 g protein, 3 g carbohydrates, 7 g total fat, 1 g saturated fat, 1 g fiber, 41 mg sodium

Sautéed Spinach with Lemon and Pine Nuts

TOTAL TIME: 15 minutes *Makes 4 servings*

- 1 large bunch (12 ounces) spinach
- 1 tablespoon extra-virgin olive oil
- 1–2 cloves garlic, minced
- 2 teaspoons fresh lemon juice
- Salt
- Ground black pepper
- 1 tablespoon toasted pine nuts

Wash the spinach with cold water. If it's sandy, wash it at least twice and spin it dry.

In a large skillet, heat the oil over medium-high heat. Add the garlic and lemon juice and cook, stirring frequently, for 1 minute. Increase the heat to high and add the spinach and a few pinches of salt and pepper. Using tongs, coat the spinach leaves with the hot oil and garlic. Toss in the pine nuts and season with more salt and pepper to taste. Serve immediately.

Per serving: 67 calories, 3 g protein, 4 g carbohydrates, 5 g total fat, 1 g saturated fat, 2 g fiber, 104 mg sodium

Roasted Jerusalem Artichokes with Herbs

TOTAL TIME: 45 minutes

Makes 4 servings

- 2 tablespoons extra-virgin olive oil
- 1¼ pounds Jerusalem artichokes, scrubbed
- 4 cloves garlic, thinly sliced
- 4 sprigs thyme
- 4 sprigs rosemary
- Salt
- Freshly ground black pepper

Preheat the oven to 400°F. Coat a 9" pie plate with the oil. Cut the artichokes into quarters and use your hands to toss the artichokes, garlic, thyme, and rosemary in the pie plate, making sure the artichokes are coated with the oil.

Roast for 20 minutes and then turn the artichokes over. Roast for another 15 minutes, or until the tips are lightly browned. Season to taste with the salt and pepper.

Per serving: 173 calories, 3 g protein, 26 g carbohydrates, 7 g total fat, 1 g saturated fat, 3 g fiber, 43 mg sodium

Honey- and Maple-Glazed Brussels Sprouts

TOTAL TIME: 30 minutes

Makes 4 servings

- 10–12 Brussels sprouts, halved
- 2 tablespoons maple syrup
- 1 tablespoon honey
- 2 tablespoons olive oil
- Pinch of ground red pepper
- Pinch of sea salt
- Ground black pepper

Preheat the oven to 400°F. Coat a baking sheet with cooking spray.

Place the Brussels sprouts on the baking sheet, cut side up. In a small bowl, mix the maple syrup and honey. Toss the sprouts with the olive oil and season to taste with the red pepper, sea salt, and black pepper. Drizzle the Brussels sprouts with the syrup mixture and roast for 20 minutes, or until golden brown.

Per serving: 126 calories, 2 g protein, 15 g carbohydrates, 7 g total fat, 1 g saturated fat, 2 g fiber, 38 mg sodium

Curried Cauliflower

TOTAL TIME: 45 minutes

Makes 4 servings

- 3 tablespoons extra-virgin olive oil
- 2 tablespoons madras curry powder
- ¼ teaspoon ground turmeric
- 2 tablespoons chicken broth or vegetable broth
- 4 cloves garlic, minced
- 1 head cauliflower, separated into florets
- Sea salt
- Ground black pepper

Preheat the oven to 450°F. In a large bowl, whisk together the oil, curry powder, turmeric, broth, and garlic. Add the cauliflower and toss until it is evenly coated. Place the cauliflower in a single layer on a baking sheet and roast for 30 minutes, or until tender and golden brown. Season with the salt and pepper to taste.

Per serving: 147 calories, 3 g protein, 10 g carbohydrates, 11 g total fat, 2 g saturated fat, 4 g fiber, 107 mg sodium

Spicy Sweet Potato Fries

TOTAL TIME: 45 minutes

Makes 4 servings

- 1 large egg white
- 1 tablespoon water
- 3 tablespoons olive oil
- 1½ teaspoons ground cumin
- 1½ teaspoons sugar
- ½ teaspoon paprika
- ¼ teaspoon ground red pepper
- 3 large sweet potatoes, peeled and cut into wedges
- 1 teaspoon sea salt

Preheat the oven to 450°F. Line a baking pan with parchment paper and set it aside.

In a large bowl, whip the egg white and water with a fork until foamy. In another large bowl, mix the olive oil, cumin, sugar, paprika, and red pepper. Add the sweet potato wedges to the beaten egg white and toss to coat. Toss the coated sweet potato wedges with the spice mixture. Arrange the wedges in a single layer in the baking pan and roast for 20 minutes, or until tender. Sprinkle with the salt before serving.

Per serving: 225 calories, 4 g protein, 30 g carbohydrates, 11 g total fat, 2 g saturated fat, 5 g fiber, 454 mg sodium

Butternut Squash with Baby Spinach

TOTAL TIME: 1 hour 10 minutes

Makes 4 servings

- 1 package (20 ounces) precut butternut squash
- 1 large red onion, chopped
- 1½ tablespoons olive oil
- Ground black pepper
- 1 bag (6 ounces) baby spinach leaves
- ¼ cup fresh or dried sweet cherries
- ¼ cup toasted pumpkin seeds
- ¼ cup pomegranate seeds (optional)

Preheat the oven to 350°F. In a large, shallow baking pan, combine the squash and onion. Drizzle with the olive oil and season to taste with the pepper. Bake for 55 minutes, or until golden brown. Add the spinach and cherries, toss well, and top with the pumpkin seeds and pomegranate seeds, if using. Serve and enjoy.

Per serving: 190 calories, 5 g protein, 27 g carbohydrates, 9 g total fat, 1 g saturated fat, 6 g fiber, 94 mg sodium

Roasted Broccoli

TOTAL TIME: 35 minutes

Makes 4 servings

- 2 cloves garlic, crushed
- 1 tablespoon lemon juice
- ¼ cup chopped red bell pepper
- ¼ cup extra-virgin olive oil
- Ground black pepper
- 5 cups broccoli florets

Preheat the oven to 425°F. In a large bowl, combine the garlic, lemon juice, red pepper, oil, and black pepper to taste.

Add the broccoli and toss until well coated. In a large roasting pan, arrange the broccoli in a single layer. Roast for 25 minutes total, stirring after the first 15 minutes. Serve hot or warm.

Per serving: 157 calories, 3 g protein, 6 g carbohydrates, 14 g total fat, 2 g saturated fat, 3 g fiber, 25 mg sodium

Roasted Green Beans with Garlic and Thyme

TOTAL TIME: 30 minutes

Makes 4 servings

- 1 pound green beans, trimmed
- ¼ cup extra-virgin olive oil
- 3 cloves garlic, smashed
- 3 sprigs thyme, each halved
- 1½ teaspoons sea salt
- 1 teaspoon ground black pepper
- 3 teaspoons fresh lemon juice
- Finely grated peel of 1 lemon
- 3 anchovy fillets, mashed (optional)

Preheat the oven to 450°F. In a large baking dish, combine the beans, oil, garlic, and thyme. Season with the salt and pepper. Spread the beans out in a single layer and roast on the upper rack of the oven for 15 minutes, or until tender and lightly brown. Transfer the beans to a large bowl and add the lemon juice, lemon peel, and anchovies (if using). Toss well and serve warm or at room temperature.

Per serving: 159 calories, 2 g protein, 8 g carbohydrates, 14 g total fat, 2 g saturated fat, 3 g fiber, 591 mg sodium

DESSERTS

Amaretto Amore

TOTAL TIME: 15 minutes

Makes 4 servings

- ¾ cup water or almond, coconut, hemp, or soy milk
- 4 frozen bananas
- ½ cup raw cashews
- 2 tablespoons maple syrup
- 3 teaspoons amaretto liqueur, divided
- 1 cup frozen or fresh cherries

In a blender, combine the water or milk, bananas, cashews, maple syrup, and 1 teaspoon of the amaretto. Blend on high speed until smooth.

Place the cherries in a small saucepan and add the remaining 2 teaspoons of amaretto. Mash the cherries using the back of a fork. Pour the frozen banana mixture into 4 glasses, top each with 2 tablespoons of the cherry sauce, and enjoy!

Per serving: 245 calories, 4 g protein, 45 g carbohydrates, 7 g total fat, 1 g saturated fat, 4 g fiber, 6 mg sodium

Maca Date Shake

TOTAL TIME: 10 minutes

Makes 1 serving

- 1½ teaspoons maca powder
- 1 teaspoon Chinese five spice powder
- 2 tablespoons unsweetened cocoa powder
- 2 Medjool dates, chopped
- ½ cup raw almonds or cashews (or a mixture)
- 1 cup almond milk
- ¼ cup goji berries
- 1 tablespoon honey

In a blender, combine the maca powder, five spice powder, cocoa, dates, nuts, almond milk, berries, and honey. Blend on high speed until smooth. Serve immediately.

Per serving: 865 calories, 26 g protein, 108 g carbohydrates, 44 g total fat, 4 g saturated fat, 18 g fiber, 260 mg sodium

Ana's Blueberry-Cashew Treat

TOTAL TIME: 5 minutes

Makes 2 servings

- 1¼ cups frozen blueberries
- ½ cup raw cashews
- 2 tablespoons cold water or milk
- ¼ cup maple syrup

In a blender, combine the blueberries, cashews, water or milk, and maple syrup. Blend on high speed until smooth. Serve immediately.

Per serving: 310 calories, 6 g protein, 47 g carbohydrates, 13 g total fat, 2 g saturated fat, 4 g fiber, 10 mg sodium

Almond Cookies

TOTAL TIME: 35 minutes + cooling time

Makes 20 to 24 cookies

- ¼ cup almond paste
- ¾ cup sugar
- 4 large egg whites
- ½ teaspoon almond extract
- ½ cup almond flour
- ⅓ cup sliced almonds

Preheat the oven to 325°F. Line a baking sheet with parchment or lightly grease it with oil.

In a food processor, combine the almond paste, sugar, egg whites, almond extract, and flour. Pulse until the batter is smooth. Spoon 1-tablespoon portions of batter onto the baking sheet, keeping about 2" of space between cookies. Sprinkle with the almonds. Bake for 20 minutes, or until golden brown. Cool on a wire rack.

Per serving: 71 calories, 2 g protein, 10 g carbohydrates, 3 g total fat, 0 g saturated fat, 1 g fiber, 12 mg sodium

Frozen Coconut-Chia-Blueberry Parfait

TOTAL TIME: 2 hours 10 minutes *Makes 1 serving*

- 3 tablespoons canned coconut milk
- 1 tablespoon chia seeds
- 1 cup frozen blueberries
- 1 tablespoon maple syrup

In a small bowl, combine the coconut milk and chia seeds. Refrigerate for at least 2 hours or as long as overnight.

In a blender, combine the milk and seed mixture, blueberries, and maple syrup. Blend at high speed until smooth. Enjoy.

Per serving: 266 calories, 3 g protein, 38 g carbohydrates, 13 g total fat, 8 g saturated fat, 8 g fiber, 11 mg sodium

Sesame Bars

TOTAL TIME: 25 minutes + cooling time *Makes 10 bars*

- 1¼ cups almond flour
- ½ cup toasted sesame seeds
- ¼ teaspoon sea salt
- 1 teaspoon baking soda
- ½ cup honey
- ½ cup almond butter or peanut butter
- 1 tablespoon olive oil
- ½ teaspoon vanilla extract

Preheat the oven to 350°F. Coat an 8" x 8" baking pan with cooking spray. In a large bowl, combine the almond flour, sesame seeds, salt, and baking soda. In a small bowl, blend together the honey, almond or peanut butter, oil, and vanilla. Stir the syrup mixture into the flour mixture. Press the mixture into the pan. Bake for 8 minutes, or until lightly browned. Cool on a rack and cut into bars.

Per serving: 268 calories, 7 g protein, 21 g carbohydrates, 19 g total fat, 2 g saturated fat, 3 g fiber, 199 mg sodium

Apple-Blueberry Crisp

TOTAL TIME: 1 hour 10 minutes + cooling time

Makes 6 servings

FILLING

- 2–3 apples, chopped (preferably Fuji)
- 1–1½ cups fresh or frozen blueberries
- Juice of ½ lemon
- 1 tablespoon arrowroot flour
- 1½ tablespoons coconut sugar

TOPPING

- 1 cup almond flour
- ½ cup teff flour
- 2 tablespoons grape seed oil
- 2 tablespoons pumpkin seeds
- 1 teaspoon almond extract
- 1 teaspoon ground cinnamon
- ½ teaspoon ground ginger
- 1 tablespoon maple syrup
- 1 tablespoon amaretto liqueur (optional)

Preheat the oven to 350°F.

To make the filling: In a large bowl, mix the apples, blueberries, lemon juice, arrowroot flour, and sugar. Spoon the filling into a 9" pie pan.

To make the topping: In a separate large bowl, mix the almond flour, teff flour, oil, seeds, almond extract, cinnamon, ginger, maple syrup, and amaretto (if using). Pour the topping over the filling in the pan. Bake for 45 minutes, or until golden brown on top.

Per serving: 290 calories, 7 g protein, 31 g carbohydrates, 16 g total fat, 1 g saturated fat, 6 g fiber, 5 mg sodium

Ultimate Date Cake

TOTAL TIME: 1 hour 15 minutes + cooling time

Makes 4 servings

- 18 dates, pitted
- 3/4 cup almond, coconut, hemp, or soy milk
- 1/2 cup coconut sugar
- 1 teaspoon vanilla extract
- 1/2 cup grape seed oil
- 1 cup almond flour
- 1 teaspoon baking soda
- 1 tablespoon chopped walnuts
- 1 teaspoon ground cinnamon
- 1 teaspoon ground ginger
- 1/4 teaspoon ground cloves

Preheat the oven to 350°F. In a medium bowl, soak the dates in the milk for 30 minutes to 1 hour. Add the sugar and vanilla. Place the date mixture in a blender or food processor. Blend or pulse so that date pieces are still visible. In a large mixing bowl, combine the coarsely blended date mixture and the oil. Stir in the flour, baking soda, walnuts, cinnamon, ginger, and cloves. Pour into a greased 8" x 8" baking pan and bake for 35 minutes, or until golden brown. Let cool before serving to your date!

Per serving: 426 calories, 5 g protein, 59 g carbohydrates, 22 g total fat, 2 g saturated fat, 6 g fiber, 181 mg sodium

Baked Apples with Cinnamon

TOTAL TIME: 40 minutes

Makes 4 servings

- 2 pounds Fuji apples, cored
- 2 teaspoons ground cinnamon
- Juice of 1 lemon
- 2 tablespoons coconut sugar
- 2 tablespoons honey
- 2 tablespoons goji berries
- 2 tablespoons chopped walnuts

Preheat the oven to 375°F. In a small bowl, combine the cinnamon, lemon juice, sugar, honey, goji berries, and walnuts. Pack the cored apples with the mixture. Place the stuffed apples in a baking dish and bake, spooning any topping that falls out back onto the apples, for 30 minutes, or until soft and juicy. Serve warm.

Per serving: 223 calories, 2 g protein, 53 g carbohydrates, 3 g total fat, 0 g saturated fat, 7 g fiber, 18 mg sodium

Almond-Chocolate Bark

TOTAL TIME: 2 hours 15 minutes

Makes 12 bars

- ½ cup almonds
- 1½ cups dark chocolate chips (70% cacao or higher)
- ¼ teaspoon spirulina

Preheat the oven to 350°F. On a baking sheet, arrange the almonds in a single layer. Toast in the oven for 5 to 10 minutes, or until fragrant and slightly brown, stirring every 2 minutes.

Line an 8" x 8" baking dish with parchment paper. In a medium saucepan, melt the chocolate over low heat. Whisk in the spirulina. Pour the chocolate mixture into the baking dish. Scatter the almonds over the chocolate. Refrigerate the bark for 2 hours to set, then cut into bars.

Per serving: 134 calories, 2 g protein, 15 g carbohydrates, 9 g total fat, 3 g saturated fat, 1 g fiber, 6 mg sodium

Chai Hot Chocolate

TOTAL TIME: 15 minutes

Makes 2 servings

- 1½ cups almond milk
- 2 tablespoons cacao nibs
- 2 tablespoons unsweetened cocoa powder
- 2 tablespoons chai tea mix
- 2 tablespoons sugar, divided
- Dark chocolate shavings (optional)

In a small food processor or blender, combine the almond milk, cacao nibs, cocoa, and tea mix. Blend on low speed until combined.

Place the blended chocolate mixture in a small saucepan and warm it over low heat until the desired temperature is reached. Be careful not to scald the almond milk.

Place 1 tablespoon of the sugar into each of 2 mugs. Remove the mixture from the heat and divide it between the mugs. Shave some dark chocolate over the top of each cup of hot chocolate, if desired.

Per serving: 208 calories, 3 g protein, 29 g carbohydrates, 10 g total fat, 5 g saturated fat, 5 g fiber, 156 mg sodium

Chocolate Chip–Beet Cake

TOTAL TIME: 50 minutes + cooling time

Makes 8 servings

- 1 cup almond flour
- ⅔ cup coconut sugar
- ¼ cup unsweetened cocoa powder
- 1 teaspoon baking soda
- ⅛ teaspoon salt
- 3 tablespoons grape seed oil
- 1 egg
- 1 teaspoon vanilla extract
- ¼ cup orange juice
- 2 medium beets (I recommend Love Beets), cooked and shredded
- ⅓ cup dark chocolate chips

Preheat the oven to 350°F. Coat an 8" x 8" baking pan with cooking spray. In a large bowl, combine the almond flour, sugar, cocoa, baking soda, and salt.

In a smaller bowl, whisk the oil, egg, vanilla, and orange juice until blended. Stir the oil mixture into the flour mixture, using a wooden spoon. Fold in the beets and chocolate chips. Pour the batter into the baking pan. Bake for 25 minutes, or until a toothpick inserted in the middle comes out dry. Cool the cake in the pan on a rack before serving.

Per serving: 270 calories, 6 g protein, 31 g carbohydrates, 16 g total fat, 3 g saturated fat, 3 g fiber, 242 mg sodium

Cashew Butter Granola Bars

TOTAL TIME: 55 minutes + cooling time

Makes 12 bars

- 3 cups old-fashioned oats
- ½ cup sesame seeds
- ¾ cup unsweetened shredded coconut
- ¼ cup sugar
- 2 tablespoons unsweetened cocoa powder
- ½ cup dark chocolate chips
- ½ cup pecans
- ½ cup almond milk
- 2 tablespoons honey
- ¼ cup coconut oil
- 1 cup cashew butter
- 1 teaspoon vanilla extract

Preheat the oven to 350°F. Coat a 13" x 9" baking pan with cooking spray. In a large bowl, mix together the oats, seeds, coconut, sugar, cocoa, chocolate chips, and pecans.

In a medium saucepan over low heat, heat the almond milk, honey, coconut oil, cashew butter, and vanilla, stirring until well blended. Add the almond milk mixture to the oat mixture and stir to combine. Spread the batter in the baking pan and bake for 25 minutes. Cool in the pan on a wire rack. When cool, cut into bars.

Per serving: 414 calories, 10 g protein, 35 g carbohydrates, 28 g total fat, 11 g saturated fat, 5 g fiber, 109 mg sodium

Pineapple Carpaccio

TOTAL TIME: 15 minutes

Makes 8 servings

- 1 pineapple
- 5 leaves mint, finely sliced
- 1–2 tablespoons fresh lime juice
- 1 teaspoon raw honey (optional)

Peel the pineapple and remove the core. Shave the pineapple into very thin slices using a mandoline or short carving knife. Arrange the pineapple slices on a plate and fan them out. Evenly sprinkle the mint leaves over the pineapple. Drizzle the lime juice and honey, if using, on top of the pineapple.

Per serving: 57 calories, 1 g protein, 15 g carbohydrates, 0 g total fat, 0 g saturated fat, 2 g fiber, 1 mg sodium

POSITIVE EMOTIONS ELIXIRS

Violet Chakra (Crown) Elixir

TOTAL TIME: 10 minutes + resting time

Makes 2 servings

- 12 cherries, pitted and muddled
- 4 slices peeled cucumber
- 2 leaves mint, torn

In a 16-ounce mason jar, combine the cherries, cucumber, and mint. Fill the jar with ice cubes and water, shake, and refrigerate it overnight. The next morning, shake well and divide the elixir between two 8-ounce mason jars. Drink one jar in the morning and the second jar during the afternoon or evening. Refrigerate until ready to drink.

Per serving: 36 calories, 1 g protein, 9 g carbohydrates, 0 g total fat, 0 g saturated fat, 1 g fiber, 1 mg sodium

Indigo Chakra (Third-Eye) Elixir

TOTAL TIME: 10 minutes + resting time

Makes 2 servings

- 12 blackberries, muddled
- 4 slices peeled cucumber
- 2 leaves sage

In a 16-ounce mason jar, combine the blackberries, cucumber, and sage. Fill the jar with ice cubes and water, shake, and refrigerate it overnight. The next morning, shake well and divide the elixir between two 8-ounce mason jars. Drink one jar in the morning and the second jar during the afternoon or evening. Refrigerate until ready to drink.

Per serving: 19 calories, 1 g protein, 4 g carbohydrates, 0 g total fat, 0 g saturated fat, 2 g fiber, 1 mg sodium

Blue Chakra (Throat) Elixir

TOTAL TIME: 10 minutes + resting time

Makes 2 servings

- 16 blueberries, muddled
- 4 slices peeled cucumber
- 1 sprig thyme
- 1 leaf fresh mint, torn

In a 16-ounce mason jar, combine the blueberries, cucumber, thyme, and mint. Fill the jar with ice cubes and water, shake, and refrigerate it overnight. The next morning, shake well and divide the elixir between two 8-ounce mason jars. Drink one jar in the morning and the second jar during the afternoon or evening. Refrigerate until ready to drink.

Per serving: 9 calories, 0 g protein, 2 g carbohydrates, 0 g total fat, 0 g saturated fat, 0 g fiber, 1 mg sodium

Green Chakra (Heart) Elixir

TOTAL TIME: 10 minutes + resting time

Makes 2 servings

- 1 medium organic or well-washed Granny Smith apple, sliced
- 4 slices peeled cucumber
- 4 slices celery
- 1 teaspoon freshly squeezed lime juice
- 1 sprig thyme
- ⅛ teaspoon spirulina (optional)

In a 16-ounce mason jar, combine the apple slices, cucumber, celery, lime juice, thyme, and spirulina (if using). Fill the jar with ice cubes and water, shake, and refrigerate it overnight. The next morning, shake well and divide the elixir between two 8-ounce mason jars. Drink one jar in the morning and the second jar during the afternoon or evening. Refrigerate until ready to drink.

Per serving: 38 calories, 0 g protein, 10 g carbohydrates, 0 g total fat, 0 g saturated fat, 2 g fiber, 1 mg sodium

Yellow Chakra (Solar Plexus) Elixir

TOTAL TIME: 10 minutes + resting time

Makes 2 servings

- 8 chunks pineapple, cubed and muddled
- 2 slices peeled cucumber
- 1 teaspoon freshly squeezed lime juice
- 2 pinches bee pollen (optional)

In a 16-ounce mason jar, combine the pineapple, cucumber, lime juice, and bee pollen (if using). Fill the jar with ice cubes and water, shake, and refrigerate it overnight. The next morning, shake well and divide the elixir between two 8-ounce mason jars. Drink one jar in the morning and the second jar during the afternoon or evening. Refrigerate until ready to drink.

Per serving: 22 calories, 0 g protein, 6 g carbohydrates, 0 g total fat, 0 g saturated fat, 1 g fiber, 1 mg sodium

Orange Chakra (Abdomen) Elixir

TOTAL TIME: 10 minutes + resting time

Makes 2 servings

- 1 orange, quartered and gently squeezed
- 2 teaspoons freshly squeezed lemon juice
- 1 teaspoon hempseeds (optional)

In a 16-ounce mason jar, combine the orange, lemon juice, and hempseeds (if using). Fill the jar with ice cubes and water, shake, and refrigerate it overnight. The next morning, shake well and divide the elixir between two 8-ounce mason jars. Drink one jar in the morning and the second jar during the afternoon or evening. Refrigerate until ready to drink.

Per serving: 20 calories, 0 g protein, 5 g carbohydrates, 0 g total fat, 0 g saturated fat, 0 g fiber, 0 mg sodium

Red Chakra (Root) Elixir

TOTAL TIME: 10 minutes + resting time

Makes 2 servings

- 12 strawberries, muddled
- 4 slices peeled cucumber
- 2 teaspoons goji berries (optional)
- 1 teaspoon chia seeds (optional)

In a 16-ounce mason jar, combine the strawberries, cucumber, and goji berries and chia seeds (if using). Fill the jar with ice cubes and water, shake, and refrigerate it overnight. The next morning, shake well and divide the elixir between two 8-ounce mason jars. Drink one jar in the morning and the second jar during the afternoon or evening. Refrigerate until ready to drink.

Per serving: 38 calories, 1 g protein, 9 g carbohydrates, 0 g total fat, 0 g saturated fat, 2 g fiber, 2 mg sodium

Sunshine Gold Elixir

TOTAL TIME: 10 minutes + resting time

Makes 2 servings

- 6 chunks mango, muddled
- 1 teaspoon freshly squeezed lemon juice
- ⅛ teaspoon ground turmeric (optional)

In a 16-ounce mason jar, combine the mango, lemon juice, and turmeric (if using). Fill the jar with ice cubes and water, shake, and refrigerate it overnight. The next morning, shake well and divide the elixir between two 8-ounce mason jars. Drink one jar in the morning and the second jar during the afternoon or evening. Refrigerate until ready to drink.

Per serving: 25 calories, 0 g protein, 6 g carbohydrates, 0 g total fat, 0 g saturated fat, 1 g fiber, 0 mg sodium

Apple-Rosemary Elixir

TOTAL TIME: 10 minutes + resting time

Makes 2 servings

1 Fuji apple, sliced (peeled if not organic)

Pinch of rosemary

In a 16-ounce mason jar, combine the apple slices and rosemary. Fill the jar with ice cubes and water, shake, and refrigerate it overnight. The next morning, shake well and divide the elixir between two 8-ounce mason jars. Drink one jar in the morning and the second jar during the afternoon or evening. Refrigerate until ready to drink.

Per serving: 40 calories, 0 g protein, 11 g carbohydrates, 0 g total fat, 0 g saturated fat, 2 g fiber, 0 mg sodium

Pineapple Elixir

TOTAL TIME: 10 minutes + resting time

Makes 2 servings

1 cup cubed pineapple, muddled
4 slices peeled cucumber
4 slices celery
2 leaves cilantro (optional)
2 teaspoons freshly squeezed lime juice (optional)

In a 16-ounce mason jar, combine the pineapple, cucumber, celery, and cilantro and lime juice (if using). Fill the jar with ice cubes and water, shake, and refrigerate it overnight. The next morning, shake well and divide the elixir between two 8-ounce mason jars. Drink one jar in the morning and the second jar during the afternoon or evening. Refrigerate until ready to drink.

Per serving: 44 calories, 1 g protein, 11 g carbohydrates, 0 g total fat, 0 g saturated fat, 1 g fiber, 6 mg sodium

Watermelon-Mint Elixir

TOTAL TIME: 10 minutes + resting time

Makes 2 servings

1 cup cubed seedless watermelon

4 leaves fresh mint, torn

2 teaspoons freshly squeezed lime juice

In a 16-ounce mason jar, combine the watermelon, mint, and lime juice. Fill the jar with ice cubes and water, shake, and refrigerate it overnight. The next morning, shake well and divide the elixir between two 8-ounce mason jars. Drink one jar in the morning and the second jar during the afternoon or evening. Refrigerate until ready to drink.

Per serving: 24 calories, 0 g protein, 6 g carbohydrates, 0 g total fat, 0 g saturated fat, 0 g fiber, 1 mg sodium

Kumquat Elixir

TOTAL TIME: 10 minutes + resting time

Makes 2 servings

1 kumquat, thinly sliced

Juice of ½ orange

2 leaves fresh mint, torn

In a 16-ounce mason jar, combine the kumquat, orange juice, and mint. Fill the jar with ice cubes and water, shake, and refrigerate it overnight. The next morning, shake well and divide the elixir between two 8-ounce mason jars. Drink one jar in the morning and the second jar during the afternoon or evening. Refrigerate until ready to drink.

Per serving: 16 calories, 0 g protein, 4 g carbohydrates, 0 g total fat, 0 g saturated fat, 1 g fiber, 1 mg sodium

ENDNOTES

Introduction

1 A. S. Go et al., "Executive Summary: Heart Disease and Stroke Statistics—2014 Update: A Report from the American Heart Association," *Circulation* 129, no. 3 (2014): 399–410.

2 Centers for Disease Control and Prevention, "Heart Disease Facts," last updated February 19, 2014, www.cdc.gov/heartdisease/facts.htm.

3 S. Yusuf et al.; INTERHEART Study Investigators. "Effect of Potentially Modifiable Risk Factors Associated with Myocardial Infarction in 52 Countries (the INTERHEART study): Case-Control Study," *Lancet* 364 (September 2004): 937–52.

4 Z. Khayyam-Nekouei et al., "Psychological Factors and Coronary Heart Disease," *ARYA Atherosclerosis* 9, no. 1 (January 2013): 102–11.

Chapter 1

1 O. Soran, A. M. Feldman, and H. A. Cohen, "Oculostenotic Reflex and Iatrogenosis Fulminans," *Circulation* 101, no. 20 (May 2000): 198–99.

2 P. A. Tonino et al, "Angiographic versus Functional Severity of Coronary Artery Stenoses in the FAME Study: Fractional Flow Reserve versus Angiography in Multivessel Evaluation," *Journal of the American College of Cardiology* 55, no. 5 (June 2010): 2816–21.

3 B. Pitt et al.; Atorvastatin versus Revascularization Treatment Investigators, "Aggressive Lipid-Lowering Therapy Compared with Angioplasty in Stable Coronary Artery Disease," *New England Journal of Medicine* 341, no. 2 (July 1999): 70–76.

4 W. E. Boden et al.; COURAGE Trial Research Group. "Optimal Medical Therapy with or without PCI for Stable Coronary Disease," *New England Journal of Medicine* 356, no. 15 (April 2007): 1503–16.

5 J. K. Liao and U. Laufs, "Pleiotropic Effects of Statins," *Annual Review of Pharmacology and Toxicology* 45 (February 2005): 89–118.

6 I. D. Nicholl and R. Bucala, "Advanced Glycation Endproducts and Cigarette Smoking," *Cellular and Molecular Biology* 44, no. 7 (1998): 1025–33.

7 J. Smith Hopkins, "William C. Stanley, 56, Cardiovascular Physiologist," *Baltimore Sun*, November 3, 2013, http://articles.baltimoresun.com/2013-11-03/news/bs-md-ob-stanley-20131103_1_heart-failure-william-c-assistant-professor.

8 A. M. Roest et al., "Anxiety and Risk of Incident Coronary Heart Disease: A Meta-Analysis," *Journal of the American College of Cardiology* 56, no. 1 (2010): 38–46.

9 A. R. Moraska et al., “Depression, Healthcare Utilization, and Death in Heart Failure: A Community Study,” *Circulation: Heart Failure* 6, no. 3 (May 2013): 387–94.

10 C. A. Jackson and G. D. Mishra, “Depression and Risk of Stroke in Midaged Women: A Prospective Longitudinal Study,” *Stroke* 44, no. 6 (June 2013): 1555–60.

11 E. Mostofsky et al., “Relation of Outbursts of Anger and Risk of Acute Myocardial Infarction,” *American Journal of Cardiology* 112, no. 3 (August 2013): 343–48.

12 E. Mostofsky, E. A. Penner, and M. A. Mittleman, “Outbursts of Anger as a Trigger of Acute Cardiovascular Events: A Systematic Review and Meta-Analysis,” *European Heart Journal*, first published online March 3, 2014, doi:10.1093/eurheartj/ehu033.

13 N. J. Stone et al., “Treatment of Blood Cholesterol to Reduce Atherosclerotic Cardiovascular Disease Risk in Adults: Synopsis of the 2013 ACC/AHA Cholesterol Guideline,” *Annals of Internal Medicine* 160, no. 5 (March 2014): 339–43.

14 F. I. Marcus et al., “Alternate-Day Dosing with Statins,” *American Journal of Medicine* 126, no. 2 (February 2013): 99–104.

15 R. Schulz and S. R. Beach, “Caregiving as a Risk Factor for Mortality: The Caregiver Health Effects Study,” *JAMA* 282, no. 23 (1999): 2215–19.

16 W. E. Haley et al., “Caregiving Strain and Estimated Risk for Stroke and Coronary Heart Disease Among Spouse Caregivers: Differential Effects by Race and Sex,” *Stroke* 41, no. 2 (February 2010): 331–36.

Chapter 2

1 S. N. Young, “How to Increase Serotonin in the Human Brain without Drugs,” *Journal of Psychiatry and Neuroscience* 32, no. 6 (November 2007): 394–99.

2 L. E. Cahill et al., “Prospective Study of Breakfast Eating and Incident Coronary Heart Disease in a Cohort of Male US Health Professionals,” *Circulation* 128, no. 4 (July 2013): 337–43.

3 C. Le Fur et al., “Influence of Mental Stress and Circadian Cycle on Postprandial Lipemia,” *American Journal of Clinical Nutrition* 70, no. 2 (August 1999): 213–20.

4 M. Miller et al., “An NCEP II Diet Reduces Postprandial Triacylglycerol in Normocholesterolemic Adults,” *Journal of Nutrition* 128, no. 3 (March 1998): 582–86.

5 M. Miller et al., “Comparative Effects of Three Popular Diets on Lipids, Endothelial Function, and C-Reactive Protein during Weight Maintenance,” *Journal of the American Dietetic Association* 109, no. 4 (April 2009): 713–17.

6 G. Assmann et al., “The Emergence of Triglycerides as a Significant Independent Risk Factor in Coronary Artery Disease,” *European Heart Journal* 19, supplement M (October 1998): M8–M14.

7 M. Miller et al. “Triglycerides and Cardiovascular Disease: A Scientific Statement from the American Heart Association,” *Circulation* 123, no. 20 (May 2011): 2292–333.

8 M. Miller et al. "Normal Triglyceride Levels and Coronary Artery Disease Events: The Baltimore Coronary Observational Long-Term Study," *Journal of the American College of Cardiology* 31, no. 6 (May 1998): 1252–57.

9 M. Miller et al. "Incorporation of Oleic Acid and Eicosapentaenoic Acid into Glycerolipids of Cultured Normal Human Fibroblasts," *Lipids* 28, no. 1 (January 1993): 1–5.

10 N. J. Stone et al., "2013 ACC/AHA Guideline on the Treatment of Blood Cholesterol to Reduce Atherosclerotic Cardiovascular Risk in Adults: A Report of the American College of Cardiology/American Heart Association Task Force on Practice Guidelines," *Journal of the American College of Cardiology*, first published online November 7, 2013, doi: 10.1016/j.jacc.2013.11.002.

11 M. Miller et al., "Impact of Triglyceride Levels beyond Low-Density Lipoprotein Cholesterol after Acute Coronary Syndrome in the PROVE IT-TIMI 22 Trial," *Journal of the American College of Cardiology* 51, no. 7 (February 2008): 724–30.

12 M. Miller et al. "Does Low HDL-C Increase CHD Risk When TG and LDL-C Are Normal? The Framingham Offspring Study," *Journal of the American College of Cardiology* 63, no. 2 (March 2014): 12S.

13 Centers for Disease Control and Prevention, "Adult BMI Calculator: English," last updated October 24, 2013, www.cdc.gov/healthyweight/assessing/bmi/adult_bmi/english_bmi_calculator/bmi_calculator.html.

14 E. J. Jacobs et al., "Waist Circumference and All-Cause Mortality in a Large US Cohort," *Archives of Internal Medicine* 170, no. 15 (August 2010): 1293–301.

15 Mayo Clinic, "Carbohydrates: How Carbs Fit into a Healthy Diet," February 8, 2011, www.mayoclinic.org/healthy-living/nutrition-and-healthy-eating/in-depth/carbohydrates/art-20045705?pg=1.

16 E. Walderhaug et al., "Interactive Effects of Sex and 5-HTTLPR on Mood and Impulsivity during Tryptophan Depletion in Healthy People," *Biological Psychiatry* 62, no. 6 (September 2007): 593–99.

17 S. N. Young, "How to Increase Serotonin in the Human Brain without Drugs," *Journal of Psychiatry and Neuroscience* 32, no. 6 (November 2007): 394–99.

18 A. M. Spaeth, D. F. Dinges, and N. Goel, "Effects of Experimental Sleep Restriction on Weight Gain, Caloric Intake, and Meal Timing in Healthy Adults," *SLEEP* 36, no. 7 (July 2013): 981–90.

19 A. L. Miller, "The Methylation, Neurotransmitter, and Antioxidant Connections between Folate and Depression," *Alternative Medicine Review* 13, no. 3 (September 2008): 216–26.

20 K. J. Mukamal, "Understanding the Mechanisms That Link Alcohol and Lower Risk of Coronary Heart Disease," *Clinical Chemistry* 58, no. 4 (2012): 664–66.

21 C. Griffith and D. Bogart, "Alcohol Consumption: Can We Safely Toast to Our Health?" *Missouri Medicine* 109, no. 6 (2012): 459–65.

22 J. M. Mitchell et al., "Alcohol Consumption Induces Endogenous Opioid Release in the Human Orbitofrontal Cortex and Nucleus Accumbens," *Science Translational Medicine* 4, no. 116 (January 2012), doi: 10.1126/scitranslmed.3002902.

23 X. Wu et al., "Lipophilic and Hydrophilic Antioxidant Capacities of Common Foods in the United States," *Journal of Agricultural and Food Chemistry* 52, no. 12 (June 2004): 4026–37.

24 USDA Agricultural Research Service, "National Nutrient Database for Standard Reference," release 26, http://ndb.nal.usda.gov/ndb/search/list.

25 I. Slutsky et al., "Enhancement of Learning and Memory by Elevating Brain Magnesium," *Neuron* 65, no. 2 (2010): 165–77.

26 L. P. Christensen, "Galactolipids as Potential Health Promoting Compounds in Vegetable Foods," *Recent Patents on Food, Nutrition & Agriculture* 1, no. 1 (2009): 50–58.

27 R. Jasuja et al., "Protein Disulfide Isomerase Inhibitors Constitute a New Class of Antithrombotic Agents," *Journal of Clinical Investigation* 122, no. 6 (2012): 2104–13.

28 J. A. Ojewole et al., "Cardiovascular Effects of *Persea Americana* Mill (Lauraceae) (Avocado) Aqueous Leaf Extract in Experimental Animals," *Cardiovascular Journal of Africa* 18, no. 2 (2007): 69–76.

29 Z. Li et al., "Hass Avocado Modulates Postprandial Vascular Reactivity and Postprandial Inflammatory Responses to a Hamburger Meal in Healthy Volunteers," *Food & Function* 4, no. 3 (2013): 384–91.

30 S. Hulsken et al., "Food-Derived Serotonergic Modulators: Effects on Mood and Cognition," *Nutrition Research Reviews* 26, no. 2 (2013): 223–34.

31 B. C. Schwahn et al., "Betaine Supplementation Improves the Atherogenic Risk Factor Profile in a Transgenic Mouse Model of Hyperhomocysteinemia," *Atherosclerosis* 195, no. 2 (2007): 100–107.

32 University of Maryland Medical Center, "S-Adenosylmethionine," last updated June 24, 2013, http://umm.edu/health/medical/altmed/supplement/sadenosylmethionine.

33 J. R. Hoffman et al., "Effect of Betaine Supplementation on Power Performance and Fatigue," *Journal of the International Society of Sports Nutrition* 6 (2009), doi:10.1186/1550-2783-6-7.

34 A. Cassidy et al., "High Anthocyanin Intake Is Associated with a Reduced Risk of Myocardial Infarction in Young and Middle-Aged Women," *Circulation* 127, no. 2 (2013): 188–96.

35 J. K. Udani et al., "Effects of Açai (*Euterpe oleracea* Mart.) Berry Preparation on Metabolic Parameters in a Healthy Overweight Population: A Pilot Study," *Nutrition Journal* 10 (2011), doi:10.1186/1475-2891-10-45.

36 M. F. Ramadan et al., "Goldenberry (*Physalis peruviana*) Juice Rich in Health-Beneficial Compounds Suppresses High-Cholesterol Diet-Induced Hypercholesterolemia in Rats," *Journal of Food Biochemistry* 37, no. 6 (2013): 708–22.

37 J. L. Medina-Franco et al., "Chemoinformatic Analysis of GRAS (Generally Recognized as Safe) Flavor Chemicals and Natural Products," *PLOS ONE* 7, no. 11 (2012), doi: 10.1371/journal.pone.0050798.

38 M. H. Moghadam, M. Imenshahidi, and S. A. Mohajeri, "Antihypertensive Effect of Celery Seed on Rat Blood Pressure in Chronic Administration," *Journal of Medicinal Food* 16, no. 6 (2013): 558–63.

39 D. Sun et al., "Luteolin Limits Infarct Size and Improves Cardiac Function after Myocardium Ischemia/Reperfusion Injury in Diabetic Rats," *PLOS ONE* 7, no. 3 (2012), doi: 10.1371/journal.pone.0033491.

40 S. Jang, R. N. Dilger, and R. W. Johnson, "Luteolin Inhibits Microglia and Alters Hippocampal-Dependent Spatial Working Memory in Aged Mice," *Journal of Nutrition* 140, no. 10 (2010): 1892–98.

41 Q. T. Le and W. J. Elliott, "Hypotensive and Hypocholesterolemic Effects of Celery Oil May Be due to BuPh," *Clinical Research* 39 (1991): 173A.

42 L. M. McCune et al., "Cherries and Health: A Review," *Critical Reviews in Food Science and Nutrition* 51, no. 1 (2011): 1–12.

43 G. Howatson et al., "Effect of Tart Cherry Juice (*Prunus cerasus*) on Melatonin Levels and Enhanced Sleep Quality," *European Journal of Nutrition* 51, no. 8 (2012): 909–16.

44 Y. T. Liang et al., "Capsaicinoids Lower Plasma Cholesterol and Improve Endothelial Function in Hamsters," *European Journal of Nutrition* 52, no. 1 (2013): 379–88.

45 S. Patanè et al., "Capsaicin and Arterial Hypertensive Crisis," *International Journal of Cardiology* 144, no. 2 (2010): 26–27.

46 S. Langer et al., "Flavanols and Methylxanthines in Commercially Available Dark Chocolate: A Study of the Correlation with Nonfat Cocoa Solids," *Journal of Agricultural and Food Chemistry* 59, no. 15 (2011): 8435–41.

47 L. Thors, M. Belghiti, and C. J. Fowler, "Inhibition of Fatty Acid Amide Hydrolase by Kaempferol and Related Naturally Occurring Flavonoids," *British Journal of Pharmacology* 155, no. 2 (2008): 244–52.

48 M. P. Pase et al., "Cocoa Polyphenols Enhance Positive Mood States but Not Cognitive Performance: A Randomized, Placebo-Controlled Trial," *Journal of Psychopharmacology* 27, no. 5 (2013): 451–58.

49 K. A. Cooper et al., "Cocoa and Health: A Decade of Research," *British Journal of Nutrition* 99, no. 1 (2008): 1–11.

50 K. Ried et al., "Effect of Cocoa on Blood Pressure," *Cochrane Database of Systematic Reviews* 8 (August 2012), doi:10.1002/14651858.

51 J. Hlebowicz et al., "Effect of Cinnamon on Postprandial Blood Glucose, Gastric Emptying, and Satiety in Healthy Subjects," *American Journal of Clinical Nutrition* 85, no. 6 (2007): 1552–56.

52 R. Akilen et al., "Effect of Short-Term Administration of Cinnamon on Blood Pressure in Patients with Prediabetes and Type 2 Diabetes," *Nutrition* 29, no. 10 (2013): 1192–96.

53 B. Raudenbush et al., "Effects of Peppermint and Cinnamon Odor Administration on Simulated Driving Alertness, Mood, and Workload," *North American Journal of Psychology* 11, no. 2 (2009): 245–56.

54 R. B. Postuma et al., "Caffeine for Treatment of Parkinson Disease: A Randomized Controlled Trial," *Neurology* 79, no. 7 (2012): 651–58.

55 M. H. Eskelinen et al., "Midlife Coffee and Tea Drinking and the Risk of Late-Life Dementia: A Population-Based CAIDE Study," *Journal of Alzheimer's Disease* 16, no. 1 (2009): 85–91.

56 X. Jiang, D. Zhang, and W. Jiang, "Coffee and Caffeine Intake and Incidence of Type 2 Diabetes Mellitus: A Meta-Analysis of Prospective Studies," *European Journal of Nutrition* 53, no. 1 (2013): 25–38.

57 M. F. McCarty, "A Chlorogenic Acid-Induced Increase in GLP-1 Production May Mediate the Impact of Heavy Coffee Consumption on Diabetes Risk," *Medical Hypotheses* 64, no. 4 (2005): 848–53.

58 S. Meng et al., "Roles of Chlorogenic Acid on Regulating Glucose and Lipids Metabolism: A Review," *Evidence-Based Complementary and Alternative Medicine* (2013), doi:10.1155/2013/801457.

59 Harvard University Health Services, "Fiber Content of Foods in Common Portions," May 2004, http://huhs.harvard.edu/assets/File/OurServices/Service_Nutrition_Fiber.pdf.

60 Z. Wang et al., "Gut Flora Metabolism of Phosphatidylcholine Promotes Cardiovascular Disease," *Nature* 472, no. 7341 (2011): 57–63.

61 T. A. Shamliyan et al., "Are Your Patients with Risk of CVD Getting the Viscous Soluble Fiber They Need?" *Journal of Family Practice* 55, no. 9 (2006): 761–69.

62 R. K. McNamara et al. "Selective Deficits in the Omega-3 Fatty Acid Docosahexaenoic Acid in the Postmortem Orbitofrontal Cortex of Patients with Major Depressive Disorder," *Biological Psychiatry* 62 (2007): 17–24.

63 T. Komori et al., "Effects of Citrus Fragrance on Immune Function and Depressive States," *Neuroimmunomodulation* 2, no. 3 (1995): 174–80.

64 G. E. Felton, "Fibrinolytic and Antithrombotic Action of Bromelain May Eliminate Thrombosis in Heart Patients," *Medical Hypotheses* 6, no. 11 (1980): 1123–33.

65 S. Egert et al., "Quercetin Reduces Systolic Blood Pressure and Plasma Oxidised Low-Density Lipoprotein Concentrations in Overweight Subjects with a High-Cardiovascular Disease Risk Phenotype: A Double-Blinded, Placebo-Controlled Cross-Over Study," *British Journal of Nutrition* 102, no. 7 (2009): 1065–74.

66 I. C. Arts et al., "Dietary Catechins in Relation to Coronary Heart Disease among Postmenopausal Women," *Epidemiology* 12, no. 6 (2001): 668–75.

67 A. Briggs, "A Statin a Day Keeps the Doctor Away: Comparative Proverb Assessment Modeling Study," *BMJ* 347 (2013), doi:10.1136/bmj.f7267.

68 S. C. Chai et al., "Daily Apple versus Dried Plum: Impact on Cardiovascular Disease Risk Factors in Postmenopausal Women," *Journal of the Academy of Nutrition and Dietetics* 112, no. 8 (2012): 1158–68.

69 P. Knekt et al., "Quercetin Intake and the Incidence of Cerebrovascular Disease," *European Journal of Clinical Nutrition* 54, no. 5 (2000): 415–17.

70 M. Ali and M. Thomson, "Consumption of a Garlic Clove a Day Could Be Beneficial in Preventing Thrombosis," *Prostaglandins, Leukotrienes, and Essential Fatty Acids* 53, no. 3 (1995): 211–12.

71 S. Warshafsky, R. S. Kramer, and S. L. Sivak, "Effect of Garlic on Total Serum Cholesterol: A Meta-Analysis," *Annals of Internal Medicine* 119, no. 7, part 1 (October 1993): 599–605.

72 L. C. Tapsell et al., "Health Benefits of Herbs and Spices: The Past, the Present, the Future," *Medical Journal of Australia* 185, supplement 4 (2006): S4–S24.

73 J. Kleijnen, P. Knipschild, and G. ter Riet, "Garlic, Onions, and Cardiovascular Risk Factors. A Review of the Evidence from Human Experiments with Emphasis on Commercially Available Preparations," *British Journal of Clinical Pharmacology* 28, no. 5 (1989): 535–44.

74 N. Morihara et al., "Aged Garlic Extract Ameliorates Physical Fatigue," *Biological and Pharmaceutical Bulletin* 29, no. 5 (2006): 962–66.

75 H. Kikuzaki and N. Nakatani, "Antioxidant Effects of Some Ginger Constituents," *Journal of Food Science* 58, no. 6 (1993): 1407–10.

76 S. Atashak et al., "Obesity-Related Cardiovascular Risk Factors after Long-Term Resistance Training and Ginger Supplementation," *Journal of Sports Science and Medicine* 10, no. 4 (2011): 685–91.

77 A. M. Waggas, "Neuroprotective Evaluation of Extract of Ginger (*Zingiber officinale*) Root in Monosodium Glutamate-Induced Toxicity in Different Brain Areas Male Albino Rats," *Pakistan Journal of Biological Sciences* 12, no. 3 (2009): 201–12.

78 C. A. Rivera et al. "Probable Interaction Between Lycium Barbarum (Goji) and Warfarin," *Pharmacotherapy* 32, no. 3 (March 2012): e50–53.

79 A. L. Hopkins et al., "*Hibiscus sabdariffa* L. in the Treatment of Hypertension and Hyperlipidemia: A Comprehensive Review of Animal and Human Studies," *Fitoterapia* 85 (March 2013): 84–94.

80 D. L. McKay et al., "*Hibiscus Sabdariffa* L. Tea (Tisane) Lowers Blood Pressure in Prehypertensive and Mildly Hypertensive Adults," *Journal of Nutrition* 140, no. 2 (2010): 298–303.

81 R. Kuriyan et al., "An Evaluation of the Hypolipidemic Effect of an Extract of *Hibiscus sabdariffa* Leaves in Hyperlipidemic Indians: A Double Blind, Placebo Controlled Trial," *BMC Complementary and Alternative Medicine* 10 (2010), doi:10.1186/1472-6882-10-27.

82 G. Ramadan et al., "Preventive Effects of Egyptian Sweet Marjoram (*Origanum majorana* L.) Leaves on Haematological Changes and Cardiotoxicity in Isoproterenol-Treated Albino Rats," *Cardiovascular Toxicology* 13, no. 2 (2013): 100–109.

83 S. Cheung and J. Tai, "Anti-Proliferative and Antioxidant Properties of Rosemary *Rosmarinus officinalis*," *Oncology Reports* 17, no. 6 (2007): 1525–31.

84 K. P. Bhargava and N. Singh, "Anti-Stress Activity of *Ocimum sanctum* Linn," *Indian Journal of Medical Research* 73 (March 1981): 443–51.

85 C. Vanzella et al., "Antidepressant-Like Effects of Methanol Extract of *Hibiscus tiliaceus* Flowers in Mice," *BMC Complementary and Alternative Medicine* 12 (April 2012), doi:10.1186/1472-6882-12-41.

86 A. O. Mechan et al., "Monoamine Reuptake Inhibition and Mood-Enhancing Potential of a Specified Oregano Extract," *British Journal of Nutrition* 105, no. 8 (2011): 1150–63.

87 M. Moss and L. Oliver, "Plasma 1,8-Cineole Correlates with Cognitive Performance Following Exposure to Rosemary Essential Oil Aroma," *Therapeutic Advances in Psychopharmacology* 2, no. 3 (2012): 103–13.

88 D. O. Kennedy et al., "Effects of Cholinesterase Inhibiting Sage (*Salvia officinalis*) on Mood, Anxiety, and Performance on a Psychological Stressor Battery," *Neuropsychopharmacology* 31, no. 4 (2006): 845–52.

89 S. Bommer, P. Klein, and A. Suter, "First Time Proof of Sage's Tolerability and Efficacy in Menopausal Women with Hot Flushes," *Advances in Therapy* 28, no. 6 (2011): 490–500.

90 J. K. Boehm et al., "Association between Optimism and Serum Antioxidants in the Midlife in the United States Study," *Psychosomatic Medicine* 75, no. 1 (2013): 2–10.

91 Y. Tsuruta et al., "Effects of Lotus Root (the Edible Rhizome of *Nelumbo nucifera*) on the Deveolopment of Non-Alcoholic Fatty Liver Disease in Obese Diabetic Db/Db Mice," *Bioscience, Biotechnology, and Biochemistry* 76, no. 3 (2012): 462–66.

92 R. Chhabra et al., "Association of Coronary Artery Calcification with Hepatic Steatosis in Asymptomatic Individuals," *Mayo Clinic Proceedings* 88, no. 11 (2013): 1259–65.

93 G. F. Gonzales, M. Gasco, and I. Lozada-Requena, "Role of Maca (*Lepidium meyenii*) Consumption on Serum Interleukin-6 Levels and Health Status in Populations Living in the Peruvian Central Andes over 4000 M of Altitude," *Plant Foods for Human Nutrition* 68, no. 4 (2013): 347–51.

94 R. Vecera et al., "The Influence of Maca (*Lepidium meyenii*) on Antioxidant Status, Lipid and Glucose Metabolism in Rat," *Plant Foods for Human Nutrition* 62, no. 2 (2007): 59–63.

95 C. M. Dording et al., "A Double-Blind, Randomized, Pilot Dose-Finding Study of Maca Root (*L. meyenii*) for the Management of SSRI-Induced Sexual Dysfunction," *CNS Neuroscience & Therapeutics* 14, no. 3 (2008): 182–91.

96 C. C. Lau, N. Abdullah, and A. S. Shuib, "Novel Angiotensin I-Converting Enzyme Inhibitory Peptides Derived from an Edible Mushroom, *Pleurotus cystidiosus* O.K. Miller Identified by LC-MS/MS," *BMC Complementary and Alternative Medicine* 13 (November 2013), doi:10.1186/1472-6882-13-313.

97 K. H. Poddar et al., "Positive Effect of Mushrooms Substituted for Meat on Body Weight, Body Composition, and Health Parameters. A 1-Year Randomized Clinical Trial," *Appetite* 71 (December 2013): 379–87.

98 M. Nagano et al., "Reduction of Depression and Anxiety by 4 Weeks *Hericium erinaceus* Intake," *Biomedical Research* 31, no. 4 (2010): 231–37.

99 N. T. Gregersen et al., "Acute Effects of Mustard, Horseradish, Black Pepper, and Ginger on Energy Expenditure, Appetite, Ad Libitum Energy Intake, and Energy Balance in Human Subjects," *British Journal of Nutrition* 109, no. 3 (2013): 556–63.

100 S. Akbar, S. Bellary, and H. Griffiths, "Dietary Antioxidant Interventions in Type 2 Diabetes Patients: A Meta-Analysis," *British Journal of Diabetes and Vascular Disease* 11, no. 2 (2011): 62–68.

101 J. Bergman et al., "Curcumin as an Add-On to Antidepressive Treatment: A Randomized, Double-Blind, Placebo-Controlled, Pilot Clinical Study," *Clinical Neuropharmacology* 36, no. 3 (2013): 73–77.

102 J. Sabaté and G. E. Fraser, "Nuts: A New Protective Food against Coronary Heart Disease," *Current Opinion in Lipidology* 5, no. 1 (1994): 11–16.

103 P. M. Kris-Etherton et al., "The Role of Tree Nuts and Peanuts in the Prevention of Coronary Heart Disease: Multiple Potential Mechanisms," *Journal of Nutrition* 138, no. 9 (2008): S1746–S1751.

104 G. Flores-Mateo et al., "Nut Intake and Adiposity: Meta-Analysis of Clinical Trials," *American Journal of Clinical Nutrition* 97, no. 6 (2013): 1346–55.

105 Z. Li et al., "Pistachio Nuts Reduce Triglycerides and Body Weight by Comparison to Refined Carbohydrate Snack in Obese Subjects on a 12-Week Weight Loss Program," *Journal of the American College of Nutrition* 29, no. 3 (2010): 198–203.

106 S. Tulipani et al., "Metabolomics Unveils Urinary Changes in Subjects with Metabolic Syndrome following 12-Week Nut Consumption," *Journal of Proteome Research* 10, no. 11 (2011): 5047–58.

107 A. Sánchez-Villegas et al., "Mediterranean Dietary Pattern and Depression: The PREDIMED Randomized Trial," *BMC Medicine* 11 (2013), doi:10.1186/1741-7015-11-208.

108 R. Estruch et al., "Primary Prevention of Cardiovascular Disease with a Mediterranean Diet," *New England Journal of Medicine* 368, no. 14 (2013): 1279–90.

109 E. A. Thomas, M. J. Carson, and J. G. Sutcliffe, "Oleamide-Induced Modulation of 5-Hydroxytryptamine Receptor-Mediated Signaling," *Annals of the New York Academy of Sciences* 861 (December 1998): 183–89.

110 A. Kyrozis et al., "Dietary Lipids and Geriatric Depression Scale Score among Elders: The EPIC-Greece Cohort," *Journal of Psychiatric Research* 43, no. 8 (2009): 763–69.

111 B. S. Kendler, "Garlic (*Allium sativum*) and Onion (*Allium cepa*): A Review of Their Relationship to Cardiovascular Disease," *Preventive Medicine* 16, no. 5 (1987): 670–85.

112 A. K. Patel, J. T. Rogers, and X. Huang, "Flavanols, Mild Cognitive Impairment, and Alzheimer's Dementia," *International Journal of Clinical and Experimental Medicine* 1, no. 2 (2008): 181–91.

113 R. R. Huxley and H. A. Neil, "The Relation between Dietary Flavonol Intake and Coronary Heart Disease Mortality: A Meta-Analysis of Prospective Cohort Studies," *European Journal of Clinical Nutrition* 57, no. 8 (2003): 904–908.

114 H. Sakakibara et al., "Antidepressant-Like Effect of Onion (*Allium cepa* L.) Powder in a Rat Behavioral Model of Depression," *Bioscience, Biotechnology, and Biochemistry* 72, no. 1 (2008): 94–100.

115 J. R. Davidson et al., "Effectiveness of Chromium in Atypical Depression: A Placebo-Controlled Trial," *Biological Psychiatry* 53, no. 3 (2003): 261–64.

116 H. Sakakibara et al., "Antidepressant-Like Effect of Onion (*Allium cepa* L.) Powder in a Rat Behavioral Model of Depression," *Bioscience, Biotechnology, and Biochemistry* 72, no. 1 (2008): 94–100.

117 S. Gorinstein et al., "Comparative Contents of Dietary Fiber, Total Phenolics, and Minerals in Persimmons and Apples," *Journal of Agricultural and Food Chemistry* 49, no. 2 (2001): 952–57.

118 B. J. An et al., "Inhibition of Enzyme Activities and the Antiwrinkle Effect of Polyphenol Isolated from the Persimmon Leaf (*Diospyros kaki* Folium) on Human Skin," *Dermatologic Surgery* 31, no. 7, part 2 (2005): 848–54.

119 M. D. Sumner et al., "Effects of Pomegranate Juice Consumption on Myocardial Perfusion in Patients with Coronary Heart Disease," *American Journal of Cardiology* 96, no. 6 (2005): 810–14.

120 C. B. Stowe, "The Effects of Pomegranate Juice Consumption on Blood Pressure and Cardiovascular Health," *Complementary Therapies in Clinical Practice* 17, no. 2 (2011): 113–15.

121 E. Al-Dujaili and N. Smail, "Pomegranate Juice Intake Enhances Salivary Testosterone Levels and Improves Mood and Well Being in Healthy Men and Women," *Endocrine Abstracts* 28 (2012): 313.

122 S. Voutilainen et al., "Carotenoids and Cardiovascular Health," *American Journal of Clinical Nutrition* 83, no. 6 (2006): 1265–71.

123 T. Xia and Q. Wang, "Antihyperglycemic Effect of *Cucurbita ficifolia* Fruit Extract in Streptozotocin-Induced Diabetic Rats," *Fitoterapia* 77, no. 7–8 (2006): 530–33.

124 C. Hyounjeong et al., "A Water-Soluble Extract from *Cucurbita moschata* Shows Antiobesity Effects by Controlling Lipid Metabolism in a High Fat Diet–Induced Obesity

Mouse Model," *Biochemical and Biophysical Research Communications* 359, no. 3 (2007): 419–25.

125 M. N. Xanthopoulou et al., "Antioxidant and Lipoxygenase Inhibitory Activities of Pumpkin Seed Extracts," *Food Research International* 42, no. 5–6 (June–July 2009): 641–46.

126 A. S. Lee et al., "Anti-TNF-Đ Activity of *Portulaca oleracea* in Vascular Endothelial Cells," *International Journal of Molecular Sciences* 13, no. 5 (2012): 5628–44.

127 M. A. Dkhil et al., "Antioxidant Effect of Purslane (*Portulaca oleracea*) and Its Mechanism of Action," *Journal of Medicinal Plants Research* 5, no. 9 (2011): 1589–93.

128 A. Movahedian, A. Ghannadi, and M. Vashirnia, "Hypocholesterolemic Effects of Purslane Extract on Serum Lipids in Rabbits Fed with High Cholesterol Levels," *International Journal of Pharmacology* 3, no. 3 (2007): 285–89.

129 A. P. Simopoulos et al., "Common Purslane: A Source of Omega-3 Fatty Acids and Antioxidants," *Journal of the American College of Nutrition* 11, no. 4 (1992): 374–82.

130 University of Maryland Medical Center, "Alpha-Linolenic Acid," last updated June 19, 2013, http://umm.edu/health/medical/altmed/supplement/alphalinolenic-acid.

131 A. Pan et al., "Đ-Linolenic Acid and Risk of Cardiovascular Disease: A Systematic Review and Meta-Analysis," *American Journal of Clinical Nutrition* 96, no. 6 (2012): 1262–73.

132 T. D. Presley et al., "Acute Effect of a High Nitrate Diet on Brain Perfusion in Older Adults," *Nitric Oxide* 24, no. 1 (2011): 34–42.

133 M. Moss and L. Oliver, "Plasma 1,8-Cineole Correlates with Cognitive Performance following Exposure to Rosemary Essential Oil Aroma," *Therapeutic Advances in Psychopharmacology* 2, no. 3 (2012): 103–13.

134 M. Moss et al., "Aromas of Rosemary and Lavender Essential Oils Differentially Affect Cognition and Mood in Healthy Adults," *International Journal of Neuroscience* 113, no. 1 (2003): 15–38.

135 University of Maryland Medical Center, "Manganese," last updated May 7, 2013, http://umm.edu/health/medical/altmed/supplement/manganese#ixzz2pRMZwHe3; George Mateljan Foundation for the World's Healthiest Foods, "Manganese," www.whfoods.com/genpage.php?tname=nutrient&dbid=77#foodchart; and U. Rudrappa, "Saffron Nutrition Facts," Nutrition-And-You.com, www.nutrition-and-you.com/saffron.html.

136 M. Kamalipour and S. Akhondzadeh, "Cardiovascular Effects of Saffron: An Evidence-Based Review," *Journal of Tehran Heart Center* 6, no. 2 (2011): 59–61.

137 S. Akhondzadeh et al., "Saffron in the Treatment of Patients with Mild to Moderate Alzheimer's Disease: A 16-Week, Randomized and Placebo-Controlled Trial," *Journal of Clinical Pharmacy and Therapeutics* 35, no. 5 (2010): 581–88.

138 M. Agha-Hosseini et al., "*Crocus sativus* L. (Saffron) in the Treatment of Premenstrual Syndrome: A Double-Blind, Randomised and Placebo-Controlled Trial," *BJOG: An International Journal of Obstetrics and Gynaecology* 115, no. 4 (2008): 515–19.

139 A. Akhondzadeh Basti et al., "Comparison of Petal of *Crocus sativus* L. and Fluoxetine in the Treatment of Depressed Outpatients: A Pilot Double-Blind Randomized Trial," *Progress in Neuro-Psychopharmacology and Biological Psychiatry* 31, no. 2 (2007): 439–42.

140 A. V. Dwyer, D. L. Whitten, and J. A. Hawrelak, "Herbal Medicines, Other Than St. John's Wort, in the Treatment of Depression: A Systematic Review," *Alternative Medicine Review* 16, no. 1 (2011): 40–49.

141 C. Fitzgerald et al., "Heart Health Peptides from Macroalgae and Their Potential Use in Functional Foods," *Journal of Agricultural and Food Chemistry* 59, no. 13 (2011): 6829–36.

142 H. Maeda et al., "Anti-Obesity and Anti-Diabetic Effects of Fucoxanthin on Diet-Induced Obesity Conditions in a Murine Model," *Molecular Medicine Reports* 2, no. 6 (2009): 897–902.

143 D. Benton, "Selenium Intake, Mood, and Other Aspects of Psychological Functioning," *Nutritional Neuroscience* 5, no. 6 (2002): 363–74.

144 C. Berr, J. Arnaud, and T. N. Akbaraly, "Selenium and Cognitive Impairment: A Brief-Review Based on Results from the EVA Study," *Biofactors* 38, no. 2 (2012): 139–44.

145 D. Rodriguez-Leyva and G. N. Pierce, "The Cardiac and Haemostatic Effects of Dietary Hempseed," *Nutrition & Metabolism* 7 (2010), doi:10.1186/1743-7075-7-32.

146 N. Mohd Ali et al., "The Promising Future of Chia, *Salvia hispanica* L," *Journal of Biomedicine and Biotechnology* (2012), doi:10.1155/2012/171956.

147 P. Mirmiran et al., "Ardeh (*Sesamum indicum*) Could Improve Serum Triglycerides and Atherogenic Lipid Parameters in Type 2 Diabetic Patients: A Randomized Clinical Trial," *Archives of Iranian Medicine* 16, no. 11 (2013): 651–56.

148 R. Deng and T. J. Chow, "Hypolipidemic, Antioxidant, and Anti-inflammatory Activities of Microalgae Spirulina," *Cardiovascular Therapeutics* 28, no. 4 (2010): 33–45.

149 L. Arab, F. Khan, and H. Lam, "Tea Consumption and Cardiovascular Disease Risk," *American Journal of Clinical Nutrition* 98, no. 6, supplement (2013): S1651–S1659.

150 R. Hursel and M. S. Westerterp-Plantenga, "Catechin- and Caffeine-Rich Teas for Control of Body Weight In Humans," *American Journal of Clinical Nutrition* 98, no. 6, supplement (2013): S1682–S1693.

151 A. Herrera-Arellano et al., "Effectiveness and Tolerability of a Standardized Extract from *Hibiscus sabdariffa* in Patients with Mild to Moderate Hypertension: A Controlled and Randomized Clinical Trial," *Phytomedicine* 11, no. 5 (2004): 375–82.

152 S. J. Einöther and V. E. Martens, "Acute Effects of Tea Consumption on Attention and Mood," *American Journal of Clinical Nutrition* 98, no. 6, supplement (2013): S1700S–S1708.

153 B. Burton-Freeman and K. Reimers, "Tomato Consumption and Health," *American Journal of Lifestyle Medicine* 5 (2011): 182–91.

154 H. D. Sesso et al., "Plasma Lycopene, Other Carotenoids, and Retinol and the Risk of Cardiovascular Disease in Women," *American Journal of Clinical Nutrition* 79, no. 1 (2004): 47–53.

155 N. O'Kennedy et al., "Effects of Antiplatelet Components of Tomato Extract on Platelet Function In Vitro and Ex Vivo: A Time-Course Cannulation Study in Healthy Humans," *American Journal of Clinical Nutrition* 84, no. 3 (2006): 570–79.

156 W. Abebe et al., "Effects of Chromium Picolinate on Vascular Reactivity and Cardiac Ischemia-Reperfusion Injury in Spontaneously Hypertensive Rats," *Pharmacological Reports* 62, no. 4 (2010): 674–82.

157 K. Niu et al., "A Tomato-Rich Diet Is Related to Depressive Symptoms among an Elderly Population Aged 70 Years and Over: A Population-Based, Cross-Sectional Analysis," *Journal of Affective Disorders* 144, no. 1–2 (2013): 165–70.

158 B. B. Aggarwal et al., "Curcumin: The Indian Solid Gold," *Advances in Experimental Medicine and Biology* 595 (2007): 1–75.

159 R. Motterlini et al., "Curcumin, An Antioxidant and Anti-Inflammatory Agent, Induces Heme Oxygenase-1 and Protects Endothelial Cells against Oxidative Stress," *Free Radical Biology & Medicine* 28, no. 8 (2000): 1303–12.

160 B. J. Willcox and D. C. Willcox, "Caloric Restriction, Caloric Restriction Mimetics, and Healthy Aging In Okinawa: Controversies and Clinical Implications," *Current Opinion in Clinical Nutrition and Metabolic Care* 17, no. 1 (2014): 51–58.

161 A. Sahebkar, "Are Curcuminoids Effective C-Reactive Protein-Lowering Agents in Clinical Practice? Evidence from a Meta-Analysis," *Phytotherapy Research* (2013), doi: 10.1002/ptr.5045.

162 N. Akazawa et al., "Curcumin Ingestion and Exercise Training Improve Vascular Endothelial Function in Postmenopausal Women," *Nutrition Research* 32, no. 10 (2012): 795–99.

163 I. Alwi et al., "The Effect of Curcuminon Lipid Level in Patients with Acute Coronary Syndrome," *Acta Medica Indonesiana* 40, no. 4 (2008): 201–10.

164 Y. Katanasaka et al., "Application of Curcumin to Heart Failure Therapy by Targeting Transcriptional Pathway in Cardiomyocytes," *Biological and Pharmaceutical Bulletin* 36, no. 1 (2013): 13–17.

165 Y. H. Aldebasi, S. M. Aly, and A. H. Rahmani, "Therapeutic Implications of Curcumin in the Prevention of Diabetic Retinopathy via Modulation of Anti-Oxidant Activity and Genetic Pathways," *International Journal of Physiology, Pathophysiology, and Pharmacology* 5, no. 4 (2013): 194–202.

166 L. L. Wang et al., "Curcumin, A Potential Therapeutic Candidate for Retinal Diseases," *Molecular Nutrition & Food Research* 57, no. 9 (2013): 1557–68.

167 J. Sanmukhani et al., "Efficacy and Safety of Curcumin in Major Depressive Disorder: A Randomized Controlled Trial," *Phytotherapy Research* 28, no. 4 (2013): 579–85.

168 B. N. Shyamala et al., "Studies on the Antioxidant Activities of Natural Vanilla Extract and Its Constituent Compounds through In Vitro Models," *Journal of Agricultural and Food Chemistry* 55, no. 19 (2007): 7738–43.

169 W. H. Redd et al., "Fragrance Administration to Reduce Anxiety During MR Imaging," *Journal of Magnetic Resonance Imaging* 4, no. 4 (1994): 623–26.

170 Y. C. Luiking, M. P. Engelen, and N. E. Deutz, "Regulation of Nitric Oxide Production in Health and Disease," *Current Opinion in Clinical Nutrition and Metabolic Care* 13, no. 1 (2010): 97–104.

171 A. Figueroa et al., "Effects of Watermelon Supplementation on Aortic Blood Pressure and Wave Reflection in Individuals with Prehypertension: A Pilot Study," *American Journal of Hypertension* 24, no. 1 (2011): 40–44.

172 K. R. Anand Swarup et al., "Effect of Dragon Fruit Extract on Oxidative Stress and Aortic Stiffness in Streptozotocin-Induced Diabetes in Rats," *Pharmacognosy Research* 2, no. 1 (2010): 31–35.

173 C. F. Haskell et al., "A Double-Blind, Placebo-Controlled, Multi-Dose Evaluation of the Acute Behavioural Effects of Guaraná in Humans," *Journal of Psychopharmacology* 21, no. 1 (2007): 65–70.

174 L. Portella Rde et al., "Guaraná (*Paullinia cupana* Kunth) Effects on LDL Oxidation in Elderly People: An In Vitro and In Vivo Study," *Lipids in Health and Disease* 12 (2013), doi:10.1186/1476-511X-12-12.

175 M. T. Subbiah and R. Yunker, "Studies on the Nature of Anti-Platelet Aggregatory Factors in the Seeds of the Amazonian Herb Guarana (*Paullinia cupana*)," *International Journal for Vitamin and Nutrition Research* 78, no. 2 (2008): 96–101.

176 C. Costa Krewer et al., "Habitual Intake of Guaraná and Metabolic Morbidities: An Epidemiological Study of an Elderly Amazonian Population," *Phytotherapy Research* (2011), doi:10.1002/ptr.3437.

177 A. Jacob et al., "Effect of the Indian Gooseberry (Amla) on Serum Cholesterol Levels in Men Aged 35–55 Years," *European Journal of Clinical Nutrition* 42, no. 11 (1988): 939–44.

178 M. S. Akhtar et al., "Effect of Amla Fruit (*Emblica officinalis* Gaertn.) on Blood Glucose and Lipid Profile of Normal Subjects and Type 2 Diabetic Patients," *International Journal of Food Sciences and Nutrition* 62, no. 6 (2011): 609–16.

179 T. P. Rao et al., "Amla (*Emblica officinalis* Gaertn.) Extract Inhibits Lipopolysaccharide-Induced Procoagulant and Pro-Inflammatory Factors in Cultured Vascular Endothelial Cells," *British Journal of Nutrition* 110, no. 12 (2013): 2201–206.

180 N. Fatima, U. Pingali, and R. Pilli, "Evaluation of *Phyllanthus emblica* Extract on Cold Pressor Induced Cardiovascular Changes in Healthy Human Subjects," *Pharmacognosy Research* 6, no. 1 (2014): 29–35.

181 N. Fatima, U. Pingali, and N. Muralidhar, "Study of Pharmacodynamic Interaction of *Phyllanthus emblica* Extract with Clopidogrel and Ecosprin in Patients with Type II Diabetes Mellitus," *Phytomedicine* 21, no. 5 (2014): 579–85.

182 M. Mathew and S. Subramanian, "*In Vitro* Screening for Anti-Cholinesterase and Antioxidant Activity of Methanolic Extracts of Ayurvedic Medicinal Plants Used for Cognitive Disorders," *PLOS ONE* 9, no. 1 (2014), doi:10.1371/journal.pone.0086804.

183 S. Pinto Mda et al., "Evaluation of Antihyperglycemia and Antihypertension Potential of Native Peruvian Fruits Using In Vitro Models," *Journal of Medicinal Food* 12, no. 2 (2009): 278–91.

184 K. B. Ramya and S. Thaakur, "Herbs Containing L-Dopa: An Update," *Ancient Science of Life* 27, no. 1 (2007): 50–55.

185 H. Ratnawati and W. Widowati, "Anticholesterol Activity of Velvet Bean (*Mucuna pruriens* L.) towards Hypercholesterolemic Rats," *Sains Malaysiana* 40, no. 4 (2011): 317–21.

186 B. K. Sharma, "A Review on *Mucuna pruriens*: Its Phyto Constituents and Therapeutic Uses," *Novel Science International Journal of Pharmaceutical Sciences* 1, no. 6 (2012): 308–12.

187 R. Katzenschlager et al., "*Mucuna pruriens* In Parkinson's Disease: A Double Blind Clinical and Pharmacological Study," *Journal of Neurology, Neurosurgery, and Psychiatry* 75, no. 12 (2004): 1672–77.

188 M. T. Escribano-Bailón et al., "Anthocyanins in Berries of Maqui (*Aristotelia chilensis* (Mol.) Stuntz)," *Phytochemical Analysis* 17, no. 1 (2006): 8–14.

189 S. Miranda-Rottmann et al., "Juice and Phenolic Fractions of the Berry *Aristotelia Chilensis* Inhibit LDL Oxidation In Vitro and Protect Human Endothelial Cells against Oxidative Stress," *Journal of Agricultural and Food Chemistry* 50, no. 26 (2002): 7542–47.

190 M. Rubilar et al., "Extracts of Maqui (*Aristotelia chilensis*) and Murta (*Ugni molinae* Turcz.): Sources of Antioxidant Compounds and Ɖ-Glucosidase/Ɖ-Amylase Inhibitors," *Journal of Agricultural and Food Chemistry* 59, no. 5 (2011): 1630–37.

191 T. T. Chu et al., "Study of Potential Cardioprotective Effects of *Ganoderma lucidum* (Lingzhi): Results of a Controlled Human Intervention Trial," *British Journal of Nutrition* 107, no. 7 (2012): 1017–27.

192 H. Zhao et al., "Spore Powder of *Ganoderma lucidum* Improves Cancer-Related Fatigue in Breast Cancer Patients Undergoing Endocrine Therapy: A Pilot Clinical Trial," *Evidence-Based Complementary and Alternative Medicine* (2012), doi:10.1155/2012/809614.

193 P. S. Larmo et al., "Effects of Sea Buckthorn and Bilberry on Serum Metabolites Differ according to Baseline Metabolic Profiles in Overweight Women: A Randomized Crossover Trial," *American Journal of Clinical Nutrition* 98, no. 4 (2013): 941–51.

194 S. Hasani-Ranjbar, Z. Jouyandeh, and M. Abdollahi, "A Systematic Review of Anti-Obesity Medicinal Plants—An Update," *Journal of Diabetes and Metabolic Disorders* 12, no. 1 (2013), doi:10.1186/2251-6581-12-28.

Chapter 3

1 The Situational Humor Response Questionnaire was designed by R.A. Martin and H. Lefcourt (1984).

2 A. Clark, A. Seidler, and M. Miller, "Inverse Association between Sense of Humor and Coronary Heart Disease," *International Journal of Cardiology* 80, no. 1 (2001): 87–88.

3 R. Provine, *Laughter: A Scientific Investigation* (New York: Viking, 2000).

4 M. Miller et al., "Impact of Cinematic Viewing on Endothelial Function," *Heart* 92, no. 2 (2006): 261–62.

5 C. Vlachopoulos et al., "Divergent Effects of Laughter and Mental Stress on Arterial Stiffness and Central Hemodynamics," *Psychosomatic Medicine* 71, no. 4 (2009): 446–53.

6 R. I. Dunbar et al., "Social Laughter Is Correlated with an Elevated Pain Threshold," *Proceedings of the Royal Society B: Biological Sciences* 279, no. 1731 (2012): 1161–67.

7 M. Miller and W. F. Fry, "The Effect of Mirthful Laughter on the Human Cardiovascular System," *Medical Hypotheses* 73, no. 5 (2009): 636–39.

8 L. Peeples, "Laughter, Music May Lower Blood Pressure," *Health*, March 25, 2011, http://news.health.com/2011/03/25/laughter-music-blood-pressure/.

9 M. S. Chaya et al., "The Effects of Hearty Extended Unconditional (HEU) Laughter Using Laughter Yoga Techniques on Physiological, Psychological, and Immunological Parameters in the Workplace: A Randomized Control Trial" (reported at the American Society of Hypertension 2008 Annual Meeting, New Orleans, May 14, 2008).

10 L. Peeples, "Laughter, Music May Lower Blood Pressure," *Health*, March 25, 2011, http://news.health.com/2011/03/25/laughter-music-blood-pressure/.

11 J. Sugawara, T. Tarumi, and H. Tanaka, "Effect of Mirthful Laughter on Vascular Function," *American Journal of Cardiology* 106, no. 6 (2010): 856–59.

12 M. S. Buchowski et al., "Energy Expenditure of Genuine Laughter," *International Journal of Obesity* 31, no. 1 (2007): 131–37.

13 M. F. Dallman et al., "Chronic Stress and Obesity: A New View of 'Comfort Food,'" *Proceedings of the National Academy of Sciences of the United States of America* 100, no. 20 (2003): 11696–701.

14 A.D.A.M., Inc., "Sleeping Difficulty," *New York Times*, June 11, 2010, http://health.nytimes.com/health/guides/symptoms/sleeping-difficulty/causes-of-chronic-insomnia.html.

15 H. J. Ko and C. H. Youn, "Effects of Laughter Therapy on Depression, Cognition, and Sleep among the Community-Dwelling Elderly," *Geriatrics & Gerontology International* 11, no. 3 (2011): 267–74.

16 M. Takahashi and T. Inoue, "The Effects of Humor on Memory for Non-Sensical Pictures," *Acta Psychologica* 132, no. 1 (2009): 80–84.

17 D. Wildgruber et al., "Different Types of Laughter Modulate Connectivity within Distinct Parts of the Laughter Perception Network," *PLOS ONE* 8, no. 5 (2013), doi: 10.1371/journal.pone.0063441.

18 R. Provine, *Laughter: A Scientific Investigation* (New York: Viking, 2000).

19 J. Gottman, *Why Marriages Succeed or Fail: And How You Can Make Yours Last* (New York: Simon & Schuster, 1995).

20 R. Provine, *Laughter: A Scientific Investigation* (New York: Viking, 2000).

21 "'The Gift of Laughter' App Offers Contagious Belly Laughs—Only Days Left for Free App," PRWeb, April 27, 2011, www.prweb.com/releases/thegiftoflaughter/april/prweb5274454.htm.

22 www.theheart.org/article/865875/print.do

23 M. Shahidi et al., "Laughter Yoga versus Group Exercise Program in Elderly Depressed Women: A Randomized Controlled Trial," *International Journal of Geriatric Psychiatry* 26, no. 3 (2011): 322–27.

24 H. J. Ko and C. H. Youn, "Effects of Laughter Therapy on Depression, Cognition, and Sleep among the Community-Dwelling Elderly," *Geriatrics & Gerontology International* 11, no. 3 (2011): 267–74.

25 H. S. Kim and E. J. Lee, "A Study on the Relation of Laughter Index, Depression, and Anxiety in Middle-Aged Women," *Korean Journal of Rehabilitation Nursing* 9, no. 2 (2006): 126–33.

Chapter 4

1 M. Miller et al. "Divergent Effects of Joyful and Anxiety-Provoking Music on Endothelial Vasoreactivity," *Psychosomatic Medicine* 72, no. 4 (2010): 354–56.

2 M. Deljanin Ilic et al., "Effects of Music Therapy on Endothelial Function in Patients with Coronary Artery Disease Participating in Rehabilitation," *European Heart Journal* 34, supplement 1 (2013), doi:10.1093/eurheartj/eht310.P5797.

3 X. F. Teng, M. Y. Wong, and Y. T. Zhang, "The Effect of Music on Hypertensive Patients," *Conference Proceedings: 29th Annual International Conference of the IEEE Engineering in Medicine and Biology Society* (2007): 4649–51.

4 J. M. White, "Effects of Relaxing Music on Cardiac Autonomic Balance and Anxiety after Acute Myocardial Infarction," *American Journal of Critical Care* 8, no. 4 (1999): 220–30.

5 S. E. Sendelbach et al., "Effects of Music Therapy on Physiological and Psychological Outcomes for Patients Undergoing Cardiac Surgery," *Journal of Cardiovascular Nursing* 21, no. 3 (2006): 194–200.

6 M. E. Cadigan et al., "The Effects of Music on Cardiac Patients on Bed Rest," *Progress in Cardiovascular Nursing* 16, no. 1 (2001): 5–13.

7 H. J. Trappe, "The Effects of Music on the Cardiovascular System and Cardiovascular Health," *Heart* 96, no. 23 (2010): 1868–71.

8 U. Nilsson, "Soothing Music Can Increase Oxytocin Levels during Bed Rest after Open-Heart Surgery: A Randomised Control Trial," *Journal of Clinical Nursing* 18, no. 15 (2009): 2153–61.

9 M. L. Chanda and D. J. Levitin, "The Neurochemistry of Music," *Trends in Cognitive Science* 17, no. 4 (2013): 179–93.

10 L. Bernardi, C. Porta, and P. Sleight, "Cardiovascular, Cerebrovascular, and Respiratory Changes Induced by Different Types of Music in Musicians and Non-Musicians: The Importance of Silence," *Heart* 92, no. 4 (2006): 445–52.

11 L. Bernardi et al., "Dynamic Interactions between Musical, Cardiovascular, and Cerebral Rhythms in Humans," *Circulation* 119, no. 25 (2009): 3171–80.

12 E. Buccelletti et al., "Heart Rate Variability and Myocardial Infarction: Systematic Literature Review and Metanalysis," *European Review for Medical and Pharmacological Sciences* 13, no. 4 (2009): 299–307.

13 A. Raglio et al., "Effects of Music Therapy on Psychological Symptoms and Heart Rate Variability in Patients with Dementia. A Pilot Study," *Current Aging Science* 3, no. 3 (2010): 242–46.

14 D. Liao et al., "Cardiac Autonomic Function and Incident Coronary Heart Disease: A Population-Based Case-Cohort Study. The ARIC Study. Atherosclerosis Risk in Communities Study," *American Journal of Epidemiology* 145, no. 8 (1997): 696–706.

15 K. Okada et al., "Effects of Music Therapy on Autonomic Nervous System Activity, Incidence of Heart Failure Events, and Plasma Cytokine and Catecholamine Levels in Elderly Patients with Cerebrovascular Disease and Dementia," *International Heart Journal* 50, no. 1 (2009): 95–110.

16 M. Uchiyama et al., "Music Exposure Induced Prolongation of Cardiac Allograft Survival and Generated Regulatory CD4Ð Cells in Mice," *Transplantation Proceedings* 44, no. 4 (2012): 1076–79.

17 E. Twiss, J. Seaver, and R. McCaffrey, "The Effect of Music Listening on Older Adults Undergoing Cardiovascular Surgery," *Nursing in Critical Care* 11, no. 5 (2006): 224–31.

18 S. B. Hanser, "Music Therapy in Cardiac Health Care: Current Issues in Research," *Cardiology in Review* 22, no. 1 (2014): 37–42.

19 V. N. Salimpoor et al., "Anatomically Distinct Dopamine Release during Anticipation and Experience of Peak Emotion to Music," *Nature Neuroscience* 14, no. 2 (2011): 257–62.

20 N. N. Niu, M. T. Perez, and J. N. Katz, "Singing Intervention for Preoperative Hypertension prior to Total Joint Replacement: A Case Report," *Arthritis Care & Research* 63, no. 4 (2011): 630–32.

21 V. Müller and U. Lindenberger, "Cardiac and Respiratory Patterns Synchronize between Persons during Choir Singing," *PLOS ONE* 6, no. 9 (2011), doi:10.1371/journal.pone.0024893.

22 B. Vickhoff et al., "Music Structure Determines Heart Rate Variability of Singers," *Frontiers in Psychology* 4 (2013), doi:10.3389/fpsyg.2013.00334.

Chapter 5

1 P. D. Loprinzi and B. J. Cardinal, "Association between Objectively-Measured Physical Activity and Sleep, NHANES 2005–2006," *Mental Health and Physical Activity* 4, no. 2 (2011): 65–69.

2 Harvard Health Publications, "Exercise and Depression," www.health.harvard.edu /newsweek/Exercise-and-Depression-report-excerpt.htm.

3 American Psychological Association, "Exercise Fuels the Brain's Stress Buffers," www.apa.org/helpcenter/exercise-stress.aspx.

4 K. Doheny, "The Truth about Fat," WebMD, reviewed on July 13, 2009, www.webmd.com/diet/features/the-truth-about-fat.

5 S. Kajimura and M. Saito, "A New Era in Brown Adipose Tissue Biology: Molecular Control of Brown Fat Development and Energy Homeostasis," *Annual Review of Physiology* 76 (2014): 225–49.

6 J. Wu et al., "Beige Adipocytes Are a Distinct Type of Thermogenic Fat Cell in Mouse and Human," *Cell* 150, no. 2 (2012): 366–76.

7 R. De Matteis et al., "Exercise as a New Physiological Stimulus for Brown Adipose Tissue Activity," *Nutrition, Metabolism, and Cardiovascular Diseases* 23, no. 6 (2013): 582–90.

8 T. Yoneshiro et al., "Nonpungent Capsaicin Analogs (Capsinoids) Increase Energy Expenditure through the Activation of Brown Adipose Tissue in Humans," *American Journal of Clinical Nutrition* 95, no. 4 (2012): 845–50.

9 T. Yoneshiro et al., "Recruited Brown Adipose Tissue as an Antiobesity Agent in Humans," *Journal of Clinical Investigation* 123, no. 8 (2013): 3404–408.

10 S. Snitker et al., "Effects of Novel Capsinoid Treatment on Fatness and Energy Metabolism in Humans: Possible Pharmacogenetic Implications," *American Journal of Clinical Nutrition* 89, no. 1 (2009): 45–50.

11 T. A. Lee et al., "Effects of Dihydrocapsiate on Adaptive and Diet-Induced Thermogenesis with a High Protein Very Low Calorie Diet: A Randomized Control Trial," *Nutrition & Metabolism* 7 (2010), doi:10.1186/1743-7075-7-78.

12 M. Saito and T. Yoneshiro, "Capsinoids and Related Food Ingredients Activating Brown Fat Thermogenesis and Reducing Body Fat in Humans," *Current Opinion in Lipidology* 24, no. 1 (2013): 71–77.

13 V. Ouellet et al., "Brown Adipose Tissue Oxidative Metabolism Contributes to Energy Expenditure during Acute Cold Exposure in Humans," *Journal of Clinical Investigation* 122, no. 2 (2012): 545–52.

14 N. A. Shevchuk, "Adapted Cold Shower as a Potential Treatment for Depression," *Medical Hypotheses* 70, no. 5 (2008): 995–1001.

15 S. Cook et al., "High Heart Rate: A Cardiovascular Risk Factor?" *European Heart Journal* 27, no. 20 (2006): 2387–93.

16 J. Nauman et al., "Combined Effect of Resting Heart Rate and Physical Activity on Ischaemic Heart Disease: Mortality Follow-Up in a Population Study (the HUNT Study, Norway)," *Journal of Epidemiology and Community Health* 64, no. 2 (2010): 175–81.

17 S. N. Young, "How to Increase Serotonin in the Human Brain without Drugs," *Journal of Psychiatry & Neuroscience* 32, no. 6 (2007): 394–99.

18 J. B. Bartholomew, D. Morrison, and J. T. Ciccolo, "Effects of Acute Exercise on Mood and Well-Being in Patients with Major Depressive Disorder," *Medicine & Science in Sports & Exercise* 37, no. 12 (2005): 2032–37.

19 K. Knubben et al., "A Randomised, Controlled Study on the Effects of a Short-Term Endurance Training Programme in Patients with Major Depression," *British Journal of Sports Medicine* 41, no. 1 (2007): 29–33.

20 I. M. Lee et al., "Effect of Physical Inactivity on Major Non-Communicable Diseases Worldwide: An Analysis of Burden of Disease and Life Expectancy," *Lancet* 380, no. 9838 (2012): 219–29.

21 E. S. George, R. R. Rosenkranz, and G. S. Kolt, "Chronic Disease and Sitting Time in Middle-Aged Australian Males: Findings from the 45 and Up Study," *International Journal of Behavioral Nutrition and Physical Activity* 10 (2013), doi:10.1186/1479-5868-10-20.

22 E. S. Ford and C. J. Caspersen, "Sedentary Behaviour and Cardiovascular Disease: A Review of Prospective Studies," *International Journal of Epidemiology* 41, no. 5 (2012): 1338–53.

23 J. G. van Uffelen et al., "Sitting-Time, Physical Activity, and Depressive Symptoms in Mid-Aged Women," *American Journal of Preventive Medicine* 45, no. 3 (2013): 276–81.

24 Ibid.

25 R. Goel et al., "Exercise-Induced Hypertension, Endothelial Dysfunction, and Coronary Artery Disease in a Marathon Runner," *American Journal of Cardiology* 99, no. 5 (2007): 743–44.

26 N. M. Kaplan, "Exercise in the Treatment and Prevention of Hypertension," UpToDate, last updated December 2, 2013, www.uptodate.com/contents/exercise-in-the-treatment-and-prevention-of-hypertension#H5.

27 J. W. Ha et al., "Hypertensive Response to Exercise: A Potential Cause for New Wall Motion Abnormality in the Absence of Coronary Artery Disease," *Journal of the American College of Cardiology* 39, no. 2 (2002): 323–27.

28 M. G. Schultz et al., "Exercise-Induced Hypertension, Cardiovascular Events, and Mortality in Patients Undergoing Exercise Stress Testing: A Systematic Review and Meta-Analysis," *American Journal of Hypertension* 26, no. 3 (2013): 357–66.

29 S. Möhlenkamp et al., "Running: The Risk of Coronary Events: Prevalence and Prognostic Relevance of Coronary Atherosclerosis in Marathon Runners," *European Heart Journal* 29, no. 15 (2008): 1903–10.

30 J. H. O'Keefe et al., "Potential Adverse Cardiovascular Effects from Excessive Endurance Exercise," *Mayo Clinic Proceedings* 87, no. 6 (2012): 587–95.

31 C. Vlachopoulos et al., "Arterial Stiffness and Wave Reflections in Marathon Runners," *American Journal of Hypertension* 23, no. 9 (2010): 974–79.

32 B. E. Ainsworth et al., "2011 Compendium of Physical Activities: A Second Update of Codes and MET Values," *Medicine & Science in Sports & Exercise* 43, no. 8 (2011): 1575–81.

33 J. E. Manson et al., "A Prospective Study of Walking as Compared with Vigorous Exercise in the Prevention of Coronary Heart Disease in Women," *New England Journal of Medicine* 341, no. 9 (1999): 650–58.

34 P. T. Williams and P. D. Thompson, "The Relationship of Walking Intensity to Total and Cause-Specific Mortality. Results from the National Walkers' Health Study," *PLOS ONE* 8, no. 11 (2013), doi:10.1371/journal.pone.0081098.

35 P. T. Williams and P. D. Thompson, "Walking versus Running for Hypertension, Cholesterol, and Diabetes Mellitus Risk Reduction," *Arteriosclerosis, Thrombosis, and Vascular Biology* 33, no. 5 (2013): 1085–91.

36 J. Verghese et al., "Leisure Activities and the Risk of Dementia in the Elderly," *New England Journal of Medicine* 348, no. 25 (2003): 2508–16.

37 J. Verghese, "Cognitive and Mobility Profile of Older Social Dancers," *Journal of the American Geriatrics Society* 54, no. 8 (2006): 1241–44.

38 J. Panula et al., "Mortality and Cause of Death in Hip Fracture Patients Aged 65 or Older: A Population-Based Study," *BMC Musculoskeletal Disorders* 12 (2011), doi: 10.1186/1471-2474-12-105.

39 R. Belardinelli et al., "Waltz Dancing in Patients with Chronic Heart Failure: New Form of Exercise Training," *Circulation: Heart Failure* 1, no. 2 (2008): 107–14.

40 T. H. Huang et al., "Effects of Different Exercise Modes on Mineralization, Structure, and Biomechanical Properties of Growing Bone," *Journal of Applied Physiology* 95, no. 1 (2003): 300–307.

41 E. Bar-Yishay et al., "Differences between Swimming and Running as Stimuli for Exercise-Induced Asthma," *European Journal of Applied Physiology and Occupational Physiology* 48, no. 3 (1982): 387–97.

42 N. L. Chase, X. Sui, and S. N. Blair, "Swimming and All-Cause Mortality Risk Compared with Running, Walking, and Sedentary Habits in Men," *International Journal of Aquatic Research and Education* 2, no. 3 (2008): 213–23.

43 B. G. Berger and D. R. Owen, "Mood Alteration with Swimming—Swimmers Really Do 'Feel Better,'" *Psychosomatic Medicine* 45, no. 5 (1983): 425–33.

44 W. J. Kraemer et al., "Effects of Different Heavy-Resistance Exercise Protocols on Plasma Beta-Endorphin Concentrations," *Journal of Applied Physiology* 74, no. 1 (1993): 450–59.

45 A. Grøntved et al., "Muscle-Strengthening and Conditioning Activities and Risk of Type 2 Diabetes: A Prospective Study in Two Cohorts of US Women," *PLOS Medicine* 11, no. 1 (2014), doi:10.1371/journal.pmed.1001587.

46 A. Grøntved et al., "A Prospective Study of Weight Training and Risk of Type 2 Diabetes Mellitus in Men," *Archives of Internal Medicine* 172, no. 17 (2012): 1306–12.

47 M. Tanasescu et al., "Exercise Type and Intensity in Relation to Coronary Heart Disease in Men," *JAMA* 288, no. 16 (2002): 1994–2000.

48 M. P. Hoevenaar-Blom et al., "Cycling and Sports, but Not Walking, Are Associated with 10-Year Cardiovascular Disease Incidence: The MORGEN Study," *European Journal of Cardiovascular Prevention and Rehabilitation* 18, no. 1 (2011): 41–47.

49 C. M. Maresh et al., "Pituitary-Adrenal Responses to Arm versus Leg Exercise in Untrained Man," *European Journal of Applied Physiology* 97, no. 4 (2006): 471–77.

50 J. Tripette et al., "Home-Based Active Video Games to Promote Weight Loss during the Postpartum Period," *Medicine & Science in Sports & Exercise* 46, no. 3 (2014): 472–78.

51 C. O'Donovan and J. Hussey, "Active Video Games as a Form of Exercise and the Effect of Gaming Experience: A Preliminary Study in Healthy Young Adults," *Physiotherapy* 98, no. 3 (2012): 205–10.

52 American College of Sports Medicine, *ACSM'S Guidelines for Exercise Testing and Prescription*, 6th ed. (Baltimore: Lippincott Williams & Wilkins, 2000).

53 J. A. Levine, N. L. Eberhardt, and M. D. Jensen, "Role of Nonexercise Activity Thermogenesis in Resistance to Fat Gain in Humans," *Science* 283, no. 5399 (1999): 212–14.

54 J. A. Levine et al., "Non-Exercise Activity Thermogenesis: The Crouching Tiger Hidden Dragon of Societal Weight Gain," *Arteriosclerosis, Thrombosis, and Vascular Biology* 26, no. 4 (2006): 729–36.

55 E. Ravussin et al., "Determinants of 24-Hour Energy Expenditure in Man. Methods and Results Using a Respiratory Chamber," *Journal of Clinical Investigation* 78, no. 6 (1986): 1568–78.

56 K. A. McGuire and R. Ross, "Incidental Physical Activity Is Positively Associated with Cardiorespiratory Fitness," *Medicine & Science in Sports & Exercise* 43, no. 11 (2011): 2189–94.

Chapter 6

1 A. Lammintausta et al., "Prognosis of Acute Coronary Events Is Worse in Patients Living Alone: The FINAMI Myocardial Infarction Register," *European Journal of Preventive Cardiology* (2013), doi:10.1177/2047487313475893.

2 E. L. Idler, D. A. Boulifard, and R. J. Contrada, "Mending Broken Hearts: Marriage and Survival following Cardiac Surgery," *Journal of Health and Social Behavior* 53, no. 1 (2012): 33–49.

3 K. B. King and H. T. Reis, "Marriage and Long-Term Survival after Coronary Artery Bypass Grafting," *Health Psychology* 31, no. 1 (2012): 55–62.

4 E. D. Eaker et al., "Marital Status, Marital Strain, and Risk of Coronary Heart Disease or Total Mortality: The Framingham Offspring Study," *Psychosomatic Medicine* 69, no. 6 (2007): 509–13.

5 Ibid.

6 K. Orth-Gomér et al., "Marital Stress Worsens Prognosis in Women with Coronary Heart Disease: The Stockholm Female Coronary Risk Study," *JAMA* 284, no. 23 (2000): 3008–14.

7 R. De Vogli, T. Chandola, and M. G. Marmot, "Negative Aspects of Close Relationships and Heart Disease," *Archives of Internal Medicine* 167, no. 18 (2007): 1951–57.

8 Ibid.

9 D. S. Felix, W. D. Robinson, and K. J. Jarzynka, "The Influence of Divorce on Men's Health," *Journal of Men's Health* 10, no. 1 (2013): 3–7.

10 Z. Zhang and M. D. Hayward, "Gender, the Marital Life Course, and Cardiovascular Health in Late Midlife," *Journal of Marriage and Family* 68, no. 3 (2006): 639–57.

11 Ibid.

12 Z. Zhang, "Marital History and the Burden of Cardiovascular Disease in Midlife," *Gerontologist* 46, no. 2 (2006): 266–70.

13 E. Mostofsky et al., "Risk of Acute Myocardial Infarction after the Death of a Significant Person in One's Life: The Determinants of Myocardial Infarction Onset Study," *Circulation* 125, no. 3 (2012): 491–96.

14 S. S. Virani et al., "Takotsubo Cardiomyopathy, or Broken-Heart Syndrome," *Texas Heart Institute Journal* 34, no. 1 (2007): 76–79.

15 I. S. Wittstein et al., "Neurohumoral Features of Myocardial Stunning due to Sudden Emotional Stress," *New England Journal of Medicine* 352, no. 6 (2005): 539–48.

16 G. A. Kaplan et al., "Social Connections and Mortality from All Causes and from Cardiovascular Disease: Prospective Evidence from Eastern Finland," *American Journal of Epidemiology* 128, no. 2 (1988): 370–80.

17 I. Kawachi et al., "A Prospective Study of Social Networks in Relation to Total Mortality and Cardiovascular Disease in Men in the USA," *Journal of Epidemiology and Community Health* 50, no. 3 (1996): 245–51.

18 A. Rosengren, L. Wilhelmsen, and K. Orth-Gomér, "Coronary Disease in Relation to Social Support and Social Class in Swedish Men: A 15 Year Follow-Up in the Study of Men Born in 1933," *European Heart Journal* 25, no. 1 (2004): 56–63.

19 T. Rutledge et al., "Social Networks and Incident Stroke among Women with Suspected Myocardial Ischemia," *Psychosomatic Medicine* 70, no. 3 (2008): 282–87.

20 T. Rutledge et al., "Social Networks Are Associated with Lower Mortality Rates among Women with Suspected Coronary Disease: The National Heart, Lung, and Blood Institute-Sponsored Women's Ischemia Syndrome Evaluation Study," *Psychosomatic Medicine* 66, no. 6 (2004): 882–88.

21 C. A. Low, R. C. Thurston, and K. A. Matthews, "Psychosocial Factors in the Development of Heart Disease in Women: Current Research and Future Directions," *Psychosomatic Medicine* 72, no. 9 (2010): 842–54.

22 J. Wei et al., "Estrogen Protects against the Detrimental Effects of Repeated Stress on Glutamatergic Transmission and Cognition," *Molecular Psychiatry* (2013), doi:10.1038/mp.2013.83.

23 M. Ingalhalikar et al., "Sex Differences in the Structural Connectome of the Human Brain," *Proceedings of the National Academy of Sciences of the United States of America* 111, no. 2 (2014): 823–28.

24 M. Miller et al., "Lecithin: Cholesterol Acyltransferase Deficiency: Identification of Two Defective Alleles in Fibroblast cDNA," *Journal of Lipid Research* 36, no. 5 (1995): 931–38.

25 K. C. Light, K. M. Grewen, and J. A. Amico, "More Frequent Partner Hugs and Higher Oxytocin Levels Are Linked to Lower Blood Pressure and Heart Rate in Premenopausal Women," *Biological Psychology* 69, no. 1 (2005): 5–21.

26 J. P. Gouin et al., "Marital Behavior, Oxytocin, Vasopressin, and Wound Healing," *Psychoneuroendocrinology* 35, no. 7 (2010): 1082–90.

27 K. M. Grewen et al., "Effects of Partner Support on Resting Oxytocin, Cortisol, Norepinephrine, and Blood Pressure before and after Warm Partner Contact," *Psychosomatic Medicine* 67, no. 4 (2005): 531–38.

28 A. Gallace et al., "The Analgesic Effect of Crossing the Arms," *Pain* 152, no. 6 (2011): 1418–23.

29 H. Sumioka et al., "Huggable Communication Medium Decreases Cortisol Levels," *Scientific Reports* 3 (2013), doi:10.1038/srep03034.

30 R. B. Miller et al., "Marital Quality and Health Over 20 Years: A Growth Curve Analysis," *Journal of Marriage and Family* 75, no. 3 (2013): 667–80.

31 V. Morhenn, L. E. Beavin, and P. J. Zak, "Massage Increases Oxytocin and Reduces Adrenocorticotropin Hormone in Humans," *Alternative Therapies in Health and Medicine* 18, no. 6 (2012): 11–18.

Chapter 7

1 M. Miller and R. A. Vogel, *The Practice of Coronary Disease Prevention* (Baltimore: Lippincott Williams & Wilkins, 1996).

2 R. A. Karasek et al., "Job Characteristics in Relation to the Prevalence of Myocardial Infarction in the US Health Examination Survey (HES) and the Health and Nutrition Examination Survey (HANES)," *American Journal of Public Health* 78, no. 8 (1988): 910–18.

3 Ibid.

4 S. Adams, "The Most Stressful Jobs of 2014," *Forbes*, January 7, 2014, www.forbes.com/sites/susanadams/2014/01/07/the-most-stressful-jobs-of-2014/.

5 Ibid.

6 M. Kivimäki et al., "Job Strain as a Risk Factor for Coronary Heart Disease: A Collaborative Meta-Analysis of Individual Participant Data," *Lancet* 380, no. 9852 (2012): 1491–97.

7 H. Yoo and W. D. Franke, "Stress and Cardiovascular Disease Risk in Female Law Enforcement Officers," *International Archives of Occupational and Environmental Health* 84, no. 3 (2011): 279–86.

8 N. Djindjić et al., "Work Stress Related Lipid Disorders and Arterial Hypertension in Professional Drivers—A Cross-Sectional Study," *Vojnosanitetski Pregled* 70, no. 6 (2013): 561–68.

9 L. Ghiadoni et al., "Mental Stress Induces Transient Endothelial Dysfunction in Humans," *Circulation* 102, no. 20 (2000): 2473–78.

10 R. De Caterina et al., "Nitric Oxide Decreases Cytokine-Induced Endothelial Activation. Nitric Oxide Selectively Reduces Endothelial Expression of Adhesion Molecules and Proinflammatory Cytokines," *Journal of Clinical Investigation* 96, no. 1 (1995): 60–68.

11 R. T. Emeny et al., "Job Strain Associated CRP Is Mediated by Leisure Time Physical Activity: Results from the MONICA/KORA Study," *Brain, Behavior, and Immunity* 26, no. 7 (2012): 1077–84.

12 R. T. Emeny et al., "Job Strain-Associated Inflammatory Burden and Long-Term Risk of Coronary Events: Findings from The MONICA/KORA Augsburg Case-Cohort Study," *Psychosomatic Medicine* 75, no. 3 (2013): 317–25.

13 S. Poorabdian et al., "Association between Job Strain (High Demand-Low Control) and Cardiovascular Disease Risk Factors among Petrochemical Industry Workers," *International Journal of Occupational Medicine and Environmental Health* 26, no. 4 (2013): 555–62.

14 U. Kraus et al., "Individual Daytime Noise Exposure during Routine Activities and Heart Rate Variability in Adults: A Repeated Measures Study," *Environmental Health Perspectives* 121, no. 5 (2013): 607–12.

15 O. Olafiranye et al., "Anxiety and Cardiovascular Risk: Review of Epidemiological and Clinical Evidence," *Mind & Brain* 2, no. 1 (2011): 32–37.

16 M. Sørensen et al., "Road Traffic Noise and Stroke: A Prospective Cohort Study," *European Heart Journal* 32, no. 6 (2011): 737–44.

17 M. Sørensen et al., "Road Traffic Noise and Incident Myocardial Infarction: A Prospective Cohort Study," *PLOS ONE* 7, no. 6 (2012), doi:10.1371/journal.pone.0039283.

18 T. Bodin et al., "Road Traffic Noise and Hypertension: Results from a Cross-Sectional Public Health Survey In Southern Sweden," *Environmental Health* 8 (2009), doi:10.1186/1476-069X-8-38.

19 Occupational Safety and Health Administration, "Occupational Noise Exposure," www.osha.gov/pls/oshaweb/owadisp.show_document?p_table=standards&p_id=9735.

20 H. Kälsch et al., "Are Air Pollution and Traffic Noise Independently Associated with Atherosclerosis: The Heinz Nixdorf Recall Study," *European Heart Journal* 35, no. 13 (2014): 853–60.

21 M. Franchini and P. M. Mannucci, "Thrombogenicity and Cardiovascular Effects of Ambient Air Pollution," *Blood* 118, no. 9 (2011): 2405–12.

22 T. Karl et al., "Efficient Atmospheric Cleansing of Oxidized Organic Trace Gases by Vegetation," *Science* 330, no. 6005 (2010): 816–19.

23 S. Shibata and N. Suzuki, "Effects of the Foliage Plant on Task Performance and Mood," *Journal of Environmental Psychology* 22, no. 3 (2002): 265–72.

24 E. Largo-Wight et al., "Healthy Workplaces: The Effects of Nature Contact at Work on Employee Stress and Health," *Public Health Reports* 126, supplement 1 (2011): 124–30.

25 P. Wennberg, "Beyond the Established Risk Factors of Myocardial Infarction: Lifestyle Factors and Novel Biomarkers," Umeå University Library, http://umu.diva-portal.org/smash/record.jsf?pid=diva2:212031.

26 H. C. Chuang et al., "In-Car Particles and Cardiovascular Health: An Air Conditioning-Based Intervention Study," *Science of the Total Environment* 452–453 (May 2013): 309–13.

27 L. Y. Lin et al., "Reducing Indoor Air Pollution by Air Conditioning Is Associated with Improvements in Cardiovascular Health among the General Population," *Science of the Total Environment* 463–464 (October 2013): 176–81.

28 A. Nyberg et al., "Managerial Leadership and Ischaemic Heart Disease among Employees: The Swedish WOLF Study," *Occupational and Environmental Medicine* 66, no. 1 (2009): 51–55.

29 T. L. Kraft and S. D. Pressman, "Grin and Bear It: The Influence of Manipulated Facial Expression on the Stress Response," *Psychological Science* 23, no. 11 (2012): 1372–78.

30 A. Hennenlotter et al., "A Common Neural Basis for Receptive and Expressive Communication of Pleasant Facial Affect," *NeuroImage* 26, no. 2 (2005): 581–91.

31 M. Desvarieux et al., "Periodontal Microbiota and Carotid Intima-Media Thickness: The Oral Infections and Vascular Disease Epidemiology Study (INVEST)," *Circulation* 111, no. 5 (2005): 576–82.

32 B. L. Mealey and L. F. Rose, "Diabetes Mellitus and Inflammatory Periodontal Diseases," *Current Opinion in Endocrinology, Diabetes, and Obesity* 15, no. 2 (2008): 135–41.

33 M. C. Chen, S. H. Fang, and L. Fang, "The Effects of Aromatherapy in Relieving Symptoms Related to Job Stress among Nurses," *International Journal of Nursing Practice* (2013), doi:10.1111/ijn.12229.

34 National Center for Complementary and Alternative Medicine, "Lavender," last updated April 2012, http://nccam.nih.gov/health/lavender/ataglance.htm.

35 W. C. Clapp and A. Gazzaley, "Distinct Mechanisms for the Impact of Distraction and Interruption on Working Memory in Aging," *Neurobiology of Aging* 33, no. 1 (2012): 134–48.

36 L. Bey and M. T. Hamilton, "Suppression of Skeletal Muscle Lipoprotein Lipase Activity during Physical Inactivity: A Molecular Reason to Maintain Daily Low-Intensity Activity," *Journal of Physiology* 551, part 2 (2003): 673–82.

37 P. T. Katzmarzyk et al., "Sitting Time and Mortality from All Causes, Cardiovascular Disease, and Cancer," *Medicine & Science in Sports & Exercise* 41, no. 5 (2009): 998–1005.

38 G. N. Healy et al., "Sedentary Time and Cardio-Metabolic Biomarkers in US Adults: NHANES 2003-06," *European Heart Journal* 32, no. 5 (2011): 590–97.

39 J. Henson et al., "Associations of Objectively Measured Sedentary Behaviour and Physical Activity with Markers of Cardiometabolic Health," *Diabetologia* 56, no. 5 (2013): 1012–20.

40 S. Brody et al., "A Randomized Controlled Trial of High Dose Ascorbic Acid for Reduction of Blood Pressure, Cortisol, and Subjective Responses to Psychological Stress," *Psychopharmacology* 159, no. 3 (2002): 319–24.

Chapter 8

1 V. Morhenn, L. E. Beavin, and P. J. Zak, "Massage Increases Oxytocin and Reduces Adrenocorticotropin Hormone in Humans," *Alternative Therapies in Health and Medicine* 18, no. 6 (2012): 11–18.

2 N. J. Cicutti et al., "Oxytocin Receptor Binding in Rat and Human Heart," *Canadian Journal of Cardiology* 15, no. 11 (1999): 1267–73.

3 J. Gutkowska and M. Jankowski, "Oxytocin Revisited: Its Role in Cardiovascular Regulation," *Journal of Neuroendocrinology* 24, no. 4 (2012): 599–608.

4 Y. S. Kim et al., "Priming of Mesenchymal Stem Cells with Oxytocin Enhances the Cardiac Repair in Ischemia/Reperfusion Injury," *Cells Tissues Organs* 195, no. 5 (2012): 428–42.

5 M. Jankowski et al., "Oxytocin in the Heart Regeneration," *Recent Patents on Cardiovascular Drug Discovery* 7, no. 2 (2012): 81–87.

6 K. C. Light, K. M. Grewen, and J. A. Amico, "More Frequent Partner Hugs and Higher Oxytocin Levels Are Linked to Lower Blood Pressure and Heart Rate in Premenopausal Women," *Biological Psychology* 69, no. 1 (2005): 5–21.

7 M. J. Poulin, "Volunteering Predicts Health among Those Who Value Others: Two National Studies," *Health Psychology* 33, no. 2 (2014): 120–29.

8 M. Tartakovsky, "The Truth about Grief: The Myth of Its Five Stages," Psych Central, last reviewed January 30, 2013, http://psychcentral.com/lib/the-truth-about-grief-the-myth-of-its-five-stages/0006292.

9 H. N. Rasmussen, M. F. Scheier, and J. B. Greenhouse, "Optimism and Physical Health: A Meta-Analytic Review," *Annals of Behavioral Medicine* 37, no. 3 (2009): 239–56.

10 J. D. Hansen et al., "Finding the Glass Half Full? Optimism Is Protective of 10-Year Incident CHD in a Population-Based Study: The Canadian Nova Scotia Health Survey," *International Journal of Cardiology* 145, no. 3 (2010): 603–604.

11 K. W. Davidson, E. Mostofsky, and W. Whang, "Don't Worry, Be Happy: Positive Affect and Reduced 10-Year Incident Coronary Heart Disease: The Canadian Nova Scotia Health Survey," *European Heart Journal* 31, no. 9 (2010): 1065–70.

12 J. K. Boehm and L. D. Kubzansky, "The Heart's Content: The Association Between Positive Psychological Well-Being and Cardiovascular Health," *Psychological Bulletin* 138, no. 4 (2012): 655–91.

13 P. Hjemdahl and G. Olsson, "Rebound Phenomena following Withdrawal of Long-Term Beta-Adrenoceptor Blockade," *Acta Medica Scandinavica* 665 (1982): 43–47.

14 D. J. Lodge, "The Medial Prefrontal and Orbitofrontal Cortices Differentially Regulate Dopamine System Function," *Neuropsychopharmacology* 36, no. 6 (2011): 1227–36.

15 P. Favaro, *Smart Parenting during and after Divorce* (New York: McGraw Hill, 2009).

16 K. S. Masters and S. A. Hooker, "Religiousness/Spirituality, Cardiovascular Disease, and Cancer: Cultural Integration for Health Research and Intervention," *Journal of Consulting and Clinical Psychology* 81, no. 2 (2013): 206–16.

17 H. G. Koenig, "Religion, Spirituality, and Health: The Research and Clinical Implications," *ISRN Psychiatry* (2012), doi:10.5402/2012/278730.

18 G. G. Ano and E. B. Vasconcelles, "Religious Coping and Psychological Adjustment to Stress: A Meta-Analysis," *Journal of Clinical Psychology* 61, no. 4 (2005): 461–80.

19 K. I. Pargament et al., "Patterns of Positive and Negative Religious Coping with Major Life Stressors," *Journal for the Scientific Study of Religion* 37, no. 4 (1998): 710–24.

20 A. Keller et al., "Does the Perception That Stress Affects Health Matter? The Association with Health and Mortality," *Health Psychology* 31, no. 5 (2012): 677–84.

21 H. Nabi et al., "Increased Risk of Coronary Heart Disease among Individuals Reporting Adverse Impact of Stress on Their Health: The Whitehall II Prospective Cohort Study," *European Heart Journal* 34 (September 2013): 2697–705.

Chapter 9

1 M. Frass et al., "Use and Acceptance of Complementary and Alternative Medicine among the General Population and Medical Personnel: A Systematic Review," *Ochsner Journal* 12, no. 1 (2012): 45–56.

2 The Center for Integrative Medicine within the University of Maryland School of Medicine, led by my colleague, Dr. Brian Berman, has been in the forefront of academic

medical centers in the U.S. studying integrative approaches for patients with a variety of ailments. Please check out the Web site at www.compmed.umm.edu/default.asp.

3 L. S. Wieland et al., "Bibliometric and Content Analysis of the Cochrane Complementary Medicine Field Specialized Register of Controlled Trials," *Systematic Reviews* 2 (2013), doi:10.1186/2046-4053-2-51.

4 R. D. Brook et al. "Beyond Medications and Diet: Alternative Approaches to Lowering Blood Pressure: A Scientific Statement from the American Heart Association," *Hypertension* 61, no. 6 (2013): 1360–83.

5 N. A. Qureshi and A. M. Al-Bedah, "Mood Disorders and Complementary and Alternative Medicine: A Literature Review," *Neuropsychiatric Disease and Treatment* 9 (2013): 639–58.

6 J. Yin, H. Xing, and J. Ye, "Efficacy of Berberine in Patients with Type 2 Diabetes Mellitus," *Metabolism* 57, no. 5 (2008): 712–17.

7 Y. Zhang et al., "Treatment of Type 2 Diabetes and Dyslipidemia with the Natural Plant Alkaloid Berberine," *Journal of Clinical Endocrinology and Metabolism* 93, no. 7 (2008): 2559–65.

8 A. J. Basler, "Pilot Study Investigating the Effects of Ayurvedic Abhyanga Massage on Subjective Stress Experience," *Journal of Alternative and Complementary Medicine* 17, no. 5 (2011): 435–40.

9 K. D. Dhuri, P. V. Bodhe, and A. B. Vaidya, "Shirodhara: A Psycho-Physiological Profile in Healthy Volunteers," *Journal of Ayurveda and Integrative Medicine* 4, no. 1 (2013): 40–44.

10 C. Kundu et al., "The Role of Psychic Factors in Pathogenesis of Essential Hypertension and Its Management by Shirodhara and Sarpagandha Vati," *AYU* 31, no. 4 (2010): 436–41.

11 M. Ghaly and D. Teplitz, "The Biologic Effects of Grounding the Human Body during Sleep as Measured by Cortisol Levels and Subjective Reporting of Sleep, Pain, and Stress," *Journal of Alternative and Complementary Medicine* 10, no. 5 (2004): 767–76.

12 J. L. Oschman, "Can Electrons Act as Antioxidants? A Review and Commentary," *Journal of Alternative and Complementary Medicine* 13, no. 9 (2007): 955–67.

13 G. Chevalier et al., "Earthing (Grounding) the Human Body Reduces Blood Viscosity—A Major Factor in Cardiovascular Disease," *Journal of Alternative and Complementary Medicine* 19, no. 2 (2013): 102–10.

14 D. Ornish et al., "Intensive Lifestyle Changes for Reversal of Coronary Heart Disease," *JAMA* 280, no. 23 (1998): 2001–2007.

15 E. L. Morris, "The Relationship of Spirituality to Coronary Heart Disease," *Alternative Therapies in Health and Medicine* 7, no. 5 (2001): 96–98.

16 A. L. Ai et al., "Prayer and Reverence in Naturalistic, Aesthetic, and Socio-Moral Contexts Predicted Fewer Complications following Coronary Artery Bypass," *Journal of Behavioral Medicine* 32, no. 6 (2009): 570–81.

17 R. J. Contrada et al., "Psychosocial Factors in Outcomes of Heart Surgery: The Impact of Religious Involvement and Depressive Symptoms," *Health Psychology* 23, no. 3 (2004): 227–38.

18 T. E. Oxman, D. H. Freeman Jr., and E. D. Manheimer, "Lack of Social Participation or Religious Strength and Comfort as Risk Factors for Death after Cardiac Surgery in the Elderly," *Psychosomatic Medicine* 57, no. 1 (1995): 5–15.

19 D. B. Bekelman et al., "Spiritual Well-Being and Depression in Patients with Heart Failure," *Journal of General Internal Medicine* 22, no. 4 (2007): 470–77.

20 W. Jiang et al., "Relationship of Depression to Increased Risk of Mortality and Re-Hospitalization in Patients with Congestive Heart Failure," *Archives of Internal Medicine* 161, no. 15 (2001): 1849–56.

21 P. Potter, "What Are the Distinctions between Reiki and Therapeutic Touch?" *Clinical Journal of Oncology Nursing* 7, no. 1 (2003): 89–91.

22 M. Zolfaghari, S. Eybpoosh, and M. Hazrati, "Effects of Therapeutic Touch on Anxiety, Vital Signs, and Cardiac Dysrhythmia in a Sample of Iranian Women Undergoing Cardiac Catheterization: A Quasi-Experimental Study," *Journal of Holistic Nursing* 30, no. 4 (2012): 225–34.

23 A. Vitale, "An Integrative Review of Reiki Touch Therapy Research," *Holistic Nursing Practice* 21, no. 4 (2007): 167–79.

24 L. Díaz-Rodríguez et al., "Immediate Effects of Reiki on Heart Rate Variability, Cortisol Levels, and Body Temperature in Health Care Professionals with Burnout," *Biological Research for Nursing* 13, no. 4 (2011): 376–82.

25 R. S. Friedman et al., "Effects of Reiki on Autonomic Activity Early after Acute Coronary Syndrome," *Journal of the American College of Cardiology* 56, no. 12 (2010): 995–96.

26 L. Rosa et al., "A Close Look at Therapeutic Touch," *JAMA* 279, no. 13 (1998): 1005–10.

27 H. Benson and M. D. Epstein, "The Placebo Effect. A Neglected Asset in the Care of Patients," *JAMA* 232, no. 12 (1975): 1225–27.

28 F. M. Sacks et al., "The Effect of Pravastatin on Coronary Events after Myocardial Infarction in Patients with Average Cholesterol Levels. Cholesterol and Recurrent Events Trial Investigators," *New England Journal of Medicine* 335, no. 14 (1996): 1001–1009.

29 D. A. Morrow, "Cardiovascular Risk Prediction in Patients with Stable and Unstable Coronary Heart Disease," *Circulation* 121, no. 24 (2010): 2681–91.

30 D. D. Price, D. G. Finniss, and F. Benedetti, "A Comprehensive Review of the Placebo Effect: Recent Advances and Current Thought," *Annual Review of Psychology* 59 (2008): 565–90.

31 J. Li et al., "Acupuncture for Patients with Mild Hypertension: Study Protocol of an Open-Label Multicenter Randomized Controlled Trial," *Trials* 14 (2013), doi:10.1186/1745-6215-14-380.

32 J. C. Longhurst and S. Tjen-A-Looi, "Acupuncture Regulation of Blood Pressure: Two Decades of Research," *International Review of Neurobiology* 111 (2013): 257–71.

33 S. Kaneko et al., "Heart Rate Variability and Hemodynamic Change in the Superior Mesenteric Artery by Acupuncture Stimulation of Lower Limb Points: A Randomized Crossover Trial," *Evidence-Based Complementary and Alternative Medicine* (2013), doi:10.1155/2013/315982.

34 M. T. Cabioglu, N. Gündogan, and N. Ergene, "The Efficacy of Electroacupuncture Therapy for Weight Loss Changes Plasma Lipoprotein A, Apolipoprotein A, and Apolipoprotein B Levels In Obese Women," *American Journal of Chinese Medicine* 36, no. 6 (2008): 1029–39.

35 M. T. Cabioglu and N. Ergene, "Electroacupuncture Therapy for Weight Loss Reduces Serum Total Cholesterol, Triglycerides, and LDL Cholesterol Levels in Obese Women," *American Journal of Chinese Medicine* 33, no. 4 (2005): 525–33.

36 C. H. Hsu et al., "Effects of Electroacupuncture in Reducing Weight and Waist Circumference in Obese Women: A Randomized Crossover Trial," *International Journal of Obesity* 29, no. 11 (2005): 1379–84.

37 M. Belivani et al., "Acupuncture in the Treatment of Obesity: A Narrative Review of the Literature," *Acupuncture in Medicine* 31, no. 1 (2013): 88–97.

38 J. Wu et al., "Acupuncture for Depression: A Review of Clinical Applications," *Canadian Journal of Psychiatry* 57, no. 7 (2012): 397–405.

39 M. Frass et al., "Use and Acceptance of Complementary and Alternative Medicine among the General Population and Medical Personnel: A Systematic Review," *Ochsner Journal* 12, no. 1 (2012): 45–56.

40 R. Nahas, "Complementary and Alternative Medicine Approaches to Blood Pressure Reduction: An Evidence-Based Review," *Canadian Family Physician* 54, no. 11 (2008): 1529–33.

41 C. E. Rogers, L. K. Larkey, and C. Keller, "A Review of Clinical Trials of Tai Chi and Qigong in Older Adults," *Western Journal of Nursing Research* 31, no. 2 (2009): 245–79.

42 C. Lan et al., "Effect of T'ai Chi Chuan Training on Cardiovascular Risk Factors in Dyslipidemic Patients," *Journal of Alternative and Complementary Medicine* 14, no. 7 (2008): 813–19.

43 C. Lan et al., "Tai Chi Chuan Exercise for Patients with Cardiovascular Disease," *Evidence-Based Complementary and Alternative Medicine* (2013), doi:10.1155/2013/983208.

44 J. Sun, N. Buys, and R. Jayasinghe, "Effects of Community-Based Meditative Tai Chi Programme on Improving Quality of Life, Physical and Mental Health in Chronic Heart Failure Participants," *Aging & Mental Health* 18, no. 3 (2014): 289–95.

45 G. Y. Yeh et al., "Tai Chi Exercise in Patients with Chronic Heart Failure: A Randomized Clinical Trial," *Archives of Internal Medicine* 171, no. 8 (2011): 750–57.

46 G. Y. Yeh et al., "Tai Chi in Patients with Heart Failure with Preserved Ejection Fraction," *Congestive Heart Failure* 19, no. 2 (2013): 77–84.

47 Y. Sher, S. Lolak, and J. R. Maldonado, "The Impact of Depression in Heart Disease," *Current Psychiatry Reports* 12, no. 3 (2010): 255–64.

48 J. X. Li, Y. Hong, and K. M. Chan, "Tai Chi: Physiological Characteristics and Beneficial Effects on Health," *British Journal of Sports Medicine* 35, no. 3 (2001): 148–56.

49 P. A. Balaji, S. R. Varne, and S. S. Ali, "Physiological Effects of Yogic Practices and Transcendental Meditation in Health and Disease," *North American Journal of Medical Sciences* 4, no. 10 (2012): 442–48.

50 K. E. Innes and H. K. Vincent, "The Influence of Yoga-Based Programs on Risk Profiles in Adults with Type 2 Diabetes Mellitus: A Systematic Review," *Evidence-Based Complementary and Alternative Medicine* 4, no. 4 (2007): 469–86.

51 J. G. Rioux and C. Ritenbaugh, "Narrative Review of Yoga Intervention Clinical Trials Including Weight-Related Outcomes," *Alternative Therapies in Health and Medicine* 19, no. 3 (2013): 32–46.

52 S. K. Gupta et al., "Regression of Coronary Atherosclerosis through Healthy Lifestyle in Coronary Artery Disease Patients—Mount Abu Open Heart Trial," *Indian Heart Journal* 63, no. 5 (2011): 461–69.

53 C. C. Streeter et al., Effects of Yoga Versus Walking on Mood, Anxiety, and Brain GABA Levels: A Randomized Controlled MRS Study," *Journal of Alternative and Complementary Medicine* 16, no. 11 (2010): 1145–52.

Chapter 10

1 S. Bhattacharyya et al., "Common Food Additive Carrageenan Stimulates Wnt/ß-Catenin Signaling in Colonic Epithelium by Inhibition of Nucleoredoxin Reduction," *Nutrition and Cancer* 66, no. 1 (2014): 117–27.

2 E. S. Mitchell et al., "Differential Contributions of Theobromine and Caffeine on Mood, Psychomotor Performance, and Blood Pressure," *Physiology & Behavior* 104, no. 5 (2011): 816–22.

3 A. L. Orsama et al., "Weight Rhythms: Weight Increases during Weekends and Decreases during Weekdays," *Obesity Facts* 7, no. 1 (2014): 36–47.

INDEX

Boldface page references indicate illustrations. Underscored references indicate boxed text.

A

Acupuncture, 160–61
Acute cardiac syndrome (ACS), 113
Adrenaline (epinephrine), 11–13, 18, 71
Aging process in blood vessels, 70–71, 74–75, 102–3
Air pollution, 133–34
ALA, 21
Alcohol
  Amaretto Amore, 274
  heart and mood benefits, 28
Almonds
  Almond-Chocolate Bark, 279
  Almond Cookies, 275
  Arugula-Avocado-Almond Salad, 223
  Baked Rainbow Trout with Dates and Almonds, 248
  Maca Date Shake, 274
  Orange-Spinach Salad, 227
  Peach and Blueberry Cobbler, 221
Alpha-linolenic acid (ALA), 21
Alternative therapies, 151–63
  Ayurvedic, 152–54
  breathing exercises, 152
  grounding, 154
  Positive Emotions Prescription, 163
  spirituality, 155–57
  touch therapy, 157–60
    placebo effect, 159–60
    Reiki, 158–59
  traditional Chinese medicine, 160–61
    acupuncture, 160–61
    Qigong, 161
    tai chi, 161
  yoga, 161–62
Amla (Indian gooseberry), 61–62
Amygdala, 12, 101, 136
Anger, 6–7, 68, 75
Angina, 1–2, 74, 99, 102
Angioplasty, 1–2
Antidepressants, 16, 96
Antioxidants, 27, 166. *See also specific foods*
Anxiety
  coronary heart disease and, 6
  reduction with
    berberine, 153
    exercise, 96, 108
    music, 88, 91
    oxytocin release, 123
    touch therapies, 158
Appetite, curbing evening, 26
Apples
  Apple-Blueberry Crisp, 277
  Apple-Rosemary Elixir, 287
  Apple-Spinach Salad, 233
  Baked Apples with Cinnamon, 279
  Celestial Celery Root and Apple Soup, 237
  Green Chakra (Heart) Elixir, 284
Apps, laughter, 81
Aromatherapy, 137
Arteries. *See also* Blood vessels
  compliance of, 70–71
  hardening of, 74–75
Arteriosclerosis, 74–75
Artichokes
  Artichoke Frittata, 222
  Green Bean, Artichoke, and Tuna Salad, 228
  heart and mood benefits, 28–29
  Roasted Jerusalem Artichokes with Herbs, 269
  Salmon with Asparagus and Artichoke-Mustard Sauce, 254
Arugula
  Arugula-Avocado-Almond Salad, 223
  Mouthwatering Watermelon Salad, 234
  Persimmon-Mozzarella Panini, 231
Asparagus
  heart and mood benefits, 29
  Roasted Asparagus with Shallots, 265
  Salmon with Asparagus and Artichoke-Mustard Sauce, 254
Asthma, exercise-induced, 108
Atherosclerosis, 74–75

Atorvastatin, 8
Atrial fibrillation, 103
Autonomic nervous system, 12, 88–89
Avocado
Arugula-Avocado-Almond Salad, 223
Avocado Turkey Burger Sprout Wrap, 229
Black Bean Burritos, 257
Fish Tacos, 260
Gazpacho Soup, 242
heart and mood benefits, 29–30
Ayurvedic, 152–54

B

Bagel, 25
Bananas
Almond Flour Banana Waffles, 220
Amaretto Amore, 274
Banana-Mango-Ginger Smoothie, 215
Chamomile Smoothie, 218
Ginger-Date Smoothie, 215
Orioles Orange Smash Smoothie, 219
Pumpkin-Almond Smoothie, 218
Ravens Purple Pride Smoothie, 217
Basal metabolic rate (BMR), 19
Basil, 44–45
Beans
Black Bean Burritos, 257
heart and mood benefits, 30
Heartwarming White Bean Soup, 240
Roasted Butternut Squash and Black Bean Tacos, 261
Seared Mahi Mahi with Mango Black Bean Salsa, 251
Stuffed Sweet Potatoes with Beans, 225
Beets
Chocolate Chip–Beet Cake, 281
Glazed Beet and Red Grapefruit Salad, 229
heart and mood benefits, 31
Quinoa Salad, 232
Behavioral cardiology, 5–11, 14
Berberine, 153
Berries. *See also specific berry types*
Ana's Blueberry-Cashew Treat, 275
Apple-Blueberry Crisp, 277
Frozen Coconut-Chia-Blueberry Parfait, 276
heart and mood benefits, 31–32
Pistachio-Crusted Tilapia with Strawberry Salsa, 262
Strawberry-Pineapple-Kale Smoothie, 219
Beta-blockers, rebound effect of, 145
Black beans
Black Bean Burritos, 257
Roasted Butternut Squash and Black Bean Tacos, 261
Seared Mahi Mahi with Mango Black Bean Salsa, 251
Stuffed Sweet Potatoes with Beans, 225
Blackberries
heart-health benefits of, 31
Indigo Chakra (Third-Eye) Elixir, 283
Blood pressure
diastolic, 75
exercise-induced hypertension, 102–3
pulse wave velocity, 70–71, 102
response to
acupuncture, 160
Ayurvedic, 153–54
breathing exercises, 152
exercise, 102–3
laughter, 75–76, 82
music/singing, 87–88, 92–93
oxytocin, 123
stress, 102
tai chi, 161
touch therapy, 158
weight training, 109
yoga, 161
systolic, 75–76
Blood vessels. *See also* Heart disease/attack
aging process in, 70–71, 74–75, 102–3
blockage, 1–2, 68, 74, 93
calcium in coronary vessels, 8, 101–2
hardening of arteries, 74–75
inflammation, 2–4
pulse wave velocity, 70–71, 102
response to
emotions, 7
laughter, 7, 68–71, 75–76
music, 86–87
stress, 68–69, 74–75
vasoconstriction, 66, 68–70
vasodilation, 7, 68–70, 72–74, **73**, 76
Blueberries
Almond Flour Banana Waffles, 220
Ana's Blueberry-Cashew Treat, 275
Apple-Blueberry Crisp, 277
Banana-Mango-Ginger Smoothie, 215
Blue Chakra (Throat) Elixir, 284
Frozen Coconut-Chia-Blueberry Parfait, 276
heart and mood benefits, 31–32
Peach and Blueberry Cobbler, 221
Ravens Purple Pride Smoothie, 217
Spinach-Mango Salad with Hempseeds, 226
Spinach Salad with Berries and Honey Pecans, 236
BMR, 19
Body fat, 97–98
Body mass index, 19, 97
Boss, toxic, 134

Bread, 25
Breakfast
importance of, 17
recipes, 214–22
skipping, 17
28-day Positive Emotions Prescription Nutrition Plan, 185–212
Breathing exercises, for blood pressure control, 152
Broccoli
Pesto Portobello Pizza, 249
Quinoa Salad, 232
Roasted Broccoli, 272
Broken heart, recovering from, 141–50
Broken heart syndrome, 116
Brown fat, 97–98
Brussels sprouts
Honey- and Maple-Glazed Brussels Sprouts, 269

C

Caffeine, 166
Calcium in blood vessels, 8, 101–3, 106
Caloric needs, 19
Calories, burned by
active video games, 110
brown fat, 97
cycling, 108
laughter, 76–77
nonexercise activity thermogenesis (NEAT), 110–12
rebounding, 110
Cancer, increase risk with sedentary lifestyle, 101
Capsaicin, 98
Carbohydrates
complex, 16
eating "carb smart," 25–26
insulin triggered by, 16, 25
late-night consumption, 25–26
recommended daily amount, 25
simple, 16
white, 25
Cardiology, behavioral, 5–11, 14
Cardiomyopathy, stress-induced (Takotsubo), 116
Cardiovascular health. *See also* Heart disease/attack; Heart health
benefits of exercise for, 99–100, 107–10
job-related stress, 129, 131–35
Carrageenan, 166
Carrots
Avocado Turkey Burger Sprout Wrap, 229
Gingered Carrot Soup, 241
Miso Soup, 243
Rejuvenating Red Lentil Soup, 239
Saffron Split Pea Soup, 238
Tuna with Veggies, 223
Cashew butter
Cashew Butter Granola Bars, 282
Cashews
Amaretto Amore, 274
Ana's Blueberry-Cashew Treat, 275
Apple-Spinach Salad, 233
Maca Date Shake, 274
Ravens Purple Pride Smoothie, 217
Cauliflower
Curried Cauliflower, 270
Celery
Celestial Celery Root and Apple Soup, 237
Green Chakra (Heart) Elixir, 284
Grilled Chicken and Celery Salad à la Marcella, 233
heart and mood benefits, 32
Pineapple Elixir, 287
Saffron Split Pea Soup, 238
Cereal, 26
Chakras, 184
Chamomile, 218
Cherries
Amaretto Amore, 274
Butternut Squash with Baby Spinach, 272
Deeply Satisfying Kasha Porridge, 214
heart and mood benefits, 32–33
Violet Chakra (Crown) Elixir, 283
Chia seeds
Frozen Coconut-Chia-Blueberry Parfait, 276
Ravens Purple Pride Smoothie, 217
Red Chakra (Root) Elixir, 286
in water to curb appetite, 26
Chicken
Grilled Chicken and Celery Salad à la Marcella, 233
heart and mood benefits, 52
Moroccan Chicken, 256
Sesame Chicken Stir-Fry, 244
Chickpeas
Tuna and Chickpea Salad, 230
Chilean wineberry, 62
Chile peppers
brown fat activation, 98
Gazpacho Soup, 242
heart and mood benefits, 33
Roasted Butternut Squash and Black Bean Tacos, 261
Chocolate
Almond-Chocolate Bark, 279
Cashew Butter Granola Bars, 282
Chai Hot Chocolate, 280

Chocolate (*cont.*)
Chocolate Chip–Beet Cake, 281
heart and mood benefits, 33–35
Cholesterol
guidelines, 8, 22
lecithin-cholesterol acyltransferase (LCAT) deficiency, 119–20
reduction with
acupuncture, 160
Ayurveda, 153
statins, 2, 8
tai chi, 161
Cholesterol plaque
formation, 4, 127
reduction with nitric oxide production, 72, **73**
rupture, 3–5, 74, 103
Cinnamon
Apple-Blueberry Crisp, 277
Baked Apples with Cinnamon, 279
heart and mood benefits, 35, 166
Pumpkin Pie Smoothie, 216
Clubs, laughter, 81, 82–83
Coffee, benefits of, 35–36, 166
Communication through laughter, 79
Complementary medicine. *See* Integrative medicine
Connections, facilitated by laughter, 79–80
Control, sense of, 128–29, 148
Cooldown, 106–7, 166
Coronary arteries, 2, 68, 162
calcification in, 8, 101–3, 106
oxygen delivery to, 99
Cortisol, 13, 71, 76–77, 86, 124
Cravings, reduced with laughter, 77
C-reactive protein (CRP), 3, 8, 22, 24, 90, 132, 148
Cruciferous vegetables, heart and mood benefits of, 36
Cucumber
Gazpacho Soup, 242
Heavenly Hearts of Palm Salad, 224
positive emotions elixirs, 283–87
Strawberry-Pineapple-Kale Smoothie, 219
Cycling, 108, 110

D

Daily living, emotions in,
charting negative, 174–75
charting positive, 170–74
tips for maximizing positive, 167
Dancing, 107–8
Dates
Baked Rainbow Trout with Dates and Almonds, 248
Deeply Satisfying Kasha Porridge, 214
Ginger-Date Smoothie, 215
Maca Date Shake, 274
Orioles Orange Smash Smoothie, 219
Peach and Blueberry Cobbler, 221
Ultimate Date Cake, 278
Death, dealing with, 142–45
Dementia, decrease risk with
dancing, 107–8
walking, 107
Dental hygiene, 26
Depression
as heart disease risk factor, 6
increased with sitting, 101
lowering with
berberine, 153
exercise, 96
laughter, 82
spirituality, 156
SSRIs, 16, 96
Desserts
recipes, 274–82
28-day Positive Emotions Prescription Nutrition Plan, 185–212
DHA, 21
Diabetes. *See also* Insulin resistance
decrease risk with weight training, 109
heart disease risk increase with, 4
increase risk with waist size, 23
Dinners
eating light, 17–18
recipes, 244–62
28-day Positive Emotions Prescription Nutrition Plan, 185–212
Divorce, 79–80, 115–16, 146–47
Docosahexaenoic acid (DHA), 21
Dopamine
foods and, 28
frisson effect and, 91–92
increase with joyful music, 86
roles in the body, 95–96
Dragon fruit, 60–61
Drivers, stress in, 132

E

Eating. *See also* Food(s)
binge-eating reduced with laughter, 77
"carb smart," 25–26
emotional, 16
late-night, 17
principles of healthy, 17–26
sensibly, 23–24
28-day Positive Emotions Prescription Nutrition Plan, 182–212

Eicosapentaenoic acid (EPA), 21
Electroacupuncture, 160
Elixirs. *See* Positive emotions elixirs
Emotional eating, 16
Emotions. *See also* Mood; Positive emotions
  charting in daily life, 168–76
  exercise for emotional health, 95–98, 100–101
  heart disease/attack risk with negative, 5–8
  relationships and, 113–25
Endorphins, 86
  effects of, 95
  foods and, 28
  increase with
    doing what you love, 112
    exercise, 107–8, 110
    laughter, 71–72, **73**
    weight training, 109
Endothelium. *See also* Blood vessels
  foods to maintain health, 19
  impairment by high-fat diet, 18
  injury to, 2
  nitric oxide production, 72–74, **73**
  response to
    music, 87, 92
    stress, 3
Energy therapy, 157–58
EPA, 21
Epinephrine (adrenaline), 11–13, 18, 71
Estrogen, 117
Exercise, 95–112
  amount needed, 100–103, 106
  benefits of
    browning of white fat, 97–98
    cardiovascular effects, 99–100
    mood improvement, 95–98
  laughter as, 76–77
  Metabolic Equivalent of Task (MET), 104–5, 106
  overactivity, 101–3, 106
  positive emotions and
    charting, 169–70
    tips for maximizing, 166
  Positive Emotions Prescription, 112
  types, 106–12
    active video games, 110
    cycling, 108, 110
    dancing, 107–8
    NEAT, 110–12
    rebounding, 110
    swimming, 108
    walking, brisk, 107
    weight training, 109
  warmup and cooldown, 106–7, 166

F

Fat. *See* Body fat
Fats, dietary, 18–19
Fear, 71
Fermented foods
  Avocado Turkey Burger Sprout Wrap, 229
  Fish Tacos, 260
  heart and mood benefits, 37
Fiber (soluble)
  heart and mood benefits, 37–38
  sources, 38–39
Fight-or-flight response, 3, 12–14, 18, 117
Fish
  Asian Baked Halibut, 259
  Baked Rainbow Trout with Dates and Almonds, 248
  Cedar-Planked Wild Salmon, 247
  Fish Tacos, 260
  Flounder in Garlic White Wine Sauce, 245
  Green Bean, Artichoke, and Tuna Salad, 228
  heart and mood benefits, 38–40
  Mediterranean Salmon with Sun-Dried Tomatoes, Capers, and Olives, 252
  Moroccan-Seasoned Wild Salmon, 245
  Pistachio-Crusted Tilapia with Strawberry Salsa, 262
  Roasted Salmon with Orange-Herb Sauce, 258
  Rockfish Cakes, 246
  Salmon with Asparagus and Artichoke-Mustard Sauce, 254
  Seared Mahi Mahi with Mango Black Bean Salsa, 251
  Sesame Miso Cod, 253
  Super-Easy Steelhead Trout Teriyaki, 253
  Tuna and Chickpea Salad, 230
  Tuna with Veggies, 223
Foam cells, 4
Food(s). *See also* Eating
  cravings reduced with laughter, 77
  GMOs and, 165–66
  heart healthy, 28–60
  mood elevating, 28–60
  organic, 27, 165–66
  recipes, 213–88
    breakfast, 214–22
    desserts, 274–82
    dinners, 244–62
    lunch, 223–36
    positive emotions elixirs, 283–88
    sides, 263–73
    soups, 237–43
  top 50 foods and food groups, 26–60
  trending positive emotion foods, 60–64

Food(s) (*cont.*)
28-day Positive Emotions Prescription Nutrition Plan, 182–212
vitamin C–rich, 139
Food labels, 26
Free radicals, 154
Frisson effect, 91–92, 93–94
Fruits
Almond Flour Banana Waffles, 220
Amaretto Amore, 274
Ana's Blueberry-Cashew Treat, 275
Apple-Blueberry Crisp, 277
Apple-Rosemary Elixir, 287
Apple-Spinach Salad, 233
Baked Apples with Cinnamon, 279
Banana-Mango-Ginger Smoothie, 215
Blue Chakra (Throat) Elixir, 284
Celestial Celery Root and Apple Soup, 237
Chamomile Smoothie, 218
Deeply Satisfying Kasha Porridge, 214
Frozen Coconut-Chia-Blueberry Parfait, 276
Ginger-Date Smoothie, 215
Glazed Beet and Red Grapefruit Salad, 229
Green Chakra (Heart) Elixir, 284
Grilled Chicken and Celery Salad à la Marcella, 233
heart and mood benefits, 40–43
Indigo Chakra (Third-Eye) Elixir, 283
Kumquat Elixir, 288
less likely to be sprayed with pesticide, 27
Moroccan Chicken, 256
Mouthwatering Watermelon Salad, 234
Orange, Lime, and Grapefruit Salad with Honey Mint Dressing, 235
Orange Chakra (Abdomen) Elixir, 285
Orange-Spinach Salad, 227
Orioles Orange Smash Smoothie, 219
Peach and Blueberry Cobbler, 221
Persimmon-Mozzarella Panini, 231
Pineapple Carpaccio, 282
Pineapple Elixir, 287
Pistachio-Crusted Tilapia with Strawberry Salsa, 262
positive emotions elixirs, 283–88
Pumpkin-Almond Smoothie, 218
Ravens Purple Pride Smoothie, 217
Red Chakra (Root) Elixir, 286
Roasted Salmon with Orange-Herb Sauce, 258
Seared Mahi Mahi with Mango Black Bean Salsa, 251
Spinach-Mango Salad with Hempseeds, 226
Strawberries and Watercress Salad, 234
Strawberry-Pineapple-Kale Smoothie, 219
Sunshine Gold Elixir, 286
Violet Chakra (Crown) Elixir, 283
Watermelon-Mint Elixir, 288
Yellow Chakra (Solar Plexus) Elixir, 285

G

GABA, 28, 96, 162
Gallstone, 20
Gamma-aminobutyric acid (GABA), 28, 96, 162
Garlic
Curried Cauliflower, 270
heart and mood benefits, 43
Roasted Broccoli, 272
Roasted Green Beans with Garlic and Thyme, 273
Roasted Jerusalem Artichokes with Herbs, 269
Sautéed Spinach with Lemon and Pine Nuts, 268
Genetically modified organisms (GMOs), 165–66
Ginger
Asian Baked Halibut, 259
Banana-Mango-Ginger Smoothie, 215
Ginger-Date Smoothie, 215
heart and mood benefits, 43–44
GMOs, 165–66
Goji berries
Baked Apples with Cinnamon, 279
heart and mood benefits, 44
Maca Date Shake, 274
Red Chakra (Root) Elixir, 286
Grapefruit
Glazed Beet and Red Grapefruit Salad, 229
Orange, Lime, and Grapefruit Salad with Honey Mint Dressing, 235
Gratitude, expressing, 146
Green beans
Green Bean, Artichoke, and Tuna Salad, 228
Green Beans with Walnuts and Thyme, 264
Roasted Green Beans with Garlic and Thyme, 273
Grief, 143–45
Grounding, 154
Guarana, 61

H

Hardening of arteries, 74–75
HDL, 22, 119
Healing Touch, 157–58
Heart disease/attack
cardiomyopathy, stress-induced (Takotsubo), 116
causes, 4–5
risk decrease with
brisk walking, 107, 109
cycling, 110

    - dancing, 108
    - optimism, 144–45
    - spiritual/religious belief, 148
    - weight training, 109
  - risk increase with
    - arteriosclerosis, 74–75
    - decreased heart rate variability, 89–90
    - exercise lack, 101
    - failure to laugh, 67–68
    - grief, 145
    - high blood pressure, 75
    - higher resting heart rates, 99–100
    - negative emotions, 5–8
    - noise pollution, 133–34
    - overexertion, 101–3, 106
    - relationship stress, 114–16
    - sitting, 101, 138
    - social isolation, 117
    - stress, 4–8, 114–16, 129, 132, 149
    - workplace stress, 129, 131–35
  - treatment
    - angioplasty and stents, 1–2, 8
    - beta-blockers, 145
    - oxytocin, 142–43
    - statins, 2–3, 8
- Heart health
  - alternative therapies for, 151–63
  - behavioral cardiology, 5–11, 14
  - exercise and, 95–112
  - foods for, 28–60
  - heart rate variability as indicator of, 89
  - laughter and, 65–83
  - music and, 85–94
  - oxytocin and, 142–43
  - relationships and, 113–25
  - touch and, 123–24
  - triglycerides and, 4, 20
- Heart rate
  - average resting, 99
  - taking, 99
  - variability, 89–90, 133–34, 158, 160
- Hearts of palm
  - Heavenly Hearts of Palm Salad, 224
- Hempseeds
  - Banana-Mango-Ginger Smoothie, 215
  - Orange Chakra (Abdomen) Elixir, 285
  - Ravens Purple Pride Smoothie, 217
  - Spinach-Mango Salad with Hempseeds, 226
- Herbs, heart and mood benefits of, 44–45
- HGH, 25–26
- Hibiscus, 44–45
- High-density lipoprotein (HDL), 22, 119
- Hijiki, 55, 243
- Hip fracture, 108
- Histoplasmosis, 119–20
- Hostility, tendencies toward, 68
- Hot chocolate, chai, 280
- HPA axis, 13
- Hugging, 123–24, 142–43
- Human growth hormone (HGH), 25–26
- Humor. *See* Laughter
- Hypertension, 4, 75–76, 102–3. *See also* Blood pressure
- Hypothalamus, 12–13

I

- IL-6, 90
- Indian gooseberry (amla), 61–62
- Inflammation
  - macrophages and, 3–4, 19, 20
  - reduction with
    - acupuncture, 160
    - music, 90
    - nitric oxide production, 72, **73**
    - oxytocin release, 123, 142
    - statins, 3
    - tai chi, 161
  - sources of
    - free radicals, 154
    - intervention-associated, 2
    - periodontal disease, 136
    - stress, 2–4, 127, 132
- Insomnia, 77–78, 82
- Insulin, 16, 25
- Insulin resistance
  - increase in periodontal disease, 136
  - reduction with
    - acupuncture, 160
    - tai chi, 161
- Integrative medicine, 151–63. *See also* Alternative therapies
- Interleukin-6 (IL-6), 90
- Interventional therapies, 1–2, 8, 9
- Irisin, 97

J

- Journal, 14
- Juicing, 27

K

- Kale
  - heart and mood benefits, 45–46
  - Mediterranean Kale Tart, 255
  - Sautéed Kale, 265
  - Strawberry-Pineapple-Kale Smoothie, 219
- Kasha, 214
- Kindness, importance of, 122

Krill oil, 21
Kumquat elixir, 288

L

Labels, food, 26
Laughter
  blood vessel dilation with, 7, 68–71
  health benefits of, 65–83, 139
    artery health, 79–80
    author's experiences with, 65–66, 69–70
    blood pressure, 75–76, 82
    calorie burn, 76–77
    connection formation, 79–80
    memory improvement, 78–79
    sleep improvement, 77–78, 82
    studies on, 66–71
  in healthy relationships, 122
  Positive Emotions Prescription, 83
  science behind, 71–74
  tips for finding/creating, 80–83
    laughter clubs, 81, 82–83
    laughter yoga, 81–82
    online links, 80–81
Lavender, 137
LCAT deficiency, 119–20
LDL, 4, 8, 20, 22, 153
Lecithin-cholesterol acyltransferase (LCAT) deficiency, 119–20
Lemon
  Moroccan Chicken, 256
  Sautéed Spinach with Lemon and Pine Nuts, 268
Lentils
  Rejuvenating Red Lentil Soup, 239
Lettuce
  Arugula-Avocado-Almond Salad, 223
Limes
  Fish Tacos, 260
  Orange, Lime, and Grapefruit Salad with Honey Mint Dressing, 235
Links to laughter, online, 80–81
Lipoprotein lipase, 18, 138
Listening, importance of, 122
Lotus root
  heart and mood benefits, 46
  Roasted Lotus Root, 266
Low-density lipoprotein (LDL), 4, 8, 20, 22, 153
Lucuma, 62
Lunch
  recipes, 223–36
  28-day Positive Emotions Prescription Nutrition Plan, 185–212

M

Maca
  heart and mood benefits, 46
  Maca Date Shake, 274
  Pumpkin Pie Smoothie, 216
Macrophages, 3–4, 19, 20, 127
Magnesium, 41, 42
Mango
  Banana-Mango-Ginger Smoothie, 215
  Seared Mahi Mahi with Mango Black Bean Salsa, 251
  Spinach-Mango Salad with Hempseeds, 226
  Sunshine Gold Elixir, 286
Maqui berry, 62
Marriage
  divorce, 79–80, 115–16, 146–47
  heart health increase with, 113–15, 118–19
Massage
  Ayurvedic Abhyanga, 153–54
  oxytocin release with, 142
Meals
  cheat, 24, 183
  recipes, 213–88
  in 28-day Positive Emotions Prescription plan, 182–212
Meat
  Avocado Turkey Burger Sprout Wrap, 229
  Grilled Chicken and Celery Salad à la Marcella, 233
  Moroccan Chicken, 256
  Sesame Chicken Stir-Fry, 244
Meditation, 157
Mediterranean diet, 18, 213
Melatonin, 28
Melon
  Mouthwatering Watermelon Salad, 234
  Orange, Lime, and Grapefruit Salad with Honey Mint Dressing, 235
  Watermelon-Mint Elixir, 288
Memory, improvement with
  dancing, 108
  laughter, 78–79
Menus, in 28-day Positive Emotions Prescription Plan, 182–212
Metabolic Equivalent of Task (MET), 104–5, 106
Methylxanthine, 166
Midazolam, 88
Milk, 165–66
Mind, synergy with heart, 149–50
Miso
  Miso Soup, 243
  Sesame Miso Cod, 253
  Sweet Potato–Miso Spread, 267

Mitochondria, in brown fat, 97
Mood
improvement with
Ayurveda, 153
exercise, 95–98, 106–8
fat burning, 97–98, 100–101
foods, 28–60
plants, 134
yoga, 161–62
mood-food connection, 15–16
"supermood" brain chemicals, 28, 95–96, 100–101, 111
Movies
affect on blood vessels, 68–70
funny, 81
Mucuna bean, 62–63
Multitasking, 137–38
Muscles, happiness, 10
Mushrooms
Artichoke Frittata, 222
Grilled Portobello Burgers, 250
heart and mood benefits, 46–47
Pesto Portobello Pizza, 249
reishi, 63
Music
frisson effect, 91–92, 93–94
healing power of, 85–94
anti-inflammatory effects, 90
heart rate variability improvement, 89–90
hospital recovery time decrease, 90–91
studies on, 86–88
Positive Emotions Prescription, 94
singing, 92–94
tempo and loudness, 88–89
Mustard
heart and mood benefits, 47–48
Orange-Spinach Salad, 227
Rockfish Cakes, 246
Salmon with Asparagus and Artichoke-Mustard Sauce, 254
Tuna and Chickpea Salad, 230
Myocardial infarction. *See* Heart disease/attack

N

NEAT, 110–12
Negative emotions
charting in daily life, 174–75
heart disease/attack risk increase with, 5–8
Nicotine, 133
Nitric oxide, 72–74, **73**, 87, 108
Noise pollution, 133
Nonexercise activity thermogenesis (NEAT), 110–12
Norepinephrine, 28, 96
Nori, 55
Novels, comic, 81
Nutrition. *See also* Food(s)
charting positive emotions, 169
tips for maximizing positive emotions, 165–66
28-day Positive Emotions Prescription Nutrition Plan, 182–212
Nuts
Almond-Chocolate Bark, 279
Almond Cookies, 275
Amaretto Amore, 274
Ana's Blueberry-Cashew Treat, 275
Apple-Spinach Salad, 233
Baked Apples with Cinnamon, 279
Baked Rainbow Trout with Dates and Almonds, 248
Cashew Butter Granola Bars, 282
Glazed Beet and Red Grapefruit Salad, 229
Green Beans with Walnuts and Thyme, 264
heart and mood benefits, 48–49
Maca Date Shake, 274
Moroccan-Seasoned Wild Salmon, 245
Orange-Spinach Salad, 227
Pistachio-Crusted Tilapia with Strawberry Salsa, 262
Ravens Purple Pride Smoothie, 217
Seared Mahi Mahi with Mango Black Bean Salsa, 251
Spinach Salad with Berries and Honey Pecans, 236
Ultimate Date Cake, 278

O

Obesity, treatment for
brown fat stimulation, 160
electroacupuncture, 160
Oculostenotic reflex, 1
Olives
Green Bean, Artichoke, and Tuna Salad, 228
heart and mood benefits, 49
Mediterranean Kale Tart, 255
Mediterranean Salmon with Sun-Dried Tomatoes, Capers, and Olives, 252
Moroccan Chicken, 256
Omega-3 fats, 21
Onions and shallots
Butternut Squash with Baby Spinach, 272
Celestial Celery Root and Apple Soup, 237
Gingered Carrot Soup, 241
heart and mood benefits, 49–50
Lightly Sautéed Purslane, 266

Onions and shallots (*cont.*)
  Pistachio-Crusted Tilapia with Strawberry Salsa, 262
  Quinoa Salad, 232
  Roasted Asparagus with Shallots, 265
  Stuffed Sweet Potatoes with Beans, 225
Optimism, 144–45
Oral health, 136
Oranges
  Orange, Lime, and Grapefruit Salad with Honey Mint Dressing, 235
  Orange Chakra (Abdomen) Elixir, 285
  Orange-Spinach Salad, 227
  Orioles Orange Smash Smoothie, 219
  Roasted Salmon with Orange-Herb Sauce, 258
Oregano, 44–45
Organic foods, 27, 165–66
Overactivity, 101–3, 106
Oxytocin, 88, 123–24, 142–43, 146

P

Pancreatitis, 20
Parasympathetic nervous system, 90
Peaches
  Peach and Blueberry Cobbler, 221
Peas
  Saffron Split Pea Soup, 238
  Tuna with Veggies, 223
Pecans
  Cashew Butter Granola Bars, 282
  Orange-Spinach Salad, 227
  Spinach Salad with Berries and Honey Pecans, 236
PEPI (Positive Emotions Prescription Inventory), 10
PEQ, 168–76
Pericardial effusion, 24
Periodontal disease, 136
Persimmons
  heart and mood benefits, 50–51
  Persimmon-Mozzarella Panini, 231
Pesticides, 27
Pets, 124
Pineapple
  Pineapple Carpaccio, 282
  Pineapple Elixir, 287
  Strawberry-Pineapple-Kale Smoothie, 219
  Yellow Chakra (Solar Plexus) Elixir, 285
Pine nuts
  Sautéed Spinach with Lemon and Pine Nuts, 268
  Sun-Dried Tomato Dip, 267
Pistachios
  Glazed Beet and Red Grapefruit Salad, 229
  Moroccan-Seasoned Wild Salmon, 245
  Pistachio-Crusted Tilapia with Strawberry Salsa, 262
  Seared Mahi Mahi with Mango Black Bean Salsa, 251
Placebo effect, 157, 159–60
Planning for the future, 146
Plants, stress reduction with, 134
Pomegranate
  heart and mood benefits, 51
  Orange-Spinach Salad, 227
Positive emotions
  charting in daily life, 168–76
  foods
    elixir recipes, 283–88
    top 50 foods and food groups, 26–60
    trending foods, 60–64
  professional life and, 127–40
  regaining after life-altering event, 141–50
  relationships and, 113–25
  tips for maximizing
    daily living, 167
    exercise, 166
    nutrition, 165–66
Positive emotions elixirs, 283–88
  Apple-Rosemary Elixir, 287
  Blue Chakra (Throat) Elixir, 284
  Green Chakra (Heart) Elixir, 284
  Indigo Chakra (Third-Eye) Elixir, 283
  Kumquat Elixir, 288
  Orange Chakra (Abdomen) Elixir, 285
  Pineapple Elixir, 287
  Red Chakra (Root) Elixir, 286
  Sunshine Gold Elixir, 286
  Violet Chakra (Crown) Elixir, 283
  Watermelon-Mint Elixir, 288
  Yellow Chakra (Solar Plexus) Elixir, 285
Positive Emotions Prescription, 22, 165–212
  alternative therapies, 163
  applying to daily life, 177–82
    case studies, 177–80
    patient success stories, 180–82
  behavioral cardiology, 14
  exercise, 112
  laughter, 83
  music, 94
  nutrition, 64, 182–212
  recovery from loss, 150
  relational wellness, 125
  work- and job-related stress, 140
Positive Emotions Prescription Inventory (PEPI), 10

Positive Emotions Quotient (PEQ), 168–76
Positive thoughts, for stress management/ prevention, 14
Potassium, 41, 42
Potatoes. *See* Sweet potatoes
Poultry, 52. *See also* Chicken; Turkey
Prayer. *See* Spirituality
Prioritizing, 140
Professional life. *See* Work
Pulse rate, 99
Pulse wave velocity, 70–71, 102
Pumpkin
  Apple-Blueberry Crisp, 277
  Butternut Squash with Baby Spinach, 272
  heart and mood benefits, 52
  Mouthwatering Watermelon Salad, 234
  Pumpkin-Almond Smoothie, 218
  Pumpkin Pie Smoothie, 216
  Roasted Butternut Squash and Black Bean Tacos, 261
Purslane
  heart and mood benefits, 53
  Lightly Sautéed Purslane, 266

Q

Qigong, 161
Quinoa
  heart and mood benefits, 53
  Quinoa Salad, 232

R

Radishes
  Arugula-Avocado-Almond Salad, 223
  heart and mood benefits, 53–54
Raspberries, 31–32
Rebounding, 110
Recipes, 213–88. *See also specific foods and food groups*
  breakfasts, 214–22
  desserts, 274–82
  dinners, 244–62
  lunches, 223–36
  positive emotions elixirs, 283–88
  sides, 263–73
  soups, 237–43
Recovery from loss, 141–50, 150
Reiki, 158–59
Reishi mushroom, 63
Relationships
  death of spouse, 115–16
  divorce, 79–80, 115–16, 146–47
  emotional connections in women *vs.* men, 117–18
  heart health and, 113–25
  laughter in successful, 79–80
  lessons from long, 118–22
  marriage, 113–15
  pointers/tips for happy, 121–22, 124–25
  Positive Emotions Prescription, 125
  recovery from loss, 141–50
  social isolation, 116
  touch, benefits of, 123–24
Religion, 147–48, 155–57
Resting metabolic rate, 19
Rosemary
  Grilled Portobello Burgers, 250
  heart and mood benefits, 44–45, 54
  Heartwarming White Bean Soup, 240
Rosuvastatin, 8

S

Saffron
  heart and mood benefits, 54–55
  Saffron Split Pea Soup, 238
Sage, 44–45
Salmon
  Cedar-Planked Wild Salmon, 247
  Mediterranean Salmon with Sun-Dried Tomatoes, Capers, and Olives, 252
  Moroccan-Seasoned Wild Salmon, 245
  Roasted Salmon with Orange-Herb Sauce, 258
  Salmon with Asparagus and Artichoke-Mustard Sauce, 254
Saturated fats, 18–19
Sea buckthorn berry, 63–64
Seaweed
  heart and mood benefits, 55
  Miso Soup, 243
Seeds
  Butternut Squash with Baby Spinach, 272
  Cashew Butter Granola Bars, 282
  Frozen Coconut-Chia-Blueberry Parfait, 276
  heart and mood benefits, 55–56
  Mouthwatering Watermelon Salad, 234
  Orange Chakra (Abdomen) Elixir, 285
  Orange-Spinach Salad, 227
  Ravens Purple Pride Smoothie, 217
  Red Chakra (Root) Elixir, 286
  Sesame Bars, 276
  Sesame Chicken Stir-Fry, 244
  Spinach-Mango Salad with Hempseeds, 226
Selective serotonin reuptake inhibitors (SSRIs), 16, 96

Serotonin
  boosting production, 16, 25
  foods and, 28
  roles in the body, 16, 96
Serving size, 26
Sesame seeds
  Cashew Butter Granola Bars, 282
  Sesame Bars, 276
  Sesame Chicken Stir-Fry, 244
Shallots. *See* Onions and shallots
Shirodhara, 153–54
Sick building syndrome, 133
Sides, recipes for, 263–73
Sitting, health risks of, 101, 138
Sleep
  human growth hormone and, 25–26
  improvement with
    exercise, 96
    laughter, 77–78, 82
  melatonin and, 28
Sleep apnea, 77
Smiling, 136
Smoking, 4, 132–33
Smoothie recipes
  Banana-Mango-Ginger Smoothie, 215
  Chamomile Smoothie, 218
  Ginger-Date Smoothie, 215
  Orioles Orange Smash Smoothie, 219
  Pumpkin-Almond Smoothie, 218
  Pumpkin Pie Smoothie, 216
  Ravens Purple Pride Smoothie, 217
  Strawberry-Pineapple-Kale Smoothie, 219
Snacks. *See* Positive emotions elixirs
Social interaction. *See also* Relationships
  dealing with divorce, 146–47
  helping others through grieving process, 143–44
  support network, 144–45
Social isolation, 116
Sodium, 26
Soups, recipes for, 237–43
Soy milk, 165–66
Spices, 98
Spinach
  Apple-Spinach Salad, 233
  Butternut Squash with Baby Spinach, 272
  heart and mood benefits, 56
  Heavenly Hearts of Palm Salad, 224
  Miso Soup, 243
  Orange-Spinach Salad, 227
  Sautéed Spinach with Lemon and Pine Nuts, 268
  Spinach-Mango Salad with Hempseeds, 226
  Spinach Salad with Berries and Honey Pecans, 236
  Stuffed Sweet Potatoes with Beans, 225
Spirituality, 147–48, 155–57
Spirulina
  Almond-Chocolate Bark, 279
  Green Chakra (Heart) Elixir, 284
  heart and mood benefits, 56–57
Sprouts
  Avocado Turkey Burger Sprout Wrap, 229
Squash
  Butternut Squash with Baby Spinach, 272
  Roasted Butternut Squash and Black Bean Tacos, 261
SSRIs, 16, 96
Statins, 2–3, 8
Stent, 1–2
Strawberries
  heart and mood benefits, 31–32
  Pistachio-Crusted Tilapia with Strawberry Salsa, 262
  Red Chakra (Root) Elixir, 286
  Spinach Salad with Berries and Honey Pecans, 236
  Strawberries and Watercress Salad, 234
  Strawberry-Pineapple-Kale Smoothie, 219
Stress
  American lifestyle norm, 11
  behavioral cardiology and, 9–11
  dealing with death, 142–45
  of divorce, 80, 115–16, 146–47
  effects on
    blood pressure, 75–76, 102
    blood vessels, 68–70, 74–75
    fat-processing, 18
    heart attack/disease risk, 4–8, 114–16, 129, 132, 149
    inflammation, 2–4, 127, 132
    sleep, 77–78
  fight-or-flight response, 3, 12–14, 18, 117
  good and bad, 11–12
  managing with
    activities at work, 137–40
    aromatherapy, 137
    Ayurveda, 153–54
    exercise, 96–97
    humor, 139
    positive thoughts, 14
    prioritizing tasks, 140
    singing, 93
    spirituality, 157
    touch therapy, 157–59
    vitamin C, 139
    volunteering, 143
  marital-related, 114–15
  oxidative, 154, 162
  perception of, 149

quantifying, 9
relationship-related, 114–16
Takotsubo (stress-induced) cardiomyopathy, 116
workplace, 127–40
Stroke
decrease risk with walking, 107
increase risk with
arteriosclerosis, 74
high blood pressure, 75
noise pollution, 133
oral disease, 136
social isolation, 117
vasoconstriction, 68
Suicide, by divorced men, 115
Support network, 144–45
Surgery
interventional therapies, 1–2, 8
positive influences on outcome
marriage, 113–14
music, 87–88, 90–91
spirituality, 155–56
Sweet potatoes
Baked Sweet Potato Fries, 263
heart and mood benefits, 51–52
Rejuvenating Red Lentil Soup, 239
Spicy Sweet Potato Fries, 271
Stuffed Sweet Potatoes with Beans, 225
Sweet Potato–Miso Spread, 267
Swimming, 108
Sympathetic nervous system, 89
Synergy of mind and heart, 149–50

T

Tai chi, 161
Takotsubo cardiomyopathy, 116
Tea, heart and mood benefits of, 57, 166
Therapeutic Touch, 157–58
Time-outs, 137
Tomatoes
Avocado Turkey Burger Sprout Wrap, 229
Gazpacho Soup, 242
Green Bean, Artichoke, and Tuna Salad, 228
Grilled Portobello Burgers, 250
heart and mood benefits, 57–58
Heavenly Hearts of Palm Salad, 224
Mediterranean Kale Tart, 255
Mediterranean Salmon with Sun-Dried Tomatoes, Capers, and Olives, 252
Sun-Dried Tomato Dip, 267
Tuna and Chickpea Salad, 230
Touch, heart benefits of, 123–24
Touch therapy, 157–60
Traditional Chinese medicine, 160–61
Trampoline, mini, 110
Trans fats, 18–19
Transient receptor potentials (TRPs), 98
Triglycerides
heart health and, 4, 20
increase with stress, 18
optimum levels, 21
pancreatitis and, 20
postprandial, 18–19
processing remnants, 20
reduction with
acupuncture, 160
Ayurveda, 153
lifestyle choices, 21, 22
tai chi, 161
yoga, 162
Trout
Baked Rainbow Trout with Dates and Almonds, 248
Super-Easy Steelhead Trout Teriyaki, 253
TRPs, 98
Tryptophan, 16
Tuna
Green Bean, Artichoke, and Tuna Salad, 228
Tuna and Chickpea Salad, 230
Tuna with Veggies, 223
Turkey
Avocado Turkey Burger Sprout Wrap, 229
heart and mood benefits, 52
Turmeric
Apple-Rosemary Elixir, 287
heart and mood benefits, 58–59
Moroccan Chicken, 256
Sunshine Gold Elixir, 286
TV shows, funny, 81
Type A personality, 129

V

Vanilla
Amaretto Amore, 274
Cashew Butter Granola Bars, 282
Chocolate Chip–Beet Cake, 281
Ginger-Date Smoothie, 215
heart and mood benefits, 59
Peach and Blueberry Cobbler, 221
Vasoconstriction, 66, 68–70
Vasodilation
with endorphin and nitric oxide release, 72–74, **73**
laughter and, 68–70, 76
Vegetables
Artichoke Frittata, 222
Baked Sweet Potato Fries, 263
Butternut Squash with Baby Spinach, 272

Vegetables (*cont.*)
Curried Cauliflower, 270
Gazpacho Soup, 242
Gingered Carrot Soup, 241
Glazed Beet and Red Grapefruit Salad, 229
Green Bean, Artichoke, and Tuna Salad, 228
heart and mood benefits cruciferous, 36
Heavenly Hearts of Palm Salad, 224
Honey- and Maple-Glazed Brussels Sprouts, 269
less likely to be sprayed with pesticide, 27
Miso Soup, 243
Pesto Portobello Pizza, 249
Pumpkin-Almond Smoothie, 218
Pumpkin Pie Smoothie, 216
Quinoa Salad, 232
Roasted Asparagus with Shallots, 265
Roasted Broccoli, 272
Roasted Green Beans with Garlic and Thyme, 273
Roasted Jerusalem Artichokes with Herbs, 269
Saffron Split Pea Soup, 238
Salmon with Asparagus and Artichoke-Mustard Sauce, 254
Spicy Sweet Potato Fries, 271
Sweet Potato–Miso Spread, 267
Tuna with Veggies, 223
Versed, 88
Video games, active, 110
Vinegar, white, 27
Vitamin C, 139
Volunteering, benefits of, 143, 157

W

Waist size, 23
Wakame, 55
Walking
grounding, 154
health benefits of brisk, 107, <u>109</u>
Walnuts
Baked Apples with Cinnamon, 279
Green Beans with Walnuts and Thyme, 264
Ravens Purple Pride Smoothie, 217
Ultimate Date Cake, 278
Warmup, 106–7, 166
Watercress
Strawberries and Watercress Salad, 234
Watermelon
heart and mood benefits, 60
Mouthwatering Watermelon Salad, 234
Watermelon-Mint Elixir, 288
Web sites, for humor, 80–81
Weight
gain with sleep deprivation, 26
healthy, 19, 23
loss therapies
electroacupuncture, 160
tai chi, 161
yoga, 162
Weight training, <u>109</u>
Wii Fit, 110
Women, emotional connections by, 117–18
Work, stress and, 127–40
causes of stress, 128–29, 133–35
air pollution, 133–34
lack of control, 128–29
noise pollution, 133–34
toxic boss, 134–35
heart disease/attack risk, 129, 131–35
managing stress, 135–40
aromatherapy, 137
avoiding multitasking, 137–38
moving around, 138–39
prioritizing tasks, 140
time-outs, 137
vitamin C, 139
most and least stressful jobs, 129, <u>130</u>
Positive Emotions Prescription, <u>140</u>
Wound healing, oxytocin facilitation of, 123

Y

Yoga
health benefits of, 161–62
laughter, 81–82